Current Research in DNA Repair

Current Research in DNA Repair

Edited by Albert Douglas

STATES
ACADEMIC PRESS
www.statesacademicpress.com

States Academic Press,
109 South 5th Street,
Brooklyn, NY 11249, USA

Visit us on the World Wide Web at:
www.statesacademicpress.com

ISBN: 978-1-63989-135-1

Cataloging-in-Publication Data

Current research in DNA repair / edited by Albert Douglas.
p. cm.
Includes bibliographical references and index.
ISBN 978-1-63989-135-1
1. DNA repair--Research. 2. Antimutagens--Research. 3. Biochemical genetics. I. Douglas, Albert.
QH467 .C87 2022
572.864 59--dc23

Table of Contents

Preface

Every book is a source of knowledge and this one is no exception. The idea that led to the conceptualization of this book was the fact that the world is advancing rapidly; which makes it crucial to document the progress in every field. I am aware that a lot of data is already available, yet, there is a lot more to learn. Hence, I accepted the responsibility of editing this book and contributing my knowledge to the community.

DNA repair refers to all the processes through which a cell identifies the damage to the DNA molecules and corrects them. Environmental factors such as radiations and normal metabolic activities can cause damage to the DNA which results in a number of individual lesions per cell per day. These lesions can cause structural damage to the DNA molecule which in turn can lead to alteration in the cell's ability to transcribe the gene that is encoded by the affected DNA. On the basis of the type of damage in the DNA's double helical structure, there are various types of DNA repair mechanisms such as direct reversal, base excision repair, nucleotide excision repair, and mismatch repair systems, etc. The book aims to shed light on some of the unexplored aspects of DNA repair and the recent researches in this field. It studies, analyses and upholds the pillars of DNA repair research and its utmost significance in modern times. This book is a complete source of knowledge on the present status of this important field.

While editing this book, I had multiple visions for it. Then I finally narrowed down to make every chapter a sole standing text explaining a particular topic, so that they can be used independently. However, the umbrella subject sinews them into a common theme. This makes the book a unique platform of knowledge.

I would like to give the major credit of this book to the experts from every corner of the world, who took the time to share their expertise with us. Also, I owe the completion of this book to the never-ending support of my family, who supported me throughout the project.

Editor

1

Recognition and Repair Pathways of Damaged DNA in Higher Plants

Sascha Biedermann[1,2], Sutton Mooney[1] and Hanjo Hellmann[1]
[1]*Washington State University Pullman*
[2]*Angewandte Genetik, Berlin*
[1]*United States of America*
[2]*Germany*

1. Introduction

Living organisms are continuously exposed to factors that threaten the integrity of their cells. This includes structural and enzymatic components like lipids or proteins, but also their genomes. Damage to genetic material can be critical as unrecognized and unrepaired DNA damage may cause fatal mutations not only threatening the organism's immediate survival but also that of its descendants. These genotoxic factors can derive from their surrounding environment and may include chemicals or ionizing radiation; but DNA damage can also be caused by reactive oxygen species (ROS) that are byproducts of daily metabolism or result from insufficient protection against abiotic stress conditions.

UV light can cause direct DNA damage by generating 6-4 and CPD photoproducts (example given in Fig. 1 is a thymine dimer). UV like most abiotic stress conditions can also generate ROS production in the cell. ROS have a high potential to damage single bases by oxidation (example give is 8-oxoG (Fig. 1)), but are also capable of introducing single or double strand breaks.

In contrast to most animals, plants are sessile organisms that cannot change their location when exposed to unfavorable conditions such as drought or salinity. Plants also face the difficult situation that they depend on sunlight for photosynthesis, a process that on its own constitutively generates ROS (Asada, 1999; Krieger-Liszkay, 2005; Triantaphylides and Havaux, 2009). Sunlight also contains significant amounts of UV-B light, which can contribute to both ROS production in the nucleus as well as directly affecting the DNA structure. Sunlight and high production rates of ROS are two of the main factors that lead to many mutations in plants. Consequently, the current review will focus on mechanisms that plants have in place to recognize and repair damaged DNA caused by either of these factors. We will provide a brief overview on the different classifications of DNA damage that can be expected, how these damages are repaired, and what is known about regulatory and physiological mechanisms that are in place in plants to recognize and respond to DNA damage. Because plants have taken a different evolutionary path than animals and possess some unique features not found in animals, we will compare selected repair and regulatory pathways in animals and plants. Despite their differences, plants and animals share many aspects in damaged DNA recognition and repair, and for this reason we will conclude this chapter by elaborating on some opinions for using plants as powerful and valuable model organisms for animals to understand the underlying processes of DNA repair.

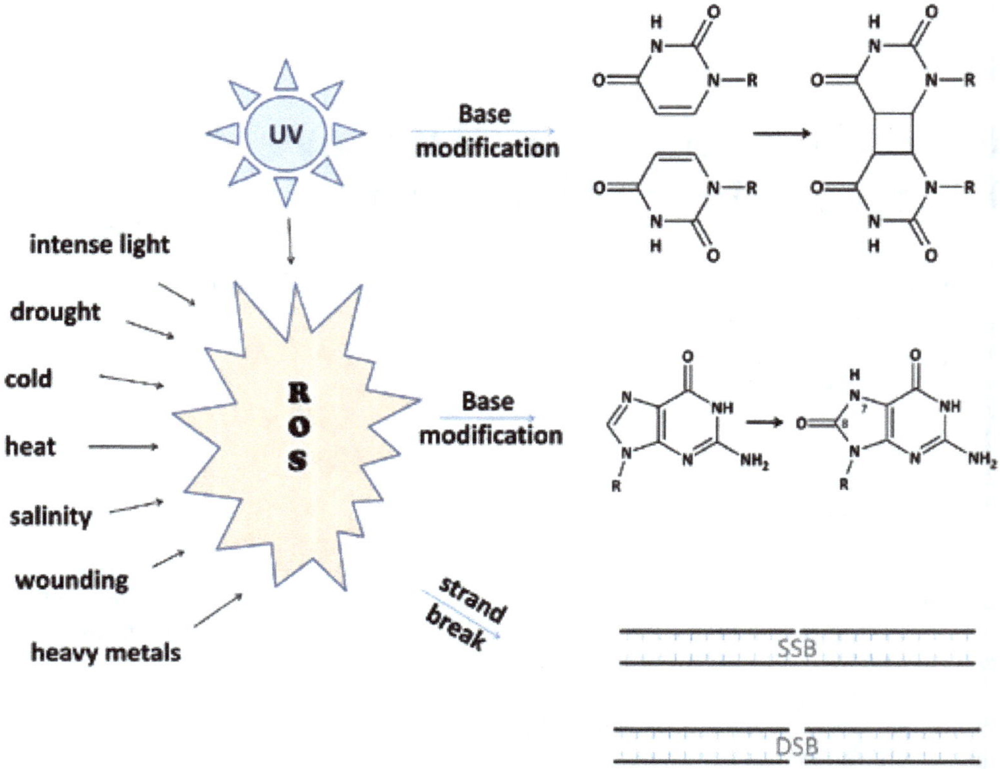

Fig. 1. UV light and ROS as genotoxic stress factors.

2. DNA damage caused by exposure to sunlight and abiotic stress

Ironically, although sunlight is obligatory for photosynthesis and survival of plants, it also represents one of the major threats to their genomic integrity. This can be ascribed to at least three reasons:

First, sunlight contains energy rich UV-C (280 to 100 nm), UV-B (290 to 320 nm) and UV-A (320–400 nm) light. Whereas UV-C is filtered out in the atmosphere, UV-B and UV-A can reach earth's surface. Although the amount strongly depends on the latitude and elevation, as well as cloud cover and canopy density, due to their sessile nature plants are exposed throughout the day to this genotoxic stress. UV-light is a strong mutagen that is absorbed by the DNA and may lead to the generation of cyclobutane pyrimidine dimers (CPD) and to a lesser extent pyrimidine (6,4) pyrimidone dimers (Friedberg EC et al., 2006). Both photoproducts are DNA lesions that affect transcriptional processes and result in error-prone replication (Fig. 1) (Friedberg EC et al., 2006). Solar UV light can also indirectly cause DNA damage by ROS production in the nucleus (Iovine et al., 2009). ROS induce a broad range of DNA damage, which includes base and nucleotide modifications, especially in sequences with a high guanosine content, and may even cause strand breaks (Wiseman and Halliwell, 1996; Tuteja et al., 2001; Tuteja and Tuteja, 2001). Although the precise nature of ROS generated by UV-light is not fully resolved, it is well established that oxygenated nucleotides like 8-oxo-guanine that can be caused by the accumulation of hydroxyl radicals (•OH) after prolonged UV exposure in the cell (Yamamoto et al., 1992; Hattori et al., 1996).

Second, ROS are commonly produced as metabolic byproducts in the chloroplasts, peroxisomes, and mitochondria (Foyer and Noctor, 2003). In fact it is estimated for mammals that per day ~180 guanines are oxidized to 8-hydroxyguanine in a single cell (Lindahl, 1993); and it is likely that this rate is even higher in photosynthetically active plants where chloroplasts continuously produce ROS. Furthermore, excessive light exposure as it may occur in mid-day under non-shaded conditions can overexcite the photosynthetic machinery. As a consequence, singlet oxygen ($^1O_2$) can be produced from triplet-state chlorophyll in the light- harvesting complex of photosystem II (PSII). In addition, byproducts of photosynthetic activities are superoxide (O_2^-) and hydrogen peroxide (H_2O_2) that can derive from water-splitting activities of the oxygen-evolving complex of PSII, and superoxide can be generated on the reducing side of PSI by the Mehler reaction (Noctor et al., 2002) (Fig. 1).

Third, heat from the sunlight can lead to failure of the structural composition and enzymatic machinery within the cell. To prevent cellular collapse, plants have developed a variety of protective mechanisms, the most important being the cooling effect of water transpiration through stomata. However, this dependency on water availability, together with their immobility, make plants highly susceptible to water stress conditions that derive from drought, salinity, or cold. Abiotic stress unbalances metabolic processes including photosynthesis, which ultimately causes a general increase in ROS concentration in the cell (Vinocur and Altman, 2005; Jaspers and Kangasjarvi, 2010). Although ROS detoxifying defense mechanisms are in place in the organelles and the cytosol, under the stress conditions described above, these mechanisms may not provide sufficient protection. To avoid excessive mutations over prolonged exposure to abiotic stress, plant cells depend on efficient repair pathways.

3. Major repair mechanisms in plants

3.1 Photoreactivation by photolyases

In plants the main repair pathway for direct DNA damage caused by UV-light that leads to the generation of CPDs and (6–4) photoproducts is based on the activity of photolyases (Jiang et al., 1997). Two types of photolyases have evolved that specifically recognize and repair either type of photodamage. Based on sequence homology, CPD photolyases are grouped into two different classes: while class I CPD photolyases are present in microorganisms, class II enzymes can be found in archaea, eubacteria, some animals (excluding placental mammals), and plants (Kanai et al., 1997). In comparison, (6-4) photolyases have been found in metazoans and plants, and they share sequence similarities with class I CPD photolyases (Kanai et al., 1997).

The structure and reaction mechanisms of photolyases have been intensively studied in the last decade, providing us with plentiful data on their function. Photolyases have two types of chromophoric co-factors that are used for photoreactivation (Huang et al., 2006; Ozturk et al., 2008; Hitomi et al., 2009). One chromophore is $FADH^-$, the two electron reduced form of FAD, while the second one can be either methenyltetrahydrofolate (MTHF) or 7,8-didemethyl-8-hydroxy-5-deazariboflavin (8-HDF). MTHF or 8-HDF function as the light harvesting chromophores that absorb blue light (300-600 nm), and transfer the energy to $FADH^-$ (Moldt et al., 2009; Li et al., 2010; Okafuji et al., 2010). Photolyases bind directly to CPD and (6-4) photoproducts, where an electron is transferred from the excited $FADH^-$ to the dimers generating pyrimidine monomers, upon which the enzyme is released (Li et al., 2010; Okafuji et al., 2010) (Fig. 2).

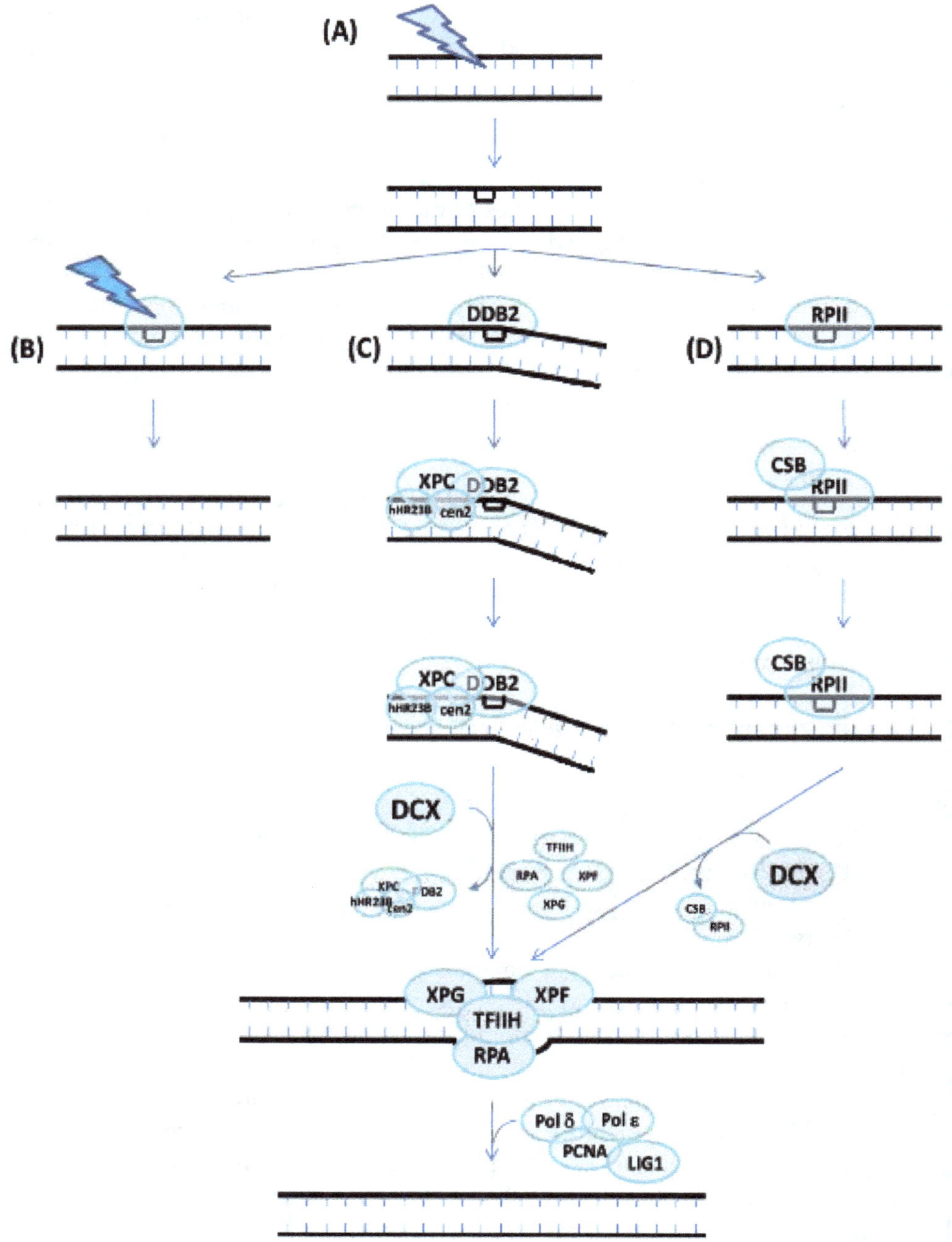

Fig. 2. Photodamage and potential repair pathways in plants.
(A) Direct DNA damage caused by UV can be recognized and repaired by **(B)** photolyases in a light-dependent reaction. Alternatively, repair can follow **(C)** the global genome nucleotide excision repair (GGR) or **(D)** the transcription coupled NER (TCR).

Photolyases have been widely described in plants and may often comprise small gene families like, for example, in *Arabidopsis,* which encodes for five members (http://www.arabidopsis.org/). While loss of single members can lead to increased UV-sensitivity (Jiang et al., 1997; Landry et al., 1997; Nakajima et al., 1998; Teranishi et al., 2004), the constitutive expression of CPD photolyases has been demonstrated to markedly improve UV tolerance in higher plants (Hidema et al., 2007; Kaiser et al., 2009). Although not much is known about their regulatory aspects, it has been demonstrated in rice that phosphorylation may play a role in regulating photolyase activities (Teranishi et al., 2008) and a few reports show that light increases photolyase expression (Chen et al., 1994; Waterworth et al., 2002). It was recently indicated that in darkness basal transcription of the photolyase genes *UVR3* and *PHR1* is sustained by the light signaling transcription factors HY5 and HYH and is limited by the actions of COP1 and DET1 dependent E3 ligases (Castells et al., 2010). Upon light exposure and during photomorphogenesis, COP1 leaves the nucleus and expression of *PHR1* is greatly induced by HY5 and HYH while the repression through DET1 remains in place. These observations suggest that photoreactivation is controlled by the photomorphogenisis pathway, and the activation of the PHR1 is dependent on photomorphogenetic regulators.

3.2 Nucleotide excision repair

A mechanism that can substitute for photolyase activities in plants, and which is required for photodamage repair in mammals, is the nucleotide excision repair (NER) pathway. NER is light-independent and, hence, sometimes referred to as dark repair. In contrast to photoreactivation, which reduces CPDs and 6-4 photoproducts back to pyrimidine monomers, NER is based on a complex recognition and repair machinery that excises and *de novo* synthesizes single DNA strands between 24-32 bp around the lesions. NER is highly conserved among eukaryotes and has two sub-pathways: transcription coupled NER (TCR) and global genome NER (GGR). NER has been intensively studied in animals, but the findings are a model for what is being found in plants, and will be briefly summarized in the following paragraph.

GGR and TCR recruit the same repair proteins; however, they mainly differ in their initial steps of damaged DNA recognition. GGR is genome-wide active, and its initial steps include the xeroderma pigmentosum group C factor (XPC), which is able to sense thermodynamic destabilizations of the Watson-Crick duplex caused by a flipping-out of the affected bases from the strands (Min and Pavletich, 2007). XPC in itself is capable of detecting most bulky DNA lesions, but for the recognition of CPDs it is supported by WD-40 protein Damaged DNA Binding 2 (DDB2) (Aboussekhra et al., 1995; Mu et al., 1995; Mu et al., 1996; Moser et al., 2005; Min and Pavletich, 2007; Scrima et al., 2008). DDB2 binds with high affinity to photoproducts, induces a bending of the DNA to approximately 40° and facilitates the flipping of the affected bases that are recognized and bound by the XPC/hHR23B complex, which further introduces structural changes into the DNA (Min and Pavletich, 2007; Scrima et al., 2008). DDB2 is part of a DDB1-CUL4-RBX1 (DCX) E3 ligase that mediates the polyubiquitination of histones, XPC and DDB2 itself (Rapic-Otrin et al., 2002; Fitch et al., 2003; Sugasawa et al., 2005; Chen et al., 2006; Kapetanaki et al., 2006; Wang et al., 2006). As a consequence, DDB2 is degraded via the 26S proteasome clearing the way for later repair stages (Rapic-Otrin et al., 2002; Fitch et al., 2003; Chen et al., 2006). Interestingly ubiquitination has the opposite effect on XPC leading to its stabilization and activation (Sugasawa et al., 2005). The DDB2-dependent ubiquitination of histones H2A, H3, and H4 may be necessary for the loosening of the DNA structure to allow the binding of other repair proteins (Kapetanaki et al., 2006; Wang et al., 2006). In a similar way the recently observed ability of DDB2 to recruit histone modifying proteins to specific DNA sequences could contribute to accessibility of the DNA for XPC and other factors (Minig et al., 2009; Roy et al., 2010). XPC is then needed for the recruitment of the core NER repair factors XPA, TFIIH, and RPA (Evans et al., 1997; Araujo et al., 2001; Thoma and Vasquez, 2003). XPA and the basal transcription factor complex TFIIH bind to the damaged site and unwind the DNA around the lesion (Reardon and Sancar, 2003; Maltseva et al., 2006; Yang et al., 2006; Kesseler et al., 2007; Krasikova et al., 2008). Unwinding is specifically performed by two subunits of TFIIH, the helicases XPB (ERCC3) and XPD (ERCC2). RPA is a heterotrimeric DNA binding protein, and while it prevents incision of the non-damaged DNA strand, together with XPA, it stabilizes the opened double helix (Blackwell et al., 1996; Camenisch et al., 2006; Maltseva et al., 2006; Yang et al., 2006). Incisions are performed by the endonucleases XPF (ERCC1) and XPG which nick the damaged DNA strand 5′ and 3′ around the lesion. After the damaged strand is excised, the gap is filled and ligated by the concerted activities of replication factors Proliferating Cell Nuclear Antigen (PCNA), Replication Factor C (RFC), Replication Protein A (RPA), DNA polymerases δ and ε, and DNA ligase 1 (LIG1) (Nichols and Sancar, 1992; Shivji et al., 1992; Green and Almouzni, 2003; Ogi et al., 2010). In contrast to GGR, TCR is specifically connected to DNA lesions in transcriptionally active regions. Here, RNA polymerase 2 (RP2) becomes stalled at CPD or (6-4) photoproduct containing sites (Selby and Sancar, 1997; Tornaletti and Hanawalt, 1999). Recognition of stalled RP2 has not been fully resolved. However, a critical role has been shown for Cockayne Syndrome factor B (CSB), a member of the SWI/SNF family of helicases (Selby and Sancar, 1997; van Gool et al., 1997; Citterio et al., 2000; Kamiuchi et al., 2002; Fousteri et al., 2006; Cazzalini et al., 2008). CSB binds to the stalled RP2, and this binding is a necessary trigger for recruitment of the same core repair proteins as described for GGR. Comparable to DDB2, CSB becomes a target of the DCX E3 ligase, which is mediated by another WD-40 protein, CSA. This interaction ultimately results in degradation of CSA, CSB and possibly also RP2 (Groisman et al., 2006).

Most of the proteins that play a role in GGR or TCR can be found in animals and plants, while only a few members, like XPA and TF2H3, a subunit of TFIIH, appear to be absent in plants (Kimura and Sakaguchi, 2006). It is currently open whether plants encode for functional analogs of XPA and TF23H that would perform tasks similar to these proteins. For most of the other NER proteins that are conserved among animals and plants, a role in DNA repair has been demonstrated, frequently by reverse genetic studies in *Arabidopsis thaliana*. Here, proteins shown to be involved in damaged DNA recognition in animals, such as DCX-E3 ligases, DDB2 and CSA, have also been recently described by several groups in plants (Bernhardt et al., 2006; Molinier et al., 2008; Al Khateeb and Schroeder, 2009; Bernhardt et al., 2010; Biedermann and Hellmann, 2010; Zhang et al., 2010; Zhang and Schroeder, 2010; Castells et al., 2011). While plants affected in ATCSA-1, the Arabidopsis CSA ortholog, do not display an abnormal development (Biedermann and Hellmann, 2010), loss of CUL4 or DDB2 cause a dwarf-like phenotype (Bernhardt et al., 2006; Koga et al., 2006). Interestingly, Arabidopsis *ddb2* or *atcsa-1* mutants are UV-hypersensitive but only when brought into the dark right after UV treatment, demonstrating that plants primarily rely on photoreactivation rather than NER (Biedermann and Hellmann, 2010). However, when kept in the dark both mutants have reduced repair activities when compared to wild type (Biedermann and Hellmann, 2010). CSB-like helicases are also present in plants

(Kimura et al., 2004; Shaked et al., 2006), and although they are not biochemically characterized, studies in Arabidopsis demonstrate their critical role for UV tolerance (Shaked et al., 2006). Other mutants directly affected in NER factors such as Arabidopsis mutants *atcen2* and *uvh3-1/xpg,* also show decreased repair activities *in vitro* and behave hypersensitive towards UV-C exposure, respectively (Liu et al., 2000; Molinier et al., 2004b). Loss of the TFIIH transcription factor complex subunits XPB/UVH6 and XPD is lethal; however, *uvh6-1* plants expressing a mutated but potentially partially functional XPB protein already show decreased repair rates of UV-induced 6-4 photoproducts (Liu et al., 2003). Overall the current findings strongly indicate that the basic mechanisms of UV-induced damaged DNA recognition and NER based repair are comparable and highly conserved among plants and animals.

3.3 Base excision repair

Not all nucleotide modifications can be repaired by NER, and many DNA lesions generated by reactive oxygen species (ROS) are not recognized by the NER proteins. Thus as an additional mechanism to ensure genomic integrity, cells utilize other repair mechanisms like base excision repair (BER). Because ROS are continuously produced as metabolic byproducts or by ionizing radiation, they represent a considerable source of the daily DNA damage. ROS-induced DNA lesions include for example 8-hydroxyguanine (8-oxoG), formamidopyrimidines, and 5-hydroxyuracil, which can potentially lead to miscoding during replication and transcription.

As a general rule BER requires the activities of DNA glycosylases, which cleave the N-glycosyl bond between the base and the sugar at the lesion site. This releases the base and leaves an abasic or apurinic/apyrimidinic (AP) site. In bacteria, fungi, plants and animals, several DNA glycosylases have been described that either specifically or broadly recognize certain lesions. For example, the mammalian DNA glycosylase OGG1 has a high affinity to 8-oxoG and some formamidopyrimidines, while another mammalian DNA glycosylase, NEIL1, efficiently repairs formamidopyrimidines but only poorly 8-oxoG (Morland et al., 2002; Parsons et al., 2005). DNA glycosylases are classified as either being mono- or bifunctional. Monofunctionally they only perform the cleavage reaction of the glycosylic bond between the deoxyribose and the target base to generate an AP site. Bifunctional DNA glycosylases/lyases, to which OGG1 and NEIL1 belong, are able to catalyze the release of the oxidized base and the cleavage of the DNA backbone at the AP site (Hazra et al., 2001).

Although there is currently no evidence that plants have NEIL1 orthologs, which are common in bacteria and animals and required in part for excision of oxidized purines and pyrimidines, most other DNA glycosylases have been found. For example, plants encode for orthologs of OGG1 (Roldan-Arjona and Ariza, 2009), and their activity in excising oxidized purines has been demonstrated for the *Arabidopsis* AtOGG1 (Dany and Tissier, 2001; Garcia-Ortiz et al., 2001; Morales-Ruiz et al., 2003). In addition to OGG1, plants also encode for proteins related to the bifunctional Endonuclease III/Nth from *E. coli*, yeast, and animals, which remove a broad range of damaged pyrimidines (Breimer and Lindahl, 1980; Boorstein et al., 1989; Hatahet et al., 1994; Phadnis et al., 2006; Guay et al., 2008). Like their bacterial counterparts, *Arabidopsis* AtNTH1 also shows a broad substrate specificity and DNA glycosylase activity for DNA lesions containing modified pyrimidines (Krokan et al., 1997; Roldan-Arjona et al., 2000). Furthermore, plants encode for proteins related to MutM/Fpg, an original model DNA glycosylase/lyase from *E. coli* that excises 8-oxo-guanine and other oxidized purines from damaged DNA (Tchou et al., 1991; Tchou et al., 1993; Bhagwat and

Gerlt, 1996; Ohtsubo et al., 1998; Murphy and Gao, 2001; Roldan-Arjona and Ariza, 2009). Although enzymatic function for all three types of plant DNA glycosylases is established, there is unfortunately no information available on how loss of these proteins affects development or ROS sensitivity of mutant plants.

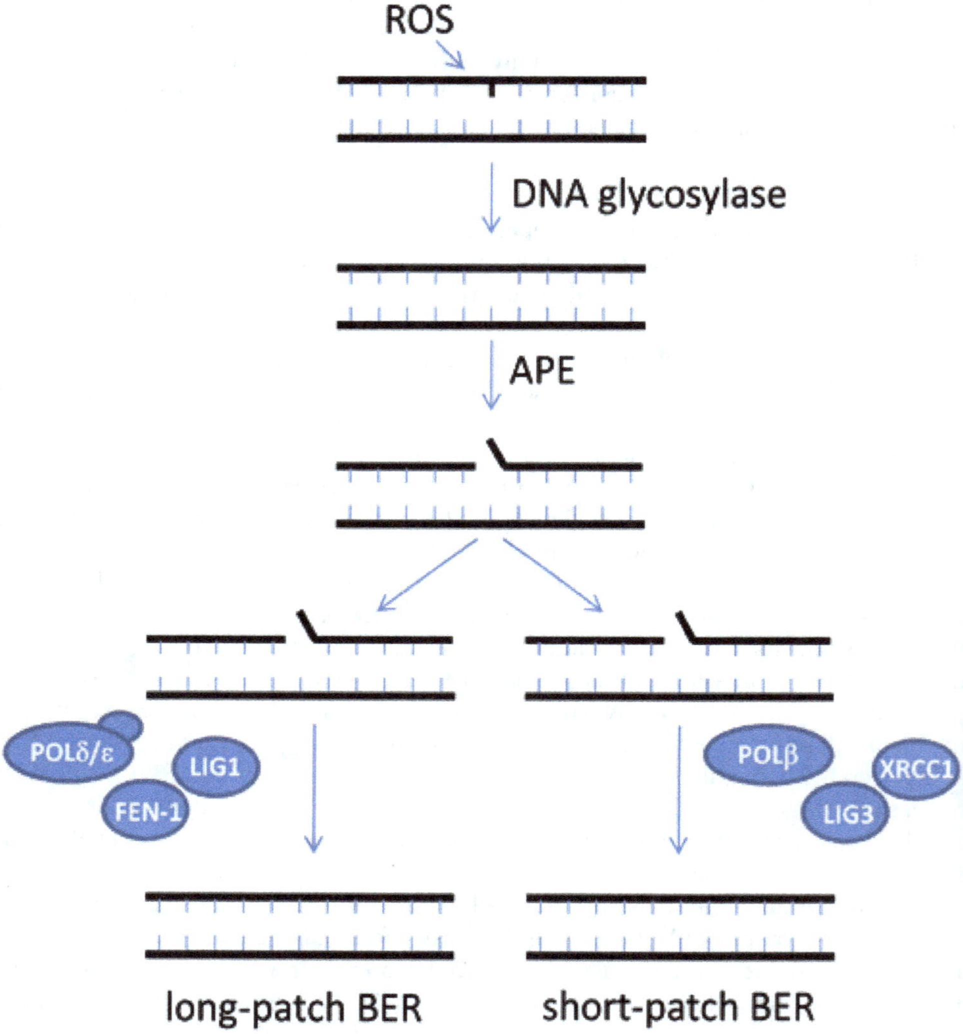

Fig. 3. Schematic model for base excision repair (BER).

DNA lesions caused by ROS are recognized and modified by the concerted activities of a DNA glycosylase and APE, after which cells can either take the route of long-patch repair or alternatively the short-patch repair pathway. Currently evidence indicates for plants that the long-patch repair is employed for BER.

Plant OGG1 and NTH proteins generate 3′ phospho α,β-unsaturated aldehydes (3′ dRP) at the strand breaks, and these need to be removed to generate free 3′ hydroxyl ends to allow gap-filling repair mediated by a DNA polymerase (Demple and Harrison, 1994; Roldan-Arjona et al., 2000; Garcia-Ortiz et al., 2001). Removal of 3′dRP is mediated in plants and animals by AP endonucleases (APE) which also work on AP sites generated by either monofunctional DNA glycosylases or those that occurred through spontaneous degradation of the DNA (Babiychuk et al., 1994; Demple et al., 1997; Pascucci et al., 2002) (Fig. 3).

Subsequently to APE, two separate BER repair pathways can become active in mammalian cells. First, the short-patch repair pathway, which relies on the concerted activities of DNA polymerase β (Polβ), X-ray repair cross-complementing protein 1 (XRCC1), and the DNA ligase 3 (LIG3). Polβ has an intrinsic 3′dRP activity and can remove deoxyribose sugar itself if required (Caldecott, 2001). XRCC1 interacts with LIG3 and other BER proteins and may function as a repair coordinating protein (Vidal et al., 2001) (Fig. 3). Alternatively, the long patch-repair pathway can be employed in mammalian cells, which requires activities of DNA polymerases δ and ε, RFC, PCNA, and flap endonuclease 1 (FEN1) to remove and resynthesize up to 10 nucleotides 3′ to the AP site, while the nick is ligated by LIG1 (Matsumoto, 2001) (Fig. 3).

While most proteins are present in plants that can participate in long-patch repair (Kimura and Sakaguchi, 2006), it is currently open whether a short-patch pathway exists in plants since no obvious homologs of POLβ and LIG3 are identified so far (Kimura and Sakaguchi, 2006; Roldan-Arjona and Ariza, 2009). In addition, plant XRCC1-like proteins lack domains that are necessary for complex assembly with POLβ and LIG3, and it is therefore currently open whether the protein participates in BER (Vidal et al., 2001; Taylor et al., 2002). Although no POLβ proteins are described in plants so far, it is possible that their function is conducted by POLλ. Both polymerases belong to the X superfamily of DNA polymerases and several amino acid residues are conserved between POLβ and λ (Garcia-Diaz et al., 2000; Uchiyama et al., 2004). In addition, POLλ has been demonstrated in rice to possess intrinsic 3′dRP activity and its expression is mainly found in meristematic and proliferating tissues (Uchiyama et al., 2004).

An important role in the recognition and repair of SSB and activation of BER involves poly(ADP-ribose) polymerases (PARP). PARP proteins belong to small protein families with, for example, 18 members in human, and they are highly conserved among eukaryotes (Ame et al., 2004); however, it is PARP1 and PARP2 that have been brought in context with damaged DNA recognition and DNA repair processes. PARP1 is a 113 kDa protein that contains a modular set of domains that enable it to fulfill multiple functions in the cell. At its N-terminal region PARP1 contains a DNA break recognition fold that is composed of a duplicated zinc finger similar to DNA ligase III. A BRCT motif is present in the center that can be found in many proteins connected with maintenance of genomic integrity and cell cycle checkpoints. The motif also functions as the main interface for protein–protein interactions. Finally, at its COOH-terminal region, PARP1 has motifs with different catalytic activities including NAD^+ hydrolysis as well as initiation, elongation, branching and termination of ADP-ribose polymers (Citarelli et al., 2010). It has been shown in mammalian cells that, upon binding a DNA lesion PARP1 poly(ADP)ribosylates itself as well as nearby histones (H1 and H2B), which relaxes the chromatin structure allowing better access for XRCC1 and other repair proteins to the damaged site (Poirier et al., 1982; Masson et al., 1998; Pleschke et al., 2000). Plant PARP1 and PARP2 are nuclear localized like their animal counterparts, and they become transcriptionally activated upon genotoxic stress conditions such as ionizing radiation or oxidative stress (Puchta et al., 1995; Babiychuk et al., 1998;

Doucet-Chabeaud et al., 2001; Chen et al., 2003). However, although a similar role of plant PARP1 and PARP2 in damaged DNA recognition and initiation of DNA repair is likely, a detailed *in planta* functional description is still missing for these proteins.

3.4 DSB repair: Nonhomologous end joining and homologous recombination

ROS, especially •OH generated by ionizing radiation or via the Fenton reaction (Karanjawala et al., 2003; Clark, 2008), also have a high potential to cause double-strand breaks (DSB) (Karanjawala et al., 2002; Karanjawala et al., 2003). DSB require repair mechanisms distinct from photolyases, NER and BER. Therefore cells primarily depend on either the nonhomologous DNA end joining pathway (NHEJ) or homologous recombination (HR). NHEJ is an error-prone repair pathway, which directly ligates the free DNA ends together. In animals, the pathway is discussed to start with the binding of the heterodimeric Ku70/Ku80 complex to a DNA end. This step is required for employment of DNA-dependent protein kinase (DNA-PK) and Artemis endonuclease that process the DNA ends (Ma et al., 2002), while rejoining and ligation is performed by the XRCC4/LIG4/XLF complex (Grawunder et al., 1997; Barnes et al., 1998) (Fig. 4). The processing of the DNA ends can result in deletions or insertions and is the reason why NHEJ based repair often results in mutations in the repaired DNA. Current research in plants indicates that the NHEJ pathway is conserved among plants and animals. Ku70 and Ku80 related proteins as well as the Artemis-like protein SNM1/PSO1 are expressed in *Arabidopsis* and rice, and *Arabidopsis* mutants affected in these proteins become hypersensitive to γ-irradiation and the chemotherapeutic agent bleomycin, a double-strand break inducing chemical, which is in agreement with their roles in NHEJ (Tamura et al., 2002; Friesner and Britt, 2003; Gallego et al., 2003; Molinier et al., 2004a; Kimura et al., 2005; Kimura and Sakaguchi, 2006; Charbonnel et al., 2010). Likewise, XRCC4 and Lig4 homologues have been described in plants, and functionally connected to NHEJ (West et al., 2000; Friesner and Britt, 2003; Kimura and Sakaguchi, 2006; Waterworth et al., 2010).

In contrast to the error prone NHEJ pathway, HR is a more accurate repair mechanism that uses homologous DNA strands as templates for repair activities (Boyko et al., 2006a; Boyko et al., 2006b; Li and Ma, 2006; Osman et al., 2011). Several alternative pathways may exist that allow HR based repair of DSBs, however, good evidence is provided for at least two alternative pathways in plants. One is the synthesis-dependent strand annealing (SDSA) mechanism which involves the meiotic recombination11/Rad50/X-ray sensitive 2 (MRN) complex (Waterworth et al., 2007; Ronceret et al., 2009; Amiard et al., 2010). The MRN complex is discussed to function as a first sensor of double strand breaks. It generates single strand DNA at the DSB sites that can be used as templates to mediate HR by RecA and Rad51 homologues (Lin et al., 2006; Li et al., 2007; Markmann-Mulisch et al., 2007; Odahara et al., 2007; Vignard et al., 2007; Waterworth et al., 2007; Odahara et al., 2009; Ronceret et al., 2009; Amiard et al., 2010; Chittela and Sainis, 2010; Devisetty et al., 2010; Ko et al., 2010; Schaefer et al., 2010; Wang et al., 2010; Ko et al., 2011) (Fig. 4). However, the precise subsequent steps of Holliday structure formation, cleavage by endonucleases and dissociation into two DNA chains is only poorly understood in plants. Alternatively to SDSA, plants also use the single strand annealing (SSA) mechanism (Tissier et al., 1995; Ayora et al., 2002; Blanck et al., 2009; Mannuss et al., 2010). SSA requires a double strand break between two repeated sequences that are oriented in the same direction. Adjacent to the break, single-stranded DNA is created so that the repeated sequences can be used as complementary strands to anneal the ends of the break, after which non-homologous tails are detached and nicks can be ligated (Tissier et al., 1995; Puchta, 2005; Blanck et al., 2009; Mannuss et al., 2010). Because HR is less likely to cause changes in the genetic information than NHEJ, it is likely that the extent to which either NHEJ or HR repair pathways are employed in DSB repair may impact genome evolution in living organisms.

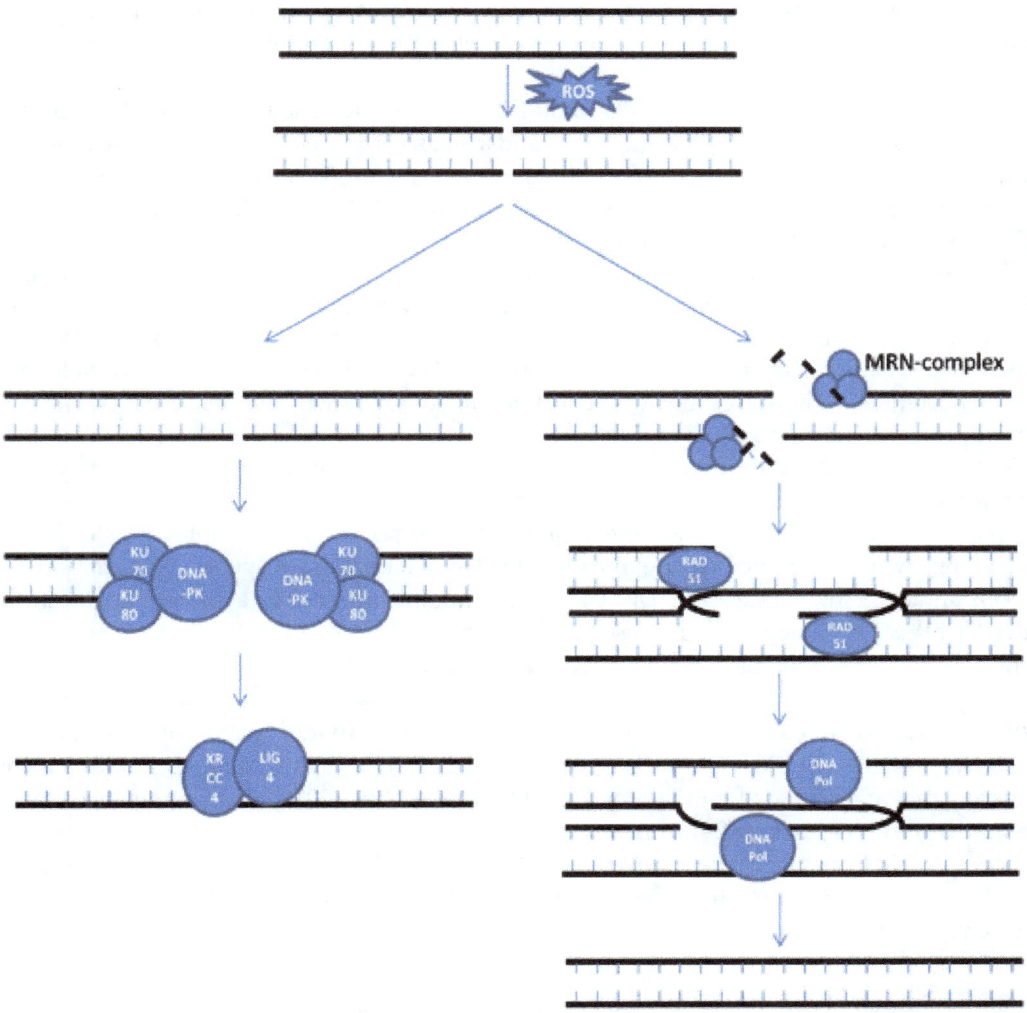

Fig. 4. ROS induced repair of double-strand breaks.

Two alternative pathways for which strong evidence is present to exist in plants are shown. Double-strand breaks can either be repaired by nonhomologous DNA end joining pathway (NHEJ; left hand side), or by homologous recombination (HR; right hand side).

3.5 DNA repair in chloroplasts

Based on their high metabolic activities in respiration and photosynthesis, organelles are centers of ROS production. Both mitochondria and chloroplasts possess their own repair pathways, and it appears to be that they have most of the repair pathways that are also found in the nucleus (for an excellent review about mitochondrial repair see (Boesch et al., 2011). We will focus here on chloroplast repair and briefly summarize recent findings.

The chloroplast genome is in general relative small, but gene numbers can vary significantly between species ranging from, for example, 54 in *Helicosporidium sp. ex Simulium jonesii* and up to 301 in *Pinus koraiensis* (http://chloroplast.cbio.psu.edu/); (Cui et al., 2006). These genes and their corresponding proteins are crucial for proper functioning of the organelle and hence survival of the plant and it is not surprising that chloroplasts have several repair pathways.

A recent report described a rice CPD photolyase to mediate repair of direct DNA damage caused by UV light (Takahashi et al., 2011), and also an earlier report describes PHR2, a class II photolyase predicted to be in chloroplasts of *C. reinhardtii* (Petersen et al., 1999). There is also strong evidence in *Arabidopsis* for two bifunctional DNA glycosylase/lyase of the *E. coli* Endonuclease III/Nth type and an APE to be involved in repair of ROS based DNA damage (Gutman and Niyogi, 2009). The authors can show specific localization of the three proteins to the chloroplast and specific activities *in vitro*. However, single or even triple mutants affected in the three proteins do not display any apparent developmental defects or increased sensitivities to photo-oxidative stress (e.g. UV- and high light or methyl viologen), from which the authors concluded that additional, yet unknown BER repair pathways exist in chloroplast (Gutman and Niyogi, 2009).

Currently no clear data are available for NER activities in the chloroplasts and only poor evidence is currently present on whether or how chloroplasts repair DSBs. Work on the green algae *Chlamydomonas reinhardtii* showed presence of a chloroplast-located RecA homolog, which is inducible in expression by DNA-damaging reagents (Nakazato et al., 2003). In addition, *Arabidopsis* T-DNA insertion mutants affected in a chloroplast localized RecA (*cpRecA*) homolog have increased amounts of single-strand DNA, altered structures of chloroplast DNA, and chloroplasts showed signs of reduced function after four generations post T-DNA insertion (Rowan et al., 2010). Yet, further data for additional repair proteins is still missing, as well as strong evidence for HR or NHEJ activities in chloroplasts of higher plants. Recent findings, however, indicate that chloroplasts repair DSBs using microhomology-mediated end joining (MMEJ) (Kwon et al., 2010). This repair mechanism requires only very short (2–14 bp) regions of homology, and is discussed as a potential backup to NHEJ in eukaryotes (Heacock et al., 2004; Bennardo et al., 2008). Although Kwon and co-workers provide strong evidence for MMEJ in chloroplasts, it is currently open which proteins mediate this repair.

3.6 Physiological responses after UV and ROS exposure

Besides immediate repair processes, it is also critical for plant cells to generate a physiological environment in which further DNA damage is prevented or at least reduced. A common physiological response to UV exposure in plants appears to be the accumulation of anthocyanin and flavonoids, potentially as a photoprotective or ROS quenching mechanism (Ng et al., 1964 ; Yatsuhashi et al., 1982; Takeda and Abe, 1992; Ye et al., 2010). It is interesting to note that some plants like grape vine (*Vitis vinifera*) or common bean (*Phaseolus vulgaris*) accumulate resveratrol or coumestrol, respectively, in response to UV exposure (Langcake and Pryce, 1977; Beggs et al., 1985). Resveratrol is a protective phytoalexin that is produced primarily under biotic stress conditions, while coumestrol is a phytoestrogen with unknown function. Both compounds are associated with effecting cell proliferation, cell cycle, and apoptosis of mammalian cells (Ndebele et al., 2010; Delmas et al., 2011) and may be signaling molecules in plants to trigger specific responses upon UV exposure.

A critical factor that is discussed as a regulator of DNA repair pathways in response to increased ROS accumulation in the cell appears to be ADP-Ribose/NADH Pyrophosphohydrolase AtNUDX7 (Ishikawa et al., 2009). AtNUDX7 belongs to the family of Nudix hydrolyases, which catalyze the hydrolysis of dinucleoside polyphosphates, nucleoside di- and triphosphates, nucleotide sugars, and coenzymes in plants and animals (McLennan, 2006; Kraszewska, 2008). AtNUDX7 substrates are ADP-Ribose (ADP-Rib) and NADH which are converted to AMP plus ribose 5-phosphate and nicotinamide mononucleotide (NMNH) plus AMP, respectively (Ogawa et al., 2005). The protein may have a central function for the homeostasis of NAD^+ pools by supplying ATP via nucleotide recycling from free ADP-Ribose molecules. This may be critical for the cell since substantial PARP activity can significantly lower NAD^+ and ATP levels; such a depletion of cellular energy can result in necrotic cell death (Ha and Snyder, 1999; Virag and Szabo, 2002; De Block et al., 2005). As discussed for BER, DNA damaged-induced, PARP-dependent poly(ADP)-ribosylation of proteins is considered a critical step for recognition of damage to be converted into intracellular signals that can trigger DNA repair programs or cell death. Consequently, AtNUDX7 is up-regulated upon abiotic stress (salinity, drought, high light, paraquat), and plants constitutively overexpressing AtNUDX7 become less susceptible to these stress conditions (Ishikawa et al., 2009).

A microarray study has shown that UV-C, bleomycin, or biotic stress factors elicit a hypersensitive response and increased H_20_2 levels in the cell (Molinier et al., 2005). Although each stress elicited specific responses, the authors could also find 209 genes that were commonly up-regulated, while 54 were similarly down-regulated by all three stress treatments. Among the commonly regulated genes were components of signaling pathways, transcription factors, and genes connected with an oxidative stress or defense response. Cell-cycle genes were also down-regulated after genotoxic stress exposure, as was earlier noted for animals (Dasika et al., 1999). However, the authors also noted that in Arabidopsis expression of only a comparably few number of repair genes was induced, and concluded that the plant must be mainly relying on existing synthesized proteins. It will be interesting to see whether results are broadly applicable to other plant species or whether the tested conditions and responses are specific for Arabidopsis.

3.7 ATM/ATR dependent regulation of DNA repair

A central regulator of the fate of damaged cells between apoptosis or cell cycle arrest and DNA repair in animals is the tumor-suppressing p53, sometimes dubbed the "guardian of the genome". This transcription factor controls not only cell cycle genes like p21 and apoptosis factors like PUMA, NOXA, and BAX but also various components of major DNA repair pathways such as CSB, DDB2 and XPC (NER); FANCC (DNA crosslink repair) and MSH2, MLH1, and PMS2 (mismatch repair) (Gatz and Wiesmuller, 2006; Brady and Attardi, 2010). There is also evidence that it has a more direct role in BER, interacting with APE1 and OGG1 and thereby enhancing the excision of oxidized DNA bases (Gatz and Wiesmuller, 2006; Vigneron and Vousden, 2010). Additionally p53 seems to recognize and bind directly to certain DNA structures e.g. Holliday junctions and mismatches where it represses the activities of HR and NHEJ (Bakalkin et al., 1994; Subramanian and Griffith, 2005; Gatz and Wiesmuller, 2006).

Activation of p53 after DNA damaging conditions is achieved by phosphorylation by the checkpoint kinases ATAXIA TELANGIECTASIA MUTATED (ATM) and ATAXIA TELANGIECTASIA AND RAD3 RELATED (ATR) (Canman et al., 1998; Tibbetts et al., 1999). While recent studies imply that ATM is a sensor for the redox state of the cell, it is mainly known to be activated by the above-mentioned DSB sensing MRN-complex (Bakkenist and Kastan, 2003; Falck et al., 2005; Kruger and Ralser, 2011; Perry and Tainer, 2011). ATR, on the other hand, is recruited to RPA-coated UV-induced lesions by the ATR INTERACTING PROTEIN (ATRIP) (Wright et al., 1998; Cortez et al., 2001; Ball and Cortez, 2005; Warmerdam et al., 2010). Once activated both kinases phosphorylate p53 and the effector kinases CHK1 and CHK2 regulating cell cycle and DNA repair (Brady and Attardi, 2010).

Curiously no plant homologues of p53 have been identified in any of the model organisms. This is probably linked to the absence of the core apoptotic machinery as we know it from animals. In contrast most of the DNA repair targets of p53, as well as ATM and ATR, are very well conserved in plants. Where loss of one of the checkpoint kinases in animals is lethal, the existence of viable *atr* and *atm* mutant plants in Arabidopsis make it an ideal model for their investigation. Both are involved in the response to ionizing radiation (IR) and necessary for the IR-induced transcription activation of many genes participating in DNA repair, cell cycle control, transcription, and replication (Culligan et al., 2006; Ricaud et al., 2007; Yoshiyama et al., 2009; Furukawa et al., 2010).

This raises the question if there is a factor that is functioning as a p53 analog mediating the DNA damage response between ATM/ATR and the downstream repair factors. An answer to that could be SUPPRESSOR OF GAMMA RESPONSE 1 (SOG1). Though unrelated to p53 and unique to plants, this transcription factor, discovered in a screen for suppressor mutants of the γ-irradiation induced cell cycle arrest of Arabidopsis *uvh1* seeds, is necessary for the activation of genes downstream of both ATM and ATR in response to γ-irradiation (Preuss and Britt, 2003; Yoshiyama et al., 2009; Furukawa et al., 2010). SOG1, ATM, and ATR were also found to trigger plant programmed cell death (PCD) in root meristems after γ- or UV-B irradiation, a mechanism that was recently shown to be distinct from animal apoptosis (Fulcher and Sablowski, 2009; Furukawa et al., 2010). Hence, SOG1 is a good candidate to control repair processes in a p53-like fashion, at least by activating transcription of the plant homologues of factors like DDB2, MSH2 and XPC in response to UV and IR stresses.

Current research indicates that plants and animals share roughly similar repair pathways. But for some repair proteins that have been described in animals no homologues have been found in plants, as yet. However, with ongoing research, it seems plausible that plant counterparts will be identified that can substitute for missing animal orthologs as it appears to be the case with p53 and SOG1.

4. Plants as model organisms to study DNA repair

Plants and animals share a surprisingly high degree of conservation among their abilities to repair damaged DNA (please also see Table 1 at the end of this passage for an overview of genes involved in DNA repair in the model plant *Arabidopsis thaliana*). While mammalian researchers have very valid and scientifically relevant reasons to use animal subjects, plants can and should be considered as excellent and viable alternatives to investigate the fundamentals of DNA repair processes. Tolerance towards mutations and abiotic stresses along with the relative ease of upkeep and propagation of the research organisms are two factors that we will briefly discuss in this final section of the review.

Due to their inability to elude many constantly damaging influences, plants need to utilize efficient ways to cope with these stresses. One strategy plants seem to have adopted to manage the higher demands on DNA repair is redundancy. For instance, genes of every pathway discussed here were found to be duplicated in Arabidopsis or rice (Singh et al., 2010). Additionally the existence of both 8-oxo-guanine glycosylases, OGG1, as well as MutM/Fpg in Arabidopsis demonstrate functional redundancy of independent, alternative repair pathways, which may have originated from the incorporation of chloroplast and mitochondrial genes into the nuclear genome (Boesch et al., 2009; Singh et al., 2010; Rowan et al., 2010).

Probably because of these gene duplications, functional redundancies, and more efficient or alternative pathways in comparison to animals, plants often have greater flexibilities in how they can respond to and potentially tolerate damaged DNA and mutations. For example a homozygous mutant in ATR kinase, which would be lethal in mammals, can in plants be investigated for the impact on DNA repair, control of apoptosis or gene expression profiles. In order to see the global effects of genotoxic stressors on a model organism, the subjects need to be exposed to different degrees of damaging agents. Here, plants are ideal models because of their sessile nature. They can be cultivated under very steady and reproducible conditions, while stress exposure is highly controlled. In addition, from an ethical point of view, plants can be taken to the edge of survival with very harsh treatments such as high levels of UV-light or toxin applications that for some may be not comfortable to perform on animals.

In comparison to animals, plants are low cost organisms that only require minimal monitoring along with water and occasionally fertilizer. Small plants like the moss *Physcomitrella patens* or *Arabidopsis thaliana* can be cultivated to great numbers within in a few square feet while by comparison animals require adequate space and regular food, water, and cleaning. While mutant lines are readily available for many animal and plant systems, shipment and propagation of plant resources can be quite straightforward. Seeds can be harvested for immediate propagation of the next generation or stored long-term, even at room temperature, before use months or even years later. Sending seed material to colleagues around the world is technically simple since no special transport accommodations need to be made. Generating transgenic *Arabidopsis* lines using *Agrobacterium* infection is a standard lab procedure, and allows for rapid complementation of mutant lines to verify protein functionality and observation of response and recovery. Also generation time of Arabidopsis plants is very short with just two months from seed to seed.

In addition to using plants as basic models to understand DNA repair processes, there are also practical reasons why this area of research urgently needs to be expanded. With the increase in food shortages for increasing populations, the recognition of environmental toxins and the growing evidence of impending and occurring climate changes across the world, it becomes critical to rapidly develop plants that can better cope with environmental stress. As such, stress tolerant crop plants generated either by genetic engineering or classical breeding will become increasingly important resources to guarantee stable food supplies to the human population in an expected changing environment.

Repair pathway	Representative Gene Model	Gene in Arabidopsis	Function	Acc. No.	Reference
Photore-activation		*PHR1/UVR2*	repair of CPDs	AT1G12370	Ahmad et al., 1997; Landry et al., 1997
		PHR2	repair of CPDs	AT2G47590	Ahmad et al., 1998; Petersen et al., 1999
		UVR3	repair of 6-4PPs	AT3G15620	Jiang et al., 1997; Nakajima et al., 1998
NER	*XPC*	*AtRAD4*	recognition of CPDs and 6-4PPs, GGR	AT5G16630	Kunz et al., 2005; Liang et al., 2006
	HHR23A,B/RAD23	*RAD23A*	recognition of CPDs and 6-4PPs, GGR	AT1G16190	Molinier et al., 2005; Kunz et al., 2005; Farmer et al., 2010
		RAD23B		AT1G79650	Molinier et al., 2004b Kunz et al., 2005; Farmer et al., 2010
		RAD23C		AT3G02540	Molinier et al., 2004b; Kunz et al., 2005; Farmer et al., 2010
		RAD23D		AT5G38470	Molinier et al., 2004b; Kunz et al., 2005; Farmer et al., 2010
	CEN2	*AtCEN2*	recognition of CPDs and 6-4PPs, GGR	AT4G37010	Molinier et al., 2004b; Liang et al., 2006
	ROC1/RBX1	*RBX1A*	activation of CUL4-dependent ligases	AT5G20570	Lechner et al., 2002; Gray et al., 2002
		RBX1B		AT3G42830	Lechner et al., 2002; Gray et al., 2002
	CUL4	*CUL4*	Ubiquitylation of targets	AT5G46210	Molinier et al., 2008; (Biedermann and Hellmann, 2010
	DDB1	*AtDDB1a*	Ubiquitylation of targets	AT4G05420	Molinier et al., 2008; (Biedermann and Hellmann, 2010
		AtDDB1b		AT4G21100	Bernhardt et al., 2006; Bernhardt et al., 2010
	DDB2	*DDB2*	recognition of CPDs and 6-4PPs, GGR, substrate recognition for CUL4-dependent ubiquitination	At5g58760	Koga et al., 2006; Molinier et al., 2008
	TFIIH1	*AtTFB1-1*	TFIIH subunit p62	At1g55750	Kunz et al., 2005; Singh et al., 2010
		AtTFB1-2		At1g55680	Kunz et al., 2005; Singh et al., 2010
		AtTFB1-3		At3g61420	Kunz et al., 2005; Singh et al., 2010

Repair pathway	Representative Gene Model	Gene in Arabidopsis	Function	Acc. No.	Reference
	TFIIH2	*AtGTF2H2*	TFIIH subunit p44	At1g05050	Kunz et al., 2005; Singh et al., 2010
	TFIIH3	*AtTFB4*	TFIIH subunit p34	AT1G18340	Kunz et al., 2005; Singh et al., 2010
	TFIIH4	*AtTFB2*	TFIIH subunit p52	At4g17020	Kunz et al., 2005; Singh et al., 2010
	TFIIH5	*AtTFB5*	TFIIH subunit	AT1G12400	Kunz et al., 2005; Singh et al., 2010
				AT1G62886	Singh et al., 2010
	CDK7	*CAK3AT/CDKD1;1*	cyclin activating kinase-subcomplex of THIIH	AT1G73690	Singh et al., 2010
		CAK4AT/CDKD1;2		AT1G66750	Singh et al., 2010
		CAK2AT/CDKD1;3		AT1G18040	Singh et al., 2010
	XPB/RAD25/ERCC3	*AtXPB1*	helicase subunit of TFIIH	AT5G41370	Costa et al., 2001
		AtXPB2		AT5G41360	Morgante et al., 2005
	XPD/RAD3/ERCC2	*AtXPD/UVH6*	helicase subunit of TFIIH	AT1G03190	Jenkins et al., 1995; Liu et al., 2003
	XPF/RAD1/ERCC4	*AtRAD1/UVH1*	5'-endonuclease	AT5G41150	Harlow et al., 1994; Jenkins et al., 1995
	XPG/RAD2/ERCC5	*UVH3/UVR1*	3'-endonuclease	AT3G28030	Jenkins et al., 1995; Liu et al., 2003
	CSA/RAD28/ERCC8	*ATCSA-1/CSAat1A*	substrate recognition for CUL4-dependent ubiquitination, TCR	AT1G27840	Biedermann and Hellmann, 2010; Zhang et al., 2010
		ATCSA-2/CSAat1B		AT1G19750	Kunz et al., 2005; Zhang et al., 2010
	CSB/RAD26/ERCC6	*CHR8*	binding of stalled RNA polymerase, recruitment of repair machinery, TCR	AT2G18760	Shaked et al., 2006
		CHR24		AT5G63950	Shaked et al., 2006
BER	*OGG1*	*AtOGG1*	8-oxoguanine DNA glycosylase	AT1G21710	Garcia-Ortiz et al., 2001; Dany and Tissier, 2001
	MutM	*AtFPG/MMH*	formamidopyrimidine DNA glycosylase	AT1G52500	Ohtsubo et al., 1998
	NTH	*AtNTH1*	DNA glycosylase and apyrimidinic (AP) lyase/endonuclease	AT2G31450	Gutman and Niyogi, 2009
		AtNTH2		AT1G05900	Gutman and Niyogi, 2009

Repair pathway	Representative Gene Model	Gene in Arabidopsis	Function	Acc. No.	Reference
	APE	*ARP/APE1*	apurinic/apyrimidinic (AP) endonuclease	AT2G41460	Babiychuk et al., 1994; Gutman and Niyogi, 2009
		APE2		AT4G36050	Singh et al., 2010
	XRCC1	*AtXRCC1*	co-factor of DNA ligase 3	AT1G80420	Petrucco et al., 2002; Singh et al., 2010
	FEN	*FEN1*	flap endonuclease	AT5G26680	Singh et al., 2010
NHEJ/HR	*KU70/XRCC6*	*AtKU70*	binding of DNA double strand break ends	AT1G16970	Riha et al., 2002
	KU80/XRCC5	*AtKU80*	binding of DNA double strand break ends	AT1G48050	Riha et al., 2002
	XRCC4	*XRCC4*	co-factor of DNA ligase 4	AT3G23100	West et al., 2000
	LIG4	*AtLIG4*	DNA ligation	AT5G57160	West et al., 2000
	MRE11	*AtMRE11*	subunit of the MRN complex, damage recognition, generation of single-stranded DNA	AT5G54260	Hartung and Puchta, 1999; Daoudal-Cotterell et al., 2002
	RAD50	*AtRAD50*	subunit of the MRN complex, damage recognition, generation of single-stranded DNA	AT2G31970	Gallego and White, 2001
	NBS1	*AtNBS1*	subunit of the MRN complex, damage recognition, generation of single-stranded DNA	AT3G02680	Bleuyard et al., 2006; Waterworth et al., 2007
	RECA (E. Coli)	*AtRECA1/cp RecA*	DNA binding, mediation of inter-strand-pairing	AT1G79050	Cerutti et al., 1992; Cao Cao et al., 1997; Shedge et al., 2007; Rowan et al., 2010
		AtRECA2		AT2G19490	Shedge et al., 2007
		AtRECA3		AT3G10140	Khazi et al., 2003; Shedge et al., 2007
				AT3G32920	Shedge et al., 2007
		DRT100		AT3G12610	Pang et al., 1992; Pang et al., 1993
	RAD51	*AtRAD51/RAD51A*	DNA binding, mediation of inter-strand-pairing	AT5G20850	Doutriaux et al., 1998
		RAD51B		AT2G28560	Bleuyard et al., 2005; Osakabe et al., 2005
		RAD51C		AT2G45280	Bleuyard et al., 2005
		RAD51D/SSN1		AT1G07745	Bleuyard et al., 2005; Osakabe et al., 2006
	BRCA1	*AtBRCA1*	supports homology pairing	AT4G21070	Lafarge and Montane, 2003

Repair pathway	Representative Gene Model	Gene in Arabidopsis	Function	Acc. No.	Reference
	BRCA2	*AtBRCA2A*	supports homology pairing	AT4G00020	Siaud et al., 2004; Dray et al., 2006
		AtBRCA2B		AT5G01630	Siaud et al., 2004; Dray et al., 2006
Other	*ATM*	*AtATM*	checkpoint kinase	AT3G48190	Garcia et al., 2000)
	ATR/RAD3	*AtATR/AtRAD3*	checkpoint kinase	AT5G40820	Culligan et al., 2004
	PCNA	*AtPCNA1*	DNA polymerase processivity factor activity	AT1G07370	Strzalka et al., 2009
		AtPCNA2		AT2G29570	Strzalka et al., 2009
	LIG1	*AtLIG1*	DNA ligation	AT1G08130	Taylor et al., 1998
				AT1G49250	Singh et al., 2010
	PARP	*AtPARP1*	damage recognition, poly(ADP)ribosylation	AT4G02390	Lepiniec et al., 1995
		AtPARP2		AT2G31320	Doucet-Chabeaud et al., 2001
		AtPARP3		AT5G22470	Singh et al., 2010
	RPA1	*AtRPA1A/AtRPA1-3/RPA70A*	stabilization of single-stranded DNA intermediates	AT2G06510	Ishibashi et al., 2005; Chang et al., 2009
		AtRPA1-1		AT4G19130	Kunz et al., 2005; Singh et al., 2010
		AtRPA1-5/RPA70B		AT5G08020	Kunz et al., 2005; Singh et al., 2010
		AtRPA1-2/RPA70C		AT5G45400	Kunz et al., 2005; Singh et al., 2010
		AtRPA1-4/RPA70D		AT5G61000	Kunz et al., 2005; Singh et al., 2010
	RPA2	*AtRPA2-1/ATRPA32A*		AT2G24490	Kunz et al., 2005
		AtRPA2-2/ATRPA32B		AT3G02920	Kunz et al., 2005
	RPA3			AT3G52630	Singh et al., 2010
				AT4G18590	Singh et al., 2010

Table 1. Overview of genes involved in DNA repair in the model plant *Arabidopsis thaliana*.

5. References

Aboussekhra, A., Biggerstaff, M., Shivji, M.K., Vilpo, J.A., Moncollin, V., Podust, V.N., Protic, M., Hubscher, U., Egly, J.M., and Wood, R.D. (1995). Mammalian DNA nucleotide excision repair reconstituted with purified protein components. Cell 80, 859-868.

Ahmad, M., Jarillo, J.A., and Cashmore, A.R. (1998). PHR2: a novel Arabidopsis gene related to the blue-light photoreceptor/photolyase family. Plant Physiol 117.

Ahmad, M., Jarillo, J.A., Klimczak, L.J., Landry, L.G., Peng, T., Last, R.L., and Cashmore, A.R. (1997). An enzyme similar to animal type II photolyases mediates photoreactivation in Arabidopsis. Plant Cell 9, 199-207.

Al Khateeb, W.M., and Schroeder, D.F. (2009). Overexpression of Arabidopsis damaged DNA binding protein 1A (DDB1A) enhances UV tolerance. Plant Mol Biol 70, 371-383.

Ame, J.C., Spenlehauer, C., and de Murcia, G. (2004). The PARP superfamily. Bioessays 26, 882-893.

Amiard, S., Charbonnel, C., Allain, E., Depeiges, A., White, C.I., and Gallego, M.E. (2010). Distinct roles of the ATR kinase and the Mre11-Rad50-Nbs1 complex in the maintenance of chromosomal stability in Arabidopsis. Plant Cell 22, 3020-3033.

Araujo, S.J., Nigg, E.A., and Wood, R.D. (2001). Strong functional interactions of TFIIH with XPC and XPG in human DNA nucleotide excision repair, without a preassembled repairosome. Mol Cell Biol 21, 2281-2291.

Asada, K. (1999). THE WATER-WATER CYCLE IN CHLOROPLASTS: Scavenging of Active Oxygens and Dissipation of Excess Photons. Annu Rev Plant Physiol Plant Mol Biol 50, 601-639.

Ayora, S., Piruat, J.I., Luna, R., Reiss, B., Russo, V.E., Aguilera, A., and Alonso, J.C. (2002). Characterization of two highly similar Rad51 homologs of Physcomitrella patens. J Mol Biol 316, 35-49.

Babiychuk, E., Kushnir, S., Van Montagu, M., and Inze, D. (1994). The Arabidopsis thaliana apurinic endonuclease Arp reduces human transcription factors Fos and Jun. Proc Natl Acad Sci U S A 91, 3299-3303.

Babiychuk, E., Cottrill, P.B., Storozhenko, S., Fuangthong, M., Chen, Y., O'Farrell, M.K., Van Montagu, M., Inze, D., and Kushnir, S. (1998). Higher plants possess two structurally different poly(ADP-ribose) polymerases. Plant J 15, 635-645.

Bakalkin, G., Yakovleva, T., Selivanova, G., Magnusson, K.P., Szekely, L., Kiseleva, E., Klein, G., Terenius, L., and Wiman, K.G. (1994). p53 binds single-stranded DNA ends and catalyzes DNA renaturation and strand transfer. Proc Natl Acad Sci U S A 91, 413-417.

Bakkenist, C.J., and Kastan, M.B. (2003). DNA damage activates ATM through intermolecular autophosphorylation and dimer dissociation. Nature 421, 499-506.

Ball, H.L., and Cortez, D. (2005). ATRIP oligomerization is required for ATR-dependent checkpoint signaling. J Biol Chem 280, 31390-31396.

Barnes, D.E., Stamp, G., Rosewell, I., Denzel, A., and Lindahl, T. (1998). Targeted disruption of the gene encoding DNA ligase IV leads to lethality in embryonic mice. Curr Biol 8, 1395-1398.

Beggs, C.J., Stolzer-Jehle, A., and Wellmann, E. (1985). Isoflavonoid formation as an indicator of UV stress in bean (Phaseolus vulgaris L.) leaves. Plant Physiol 79, 630-634.

Bennardo, N., Cheng, A., Huang, N., and Stark, J.M. (2008). Alternative-NHEJ is a mechanistically distinct pathway of mammalian chromosome break repair. PLoS Genet 4, e1000110.

Bernhardt, A., Mooney, S., and Hellmann, H. (2010). Arabidopsis DDB1a and DDB1b are critical for embryo development. Planta 232, 555-566.

Bernhardt, A., Lechner, E., Hano, P., Schade, V., Dieterle, M., Anders, M., Dubin, M.J., Benvenuto, G., Bowler, C., Genschik, P., and Hellmann, H. (2006). CUL4 associates with DDB1 and DET1 and its downregulation affects diverse aspects of development in Arabidopsis thaliana. Plant J 47, 591-603.

Bhagwat, M., and Gerlt, J.A. (1996). 3'- and 5'-strand cleavage reactions catalyzed by the Fpg protein from Escherichia coli occur via successive beta- and delta-elimination mechanisms, respectively. Biochemistry 35, 659-665.

Biedermann, S., and Hellmann, H. (2010). The DDB1a interacting proteins ATCSA-1 and DDB2 are critical factors for UV-B tolerance and genomic integrity in Arabidopsis thaliana. Plant J 62, 404-415.

Blackwell, L.J., Borowiec, J.A., and Mastrangelo, I.A. (1996). Single-stranded-DNA binding alters human replication protein A structure and facilitates interaction with DNA-dependent protein kinase. Mol Cell Biol 16, 4798-4807.

Blanck, S., Kobbe, D., Hartung, F., Fengler, K., Focke, M., and Puchta, H. (2009). A SRS2 homolog from Arabidopsis thaliana disrupts recombinogenic DNA intermediates and facilitates single strand annealing. Nucleic Acids Res 37, 7163-7176.

Bleuyard, J.Y., Gallego, M.E., and White, C.I. (2006). Recent advances in understanding of the DNA double-strand break repair machinery of plants. DNA Repair (Amst) 5, 1-12.

Boesch, P., Weber-Lotfi, F., Ibrahim, N., Tarasenko, V., Cosset, A., Paulus, F., Lightowlers, R.N., and Dietrich, A. (2011). DNA repair in organelles: Pathways, organization, regulation, relevance in disease and aging. Biochim Biophys Acta 1813, 186-200.

Boorstein, R.J., Hilbert, T.P., Cadet, J., Cunningham, R.P., and Teebor, G.W. (1989). UV-induced pyrimidine hydrates in DNA are repaired by bacterial and mammalian DNA glycosylase activities. Biochemistry 28, 6164-6170.

Boyko, A., Filkowski, J., Hudson, D., and Kovalchuk, I. (2006a). Homologous recombination in plants is organ specific. Mutat Res 595, 145-155.

Boyko, A., Zemp, F., Filkowski, J., and Kovalchuk, I. (2006b). Double-strand break repair in plants is developmentally regulated. Plant Physiol 141, 488-497.

Brady, C.A., and Attardi, L.D. (2010). p53 at a glance. J Cell Sci 123, 2527-2532.

Breimer, L., and Lindahl, T. (1980). A DNA glycosylase from Escherichia coli that releases free urea from a polydeoxyribonucleotide containing fragments of base residues. Nucleic Acids Res 8, 6199-6211.

Caldecott, K.W. (2001). Mammalian DNA single-strand break repair: an X-ra(y)ted affair. Bioessays 23, 447-455.

Camenisch, U., Dip, R., Schumacher, S.B., Schuler, B., and Naegeli, H. (2006). Recognition of helical kinks by xeroderma pigmentosum group A protein triggers DNA excision repair. Nat Struct Mol Biol 13, 278-284.

Canman, C.E., Lim, D.S., Cimprich, K.A., Taya, Y., Tamai, K., Sakaguchi, K., Appella, E., Kastan, M.B., and Siliciano, J.D. (1998). Activation of the ATM kinase by ionizing radiation and phosphorylation of p53. Science 281, 1677-1679.

Cao, J., Combs, C., and Jagendorf, A.T. (1997). The chloroplast-located homolog of bacterial DNA recombinase. Plant Cell Physiol 38, 1319-1325.

Castells, E., Molinier, J., Drevensek, S., Genschik, P., Barneche, F., and Bowler, C. (2010). det1-1-induced UV-C hyposensitivity through UVR3 and PHR1 photolyase gene over-expression. Plant J.

Castells, E., Molinier, J., Benvenuto, G., Bourbousse, C., Zabulon, G., Zalc, A., Cazzaniga, S., Genschik, P., Barneche, F., and Bowler, C. (2011). The conserved factor DE-ETIOLATED 1 cooperates with CUL4-DDB1(DDB2) to maintain genome integrity upon UV stress. EMBO J 30, 1162-1172.

Cazzalini, O., Perucca, P., Savio, M., Necchi, D., Bianchi, L., Stivala, L.A., Ducommun, B., Scovassi, A.I., and Prosperi, E. (2008). Interaction of p21(CDKN1A) with PCNA regulates the histone acetyltransferase activity of p300 in nucleotide excision repair. Nucleic Acids Res 36, 1713-1722.

Cerutti, H., Osman, M., Grandoni, P., and Jagendorf, A.T. (1992). A homolog of Escherichia coli RecA protein in plastids of higher plants. Proc Natl Acad Sci U S A 89, 8068-8072.

Chang, Y., Gong, L., Yuan, W., Li, X., Chen, G., Zhang, Q., and Wu, C. (2009). Replication protein A (RPA1a) is required for meiotic and somatic DNA repair but is dispensable for DNA replication and homologous recombination in rice. Plant Physiol 151, 2162-2173.

Charbonnel, C., Gallego, M.E., and White, C.I. (2010). Xrcc1-dependent and Ku-dependent DNA double-strand break repair kinetics in Arabidopsis plants. Plant J 64, 280-290.

Chen, H., Shen, Y., Tang, X., Yu, L., Wang, J., Guo, L., Zhang, Y., Zhang, H., Feng, S., Strickland, E., Zheng, N., and Deng, X.W. (2006). Arabidopsis CULLIN4 Forms an E3 Ubiquitin Ligase with RBX1 and the CDD Complex in Mediating Light Control of Development. Plant Cell 18, 1991-2004.

Chen, I.P., Haehnel, U., Altschmied, L., Schubert, I., and Puchta, H. (2003). The transcriptional response of Arabidopsis to genotoxic stress - a high-density colony array study (HDCA). Plant J 35, 771-786.

Chen, J.J., Mitchell, D.L., and Britt, A.B. (1994). A Light-Dependent Pathway for the Elimination of UV-Induced Pyrimidine (6-4) Pyrimidinone Photoproducts in Arabidopsis. Plant Cell 6, 1311-1317.

Chittela, R.K., and Sainis, J.K. (2010). Plant DNA recombinases: a long way to go. J Nucleic Acids 2010.

Citarelli, M., Teotia, S., and Lamb, R.S. (2010). Evolutionary history of the poly(ADP-ribose) polymerase gene family in eukaryotes. BMC Evol Biol 10, 308.

Citterio, E., Van Den Boom, V., Schnitzler, G., Kanaar, R., Bonte, E., Kingston, R.E., Hoeijmakers, J.H., and Vermeulen, W. (2000). ATP-dependent chromatin remodeling by the Cockayne syndrome B DNA repair-transcription-coupling factor. Mol Cell Biol 20, 7643-7653.

Clark, R.A.F. (2008). Oxidative Stress and "Senescent" Fibroblasts in Non-Healing Wounds as Potential Therapeutic Targets. J Invest Dermatol 128, 2361–2364.

Cortez, D., Guntuku, S., Qin, J., and Elledge, S.J. (2001). ATR and ATRIP: partners in checkpoint signaling. Science 294, 1713-1716.

Costa, R.M., Morgante, P.G., Berra, C.M., Nakabashi, M., Bruneau, D., Bouchez, D., Sweder, K.S., Van Sluys, M.A., and Menck, C.F. (2001). The participation of AtXPB1, the XPB/RAD25 homologue gene from Arabidopsis thaliana, in DNA repair and plant development. Plant J 28, 385-395.

Cui, L., Veeraraghavan, N., Richter, A., Wall, K., Jansen, R.K., Leebens-Mack, J., Makalowska, I., and dePamphilis, C.W. (2006). ChloroplastDB: the Chloroplast Genome Database. Nucleic Acids Res 34, D692-696.

Culligan, K., Tissier, A., and Britt, A. (2004). ATR regulates a G2-phase cell-cycle checkpoint in Arabidopsis thaliana. Plant Cell 16, 1091-1104.

Culligan, K.M., Robertson, C.E., Foreman, J., Doerner, P., and Britt, A.B. (2006). ATR and ATM play both distinct and additive roles in response to ionizing radiation. Plant J 48, 947-961.

Dany, A.L., and Tissier, A. (2001). A functional OGG1 homologue from Arabidopsis thaliana. Mol Genet Genomics 265, 293-301.

Daoudal-Cotterell, S., Gallego, M.E., and White, C.I. (2002). The plant Rad50-Mre11 protein complex. FEBS Lett 516, 164-166.

Dasika, G.K., Lin, S.C., Zhao, S., Sung, P., Tomkinson, A., and Lee, E.Y. (1999). DNA damage-induced cell cycle checkpoints and DNA strand break repair in development and tumorigenesis. Oncogene 18, 7883-7899.

De Block, M., Verduyn, C., De Brouwer, D., and Cornelissen, M. (2005). Poly(ADP-ribose) polymerase in plants affects energy homeostasis, cell death and stress tolerance. Plant J 41, 95-106.

Delmas, D., Aires, V., Limagne, E., Dutartre, P., Mazue, F., Ghiringhelli, F., and Latruffe, N. (2011). Transport, stability, and biological activity of resveratrol. Ann N Y Acad Sci 1215, 48-59.

Demple, B., and Harrison, L. (1994). Repair of oxidative damage to DNA: enzymology and biology. Annu Rev Biochem 63, 915-948.

Demple, B., Harrison, L., Wilson, D.M., 3rd, Bennett, R.A., Takagi, T., and Ascione, A.G. (1997). Regulation of eukaryotic abasic endonucleases and their role in genetic stability. Environ Health Perspect 105 Suppl 4, 931-934.

Devisetty, U.K., Mayes, K., and Mayes, S. (2010). The RAD51 and DMC1 homoeologous genes of bread wheat: cloning, molecular characterization and expression analysis. BMC Res Notes 3, 245.

Doucet-Chabeaud, G., Godon, C., Brutesco, C., de Murcia, G., and Kazmaier, M. (2001). Ionising radiation induces the expression of PARP-1 and PARP-2 genes in Arabidopsis. Mol Genet Genomics 265, 954-963.

Dray, E., Siaud, N., Dubois, E., and Doutriaux, M.P. (2006). Interaction between Arabidopsis Brca2 and its partners Rad51, Dmc1, and Dss1. Plant Physiol 140, 1059-1069.

Evans, E., Moggs, J.G., Hwang, J.R., Egly, J.M., and Wood, R.D. (1997). Mechanism of open complex and dual incision formation by human nucleotide excision repair factors. EMBO J 16, 6559-6573.

Falck, J., Coates, J., and Jackson, S.P. (2005). Conserved modes of recruitment of ATM, ATR and DNA-PKcs to sites of DNA damage. Nature 434, 605-611.

Farmer, L.M., Book, A.J., Lee, K.H., Lin, Y.L., Fu, H., and Vierstra, R.D. (2010). The RAD23 family provides an essential connection between the 26S proteasome and ubiquitylated proteins in Arabidopsis. Plant Cell 22, 124-142.

Fitch, M.E., Cross, I.V., Turner, S.J., Adimoolam, S., Lin, C.X., Williams, K.G., and Ford, J.M. (2003). The DDB2 nucleotide excision repair gene product p48 enhances global genomic repair in p53 deficient human fibroblasts. DNA Repair (Amst) 2, 819-826.

Fousteri, M., Vermeulen, W., van Zeeland, A.A., and Mullenders, L.H. (2006). Cockayne syndrome A and B proteins differentially regulate recruitment of chromatin remodeling and repair factors to stalled RNA polymerase II in vivo. Mol Cell 23, 471-482.

Foyer, C.H., and Noctor, G. (2003). Redox sensing and signalling associated with reactive oxygen in chloroplasts, peroxisomes and mitochondria Physiol Plant 119, 355-364.

Friedberg EC, Walker GC, Siede W, Wood RD, Schultz RA, and ., E.E. (2006). DNA repair and mutagenesis. (ASM Press, Washington, DC).

Friesner, J., and Britt, A.B. (2003). Ku80- and DNA ligase IV-deficient plants are sensitive to ionizing radiation and defective in T-DNA integration. Plant J 34, 427-440.

Fulcher, N., and Sablowski, R. (2009). Hypersensitivity to DNA damage in plant stem cell niches. Proc Natl Acad Sci U S A 106, 20984-20988.

Furukawa, T., Curtis, M.J., Tominey, C.M., Duong, Y.H., Wilcox, B.W., Aggoune, D., Hays, J.B., and Britt, A.B. (2010). A shared DNA-damage-response pathway for induction of stem-cell death by UVB and by gamma irradiation. DNA Repair (Amst) 9, 940-948.

Gallego, M.E., and White, C.I. (2001). RAD50 function is essential for telomere maintenance in Arabidopsis. Proc Natl Acad Sci U S A 98, 1711-1716.

Gallego, M.E., Bleuyard, J.Y., Daoudal-Cotterell, S., Jallut, N., and White, C.I. (2003). Ku80 plays a role in non-homologous recombination but is not required for T-DNA integration in Arabidopsis. Plant J 35, 557-565.

Garcia-Diaz, M., Dominguez, O., Lopez-Fernandez, L.A., de Lera, L.T., Saniger, M.L., Ruiz, J.F., Parraga, M., Garcia-Ortiz, M.J., Kirchhoff, T., del Mazo, J., Bernad, A., and Blanco, L. (2000). DNA polymerase lambda (Pol lambda), a novel eukaryotic DNA polymerase with a potential role in meiosis. J Mol Biol 301, 851-867.

Garcia-Ortiz, M.V., Ariza, R.R., and Roldan-Arjona, T. (2001). An OGG1 orthologue encoding a functional 8-oxoguanine DNA glycosylase/lyase in Arabidopsis thaliana. Plant Mol Biol 47, 795-804.

Garcia, V., Salanoubat, M., Choisne, N., and Tissier, A. (2000). An ATM homologue from Arabidopsis thaliana: complete genomic organisation and expression analysis. Nucleic Acids Res 28, 1692-1699.

Gatz, S.A., and Wiesmuller, L. (2006). p53 in recombination and repair. Cell Death Differ 13, 1003-1016.

Grawunder, U., Wilm, M., Wu, X., Kulesza, P., Wilson, T.E., Mann, M., and Lieber, M.R. (1997). Activity of DNA ligase IV stimulated by complex formation with XRCC4 protein in mammalian cells. Nature 388, 492-495.

Gray, W.M., Hellmann, H., Dharmasiri, S., and Estelle, M. (2002). Role of the Arabidopsis RING-H2 protein RBX1 in RUB modification and SCF function. Plant Cell 14, 2137-2144.

Green, C.M., and Almouzni, G. (2003). Local action of the chromatin assembly factor CAF-1 at sites of nucleotide excision repair in vivo. EMBO J 22, 5163-5174.

Groisman, R., Kuraoka, I., Chevallier, O., Gaye, N., Magnaldo, T., Tanaka, K., Kisselev, A.F., Harel-Bellan, A., and Nakatani, Y. (2006). CSA-dependent degradation of CSB by the ubiquitin-proteasome pathway establishes a link between complementation factors of the Cockayne syndrome. Genes Dev 20, 1429-1434.

Guay, D., Garand, C., Reddy, S., Schmutte, C., and Lebel, M. (2008). The human endonuclease III enzyme is a relevant target to potentiate cisplatin cytotoxicity in Y-box-binding protein-1 overexpressing tumor cells. Cancer Sci 99, 762-769.

Gutman, B.L., and Niyogi, K.K. (2009). Evidence for base excision repair of oxidative DNA damage in chloroplasts of Arabidopsis thaliana. J Biol Chem 284, 17006-17012.

Ha, H.C., and Snyder, S.H. (1999). Poly(ADP-ribose) polymerase is a mediator of necrotic cell death by ATP depletion. Proc Natl Acad Sci U S A 96, 13978-13982.

Harlow, G.R., Jenkins, M.E., Pittalwala, T.S., and Mount, D.W. (1994). Isolation of uvh1, an Arabidopsis mutant hypersensitive to ultraviolet light and ionizing radiation. Plant Cell 6, 227-235.

Hartung, F., and Puchta, H. (1999). Isolation of the Complete cDNA of the Mre11 Homologue of Arabidopsis (Accession No. AJ243822) Indicates Conservation of DNA Recombination Mechanisms Between Plants and Other Eucaryotes. Plant Physiol 121, 312.

Hatahet, Z., Kow, Y.W., Purmal, A.A., Cunningham, R.P., and Wallace, S.S. (1994). New substrates for old enzymes. 5-Hydroxy-2'-deoxycytidine and 5-hydroxy-2'-deoxyuridine are substrates for Escherichia coli endonuclease III and formamidopyrimidine DNA N-glycosylase, while 5-hydroxy-2'-deoxyuridine is a substrate for uracil DNA N-glycosylase. J Biol Chem 269, 18814-18820.

Hattori, Y., Nishigori, C., Tanaka, T., Uchida, K., Nikaido, O., Osawa, T., Hiai, H., Imamura, S., and Toyokuni, S. (1996). 8-hydroxy-2′-deoxyguanosine is increased in epidermal cells of hairless mice after chronic ultraviolet B exposure. J Invest Dermatol 107, 733-737.

Hazra, T.K., Hill, J.W., Izumi, T., and Mitra, S. (2001). Multiple DNA glycosylases for repair of 8-oxoguanine and their potential in vivo functions. Prog Nucleic Acid Res Mol Biol 68, 193-205.

Heacock, M., Spangler, E., Riha, K., Puizina, J., and Shippen, D.E. (2004). Molecular analysis of telomere fusions in Arabidopsis: multiple pathways for chromosome end-joining. EMBO J 23, 2304-2313.

Hidema, J., Taguchi, T., Ono, T., Teranishi, M., Yamamoto, K., and Kumagai, T. (2007). Increase in CPD photolyase activity functions effectively to prevent growth inhibition caused by UVB radiation. Plant J 50, 70-79.

Hitomi, K., DiTacchio, L., Arvai, A.S., Yamamoto, J., Kim, S.T., Todo, T., Tainer, J.A., Iwai, S., Panda, S., and Getzoff, E.D. (2009). Functional motifs in the (6-4) photolyase crystal structure make a comparative framework for DNA repair photolyases and clock cryptochromes. Proc Natl Acad Sci U S A 106, 6962-6967.

Huang, Y., Baxter, R., Smith, B.S., Partch, C.L., Colbert, C.L., and Deisenhofer, J. (2006). Crystal structure of cryptochrome 3 from Arabidopsis thaliana and its implications for photolyase activity. Proc Natl Acad Sci U S A 103, 17701-17706.

Iovine, B., Nino, M., Irace, C., Bevilacqua, M.A., and Monfrecola, G. (2009). Ultraviolet B and A irradiation induces fibromodulin expression in human fibroblasts in vitro. Biochimie 91, 364-372.

Ishibashi, T., Koga, A., Yamamoto, T., Uchiyama, Y., Mori, Y., Hashimoto, J., Kimura, S., and Sakaguchi, K. (2005). Two types of replication protein A in seed plants. FEBS J 272, 3270-3281.

Ishikawa, K., Ogawa, T., Hirosue, E., Nakayama, Y., Harada, K., Fukusaki, E., Yoshimura, K., and Shigeoka, S. (2009). Modulation of the poly(ADP-ribosyl)ation reaction via the Arabidopsis ADP-ribose/NADH pyrophosphohydrolase, AtNUDX7, is involved in the response to oxidative stress. Plant Physiol 151, 741-754.

Jaspers, P., and Kangasjarvi, J. (2010). Reactive oxygen species in abiotic stress signaling. Physiol Plant 138, 405-413.

Jenkins, M.E., Harlow, G.R., Liu, Z., Shotwell, M.A., Ma, J., and Mount, D.W. (1995). Radiation-sensitive mutants of Arabidopsis thaliana. Genetics 140, 725-732.

Jiang, C.Z., Yee, J., Mitchell, D.L., and Britt, A.B. (1997). Photorepair mutants of Arabidopsis. Proc Natl Acad Sci U S A 94, 7441-7445.

Kaiser, G., Kleiner, O., Beisswenger, C., and Batschauer, A. (2009). Increased DNA repair in Arabidopsis plants overexpressing CPD photolyase. Planta 230, 505-515.

Kamiuchi, S., Saijo, M., Citterio, E., de Jager, M., Hoeijmakers, J.H., and Tanaka, K. (2002). Translocation of Cockayne syndrome group A protein to the nuclear matrix: possible relevance to transcription-coupled DNA repair. Proc Natl Acad Sci U S A 99, 201-206.

Kanai, S., Kikuno, R., Toh, H., Ryo, H., and Todo, T. (1997). Molecular evolution of the photolyase-blue-light photoreceptor family. J Mol Evol 45, 535-548.

Kapetanaki, M.G., Guerrero-Santoro, J., Bisi, D.C., Hsieh, C.L., Rapic-Otrin, V., and Levine, A.S. (2006). The DDB1-CUL4ADDB2 ubiquitin ligase is deficient in xeroderma pigmentosum group E and targets histone H2A at UV-damaged DNA sites. Proc Natl Acad Sci U S A 103, 2588-2593.

Karanjawala, Z.E., Hsieh, C.L., and Lieber, M.R. (2003). Overexpression of Cu/Zn superoxide dismutase is lethal for mice lacking double-strand break repair. DNA Repair (Amst) 2, 285-294.

Karanjawala, Z.E., Murphy, N., Hinton, D.R., Hsieh, C.L., and Lieber, M.R. (2002). Oxygen metabolism causes chromosome breaks and is associated with the neuronal apoptosis observed in DNA double-strand break repair mutants. Curr Biol 12, 397-402.

Kesseler, K.J., Kaufmann, W.K., Reardon, J.T., Elston, T.C., and Sancar, A. (2007). A mathematical model for human nucleotide excision repair: damage recognition by random order assembly and kinetic proofreading. J Theor Biol 249, 361-375.

Khazi, F.R., Edmondson, A.C., and Nielsen, B.L. (2003). An Arabidopsis homologue of bacterial RecA that complements an E. coli recA deletion is targeted to plant mitochondria. Mol Genet Genomics 269, 454-463.

Kimura, S., and Sakaguchi, K. (2006). DNA repair in plants. Chem Rev 106, 753-766.

Kimura, S., Saotome, A., Uchiyama, Y., Mori, Y., Tahira, Y., and Sakaguchi, K. (2005). The expression of the rice (Oryza sativa L.) homologue of Snm1 is induced by DNA damages. Biochem Biophys Res Commun 329, 668-672.

Kimura, S., Tahira, Y., Ishibashi, T., Mori, Y., Mori, T., Hashimoto, J., and Sakaguchi, K. (2004). DNA repair in higher plants; photoreactivation is the major DNA repair pathway in non-proliferating cells while excision repair (nucleotide excision repair and base excision repair) is active in proliferating cells. Nucleic Acids Res 32, 2760-2767.

Ko, J.C., Su, Y.J., Lin, S.T., Jhan, J.Y., Ciou, S.C., Cheng, C.M., and Lin, Y.W. (2010). Suppression of ERCC1 and Rad51 expression through ERK1/2 inactivation is essential in emodin-mediated cytotoxicity in human non-small cell lung cancer cells. Biochem Pharmacol 79, 655-664.

Ko, J.C., Tsai, M.S., Kuo, Y.H., Chiu, Y.F., Weng, S.H., Su, Y.C., and Lin, Y.W. (2011). Modulation of Rad51, ERCC1, and thymidine phosphorylase by emodin result in synergistic cytotoxic effect in combination with capecitabine. Biochem Pharmacol 81, 680-690.

Koga, A., Ishibashi, T., Kimura, S., Uchiyama, Y., and Sakaguchi, K. (2006). Characterization of T-DNA insertion mutants and RNAi silenced plants of Arabidopsis thaliana UV-damaged DNA binding protein 2 (AtUV-DDB2). Plant Mol Biol 61, 227-240.

Krasikova, Y.S., Rechkunova, N.I., Maltseva, E.A., Petruseva, I.O., Silnikov, V.N., Zatsepin, T.S., Oretskaya, T.S., Scharer, O.D., and Lavrik, O.I. (2008). Interaction of nucleotide excision repair factors XPC-HR23B, XPA, and RPA with damaged DNA. Biochemistry (Mosc) 73, 886-896.

Kraszewska, E. (2008). The plant Nudix hydrolase family. Acta Biochim Pol 55, 663-671.

Krieger-Liszkay, A. (2005). Singlet oxygen production in photosynthesis. J Exp Bot 56, 337 - 346.

Krokan, H.E., Standal, R., and Slupphaug, G. (1997). DNA glycosylases in the base excision repair of DNA. Biochem J 325 (Pt 1), 1-16.

Kruger, A., and Ralser, M. (2011). ATM Is a Redox Sensor Linking Genome Stability and Carbon Metabolism. Sci Signal 4, pe17.

Kunz, B.A., Anderson, H.J., Osmond, M.J., and Vonarx, E.J. (2005). Components of nucleotide excision repair and DNA damage tolerance in Arabidopsis thaliana. Environ Mol Mutagen 45, 115-127.

Kwon, T., Huq, E., and Herrin, D.L. (2010). Microhomology-mediated and nonhomologous repair of a double-strand break in the chloroplast genome of Arabidopsis. Proc Natl Acad Sci U S A 107, 13954-13959.

Lafarge, S., and Montane, M.H. (2003). Characterization of Arabidopsis thaliana ortholog of the human breast cancer susceptibility gene 1: AtBRCA1, strongly induced by gamma rays. Nucleic Acids Res 31, 1148-1155.

Landry, L.G., Stapleton, A.E., Lim, J., Hoffman, P., Hays, J.B., Walbot, V., and Last, R.L. (1997). An Arabidopsis photolyase mutant is hypersensitive to ultraviolet-B radiation. Proc Natl Acad Sci U S A 94, 328-332.

Langcake, P., and Pryce, R.J. (1977). The production of resveratrol and the viniferins by grapevines in response to UV radiation. Phytochemistry 16, 1193-1196.

Lechner, E., Xie, D., Grava, S., Pigaglio, E., Planchais, S., Murray, J.A., Parmentier, Y., Mutterer, J., Dubreucq, B., Shen, W.H., and Genschik, P. (2002). The AtRbx1 protein is part of plant SCF complexes, and its down-regulation causes severe growth and developmental defects. J Biol Chem 277, 50069-50080.

Lepiniec, L., Babiychuk, E., Kushnir, S., Van Montagu, M., and Inze, D. (1995). Characterization of an Arabidopsis thaliana cDNA homologue to animal poly(ADP-ribose) polymerase. FEBS Lett 364, 103-108.

Li, J., Liu, Z., Tan, C., Guo, X., Wang, L., Sancar, A., and Zhong, D. (2010). Dynamics and mechanism of repair of ultraviolet-induced (6-4) photoproduct by photolyase. Nature 466, 887-890.

Li, J., Harper, L.C., Golubovskaya, I., Wang, C.R., Weber, D., Meeley, R.B., McElver, J., Bowen, B., Cande, W.Z., and Schnable, P.S. (2007). Functional analysis of maize RAD51 in meiosis and double-strand break repair. Genetics 176, 1469-1482.

Li, W., and Ma, H. (2006). Double-stranded DNA breaks and gene functions in recombination and meiosis. Cell Res 16, 402-412.

Liang, L., Flury, S., Kalck, V., Hohn, B., and Molinier, J. (2006). CENTRIN2 interacts with the Arabidopsis homolog of the human XPC protein (AtRAD4) and contributes to efficient synthesis-dependent repair of bulky DNA lesions. Plant Mol Biol 61, 345-356.

Lin, Z., Kong, H., Nei, M., and Ma, H. (2006). Origins and evolution of the recA/RAD51 gene family: evidence for ancient gene duplication and endosymbiotic gene transfer. Proc Natl Acad Sci U S A 103, 10328-10333.

Lindahl, T. (1993). Instability and decay of the primary structure of DNA. Nature 362, 709-715.

Liu, Z., Hossain, G.S., Islas-Osuna, M.A., Mitchell, D.L., and Mount, D.W. (2000). Repair of UV damage in plants by nucleotide excision repair: Arabidopsis UVH1 DNA repair gene is a homolog of Saccharomyces cerevisiae Rad1. Plant J 21, 519-528.

Liu, Z., Hong, S.W., Escobar, M., Vierling, E., Mitchell, D.L., Mount, D.W., and Hall, J.D. (2003). Arabidopsis UVH6, a homolog of human XPD and yeast RAD3 DNA repair genes, functions in DNA repair and is essential for plant growth. Plant Physiol 132, 1405-1414.

Ma, Y., Pannicke, U., Schwarz, K., and Lieber, M.R. (2002). Hairpin opening and overhang processing by an Artemis/DNA-dependent protein kinase complex in nonhomologous end joining and V(D)J recombination. Cell 108, 781-794.

Maltseva, E.A., Rechkunova, N.I., Petruseva, I.O., Silnikov, V.N., Vermeulen, W., and Lavrik, O.I. (2006). Interaction of nucleotide excision repair factors RPA and XPA with DNA containing bulky photoreactive groups imitating damages. Biochemistry (Mosc) 71, 270-278.

Mannuss, A., Dukowic-Schulze, S., Suer, S., Hartung, F., Pacher, M., and Puchta, H. (2010). RAD5A, RECQ4A, and MUS81 have specific functions in homologous recombination and define different pathways of DNA repair in Arabidopsis thaliana. Plant Cell 22, 3318-3330.

Markmann-Mulisch, U., Wendeler, E., Zobell, O., Schween, G., Steinbiss, H.H., and Reiss, B. (2007). Differential requirements for RAD51 in Physcomitrella patens and Arabidopsis thaliana development and DNA damage repair. Plant Cell 19, 3080-3089.

Masson, M., Niedergang, C., Schreiber, V., Muller, S., Menissier-de Murcia, J., and de Murcia, G. (1998). XRCC1 is specifically associated with poly(ADP-ribose) polymerase and negatively regulates its activity following DNA damage. Mol Cell Biol 18, 3563-3571.

Matsumoto, Y. (2001). Molecular mechanism of PCNA-dependent base excision repair. Prog Nucleic Acid Res Mol Biol 68, 129-138.

McLennan, A.G. (2006). The Nudix hydrolase superfamily. Cell Mol Life Sci 63, 123-143.

Min, J.H., and Pavletich, N.P. (2007). Recognition of DNA damage by the Rad4 nucleotide excision repair protein. Nature 449, 570-575.

Minig, V., Kattan, Z., van Beeumen, J., Brunner, E., and Becuwe, P. (2009). Identification of DDB2 protein as a transcriptional regulator of constitutive SOD2 gene expression in human breast cancer cells. J Biol Chem 284, 14165-14176.

Moldt, J., Pokorny, R., Orth, C., Linne, U., Geisselbrecht, Y., Marahiel, M.A., Essen, L.O., and Batschauer, A. (2009). Photoreduction of the folate cofactor in members of the photolyase family. J Biol Chem 284, 21670-21683.

Molinier, J., Stamm, M.E., and Hohn, B. (2004a). SNM-dependent recombinational repair of oxidatively induced DNA damage in Arabidopsis thaliana. EMBO Rep 5, 994-999.

Molinier, J., Ramos, C., Fritsch, O., and Hohn, B. (2004b). CENTRIN2 modulates homologous recombination and nucleotide excision repair in Arabidopsis. Plant Cell 16, 1633-1643.

Molinier, J., Lechner, E., Dumbliauskas, E., and Genschik, P. (2008). Regulation and role of Arabidopsis CUL4-DDB1A-DDB2 in maintaining genome integrity upon UV stress. PLoS Genet 4, e1000093.

Molinier, J., Oakeley, E.J., Niederhauser, O., Kovalchuk, I., and Hohn, B. (2005). Dynamic response of plant genome to ultraviolet radiation and other genotoxic stresses. Mutat Res 571, 235-247.

Morales-Ruiz, T., Birincioglu, M., Jaruga, P., Rodriguez, H., Roldan-Arjona, T., and Dizdaroglu, M. (2003). Arabidopsis thaliana Ogg1 protein excises 8-hydroxyguanine and 2,6-diamino-4-hydroxy-5-formamidopyrimidine from oxidatively damaged DNA containing multiple lesions. Biochemistry 42, 3089-3095.

Morgante, P.G., Berra, C.M., Nakabashi, M., Costa, R.M., Menck, C.F., and Van Sluys, M.A. (2005). Functional XPB/RAD25 redundancy in Arabidopsis genome: characterization of AtXPB2 and expression analysis. Gene 344, 93-103.

Morland, I., Rolseth, V., Luna, L., Rognes, T., Bjoras, M., and Seeberg, E. (2002). Human DNA glycosylases of the bacterial Fpg/MutM superfamily: an alternative pathway for the repair of 8-oxoguanine and other oxidation products in DNA. Nucleic Acids Res 30, 4926-4936.

Moser, J., Volker, M., Kool, H., Alekseev, S., Vrieling, H., Yasui, A., van Zeeland, A.A., and Mullenders, L.H. (2005). The UV-damaged DNA binding protein mediates efficient targeting of the nucleotide excision repair complex to UV-induced photo lesions. DNA Repair (Amst) 4, 571-582.

Mu, D., Hsu, D.S., and Sancar, A. (1996). Reaction mechanism of human DNA repair excision nuclease. J Biol Chem 271, 8285-8294.

Mu, D., Park, C.H., Matsunaga, T., Hsu, D.S., Reardon, J.T., and Sancar, A. (1995). Reconstitution of human DNA repair excision nuclease in a highly defined system. J Biol Chem 270, 2415-2418.

Murphy, T.M., and Gao, M.J. (2001). Multiple forms of formamidopyrimidine-DNA glycosylase produced by alternative splicing in Arabidopsis thaliana. J Photochem Photobiol B 61, 87-93.

Nakajima, S., Sugiyama, M., Iwai, S., Hitomi, K., Otoshi, E., Kim, S.T., Jiang, C.Z., Todo, T., Britt, A.B., and Yamamoto, K. (1998). Cloning and characterization of a gene (UVR3) required for photorepair of 6-4 photoproducts in Arabidopsis thaliana. Nucleic Acids Res 26, 638-644.

Nakazato, E., Fukuzawa, H., Tabata, S., Takahashi, H., and Tanaka, K. (2003). Identification and expression analysis of cDNA encoding a chloroplast recombination protein REC1, the chloroplast RecA homologue in Chlamydomonas reinhardtii. Biosci Biotechnol Biochem 67, 2608-2613.

Ndebele, K., Graham, B., and Tchounwou, P.B. (2010). Estrogenic activity of coumestrol, DDT, and TCDD in human cervical cancer cells. Int J Environ Res Public Health 7, 2045-2056.

Ng, Y.L., Thimann, K.V., and Gordon, S.A. (1964). The biogenesis of anthocyanins. X. The action spectrum for anthocyanin formation in *Spirodela oligorrhiza*. Arch Biochem Biophys 107, 550-558.

Nichols, A.F., and Sancar, A. (1992). Purification of PCNA as a nucleotide excision repair protein. Nucleic Acids Res 20, 2441-2446.

Noctor, G., Veljovic-Jovanovic, S., Driscoll, S., Novitskaya, L., and Foyer, C.H. (2002). Drought and oxidative load in the leaves of C3 plants: a predominant role for photorespiration? Ann Bot 89 Spec No, 841-850.

Odahara, M., Kuroiwa, H., Kuroiwa, T., and Sekine, Y. (2009). Suppression of repeat-mediated gross mitochondrial genome rearrangements by RecA in the moss Physcomitrella patens. Plant Cell 21, 1182-1194.

Odahara, M., Inouye, T., Fujita, T., Hasebe, M., and Sekine, Y. (2007). Involvement of mitochondrial-targeted RecA in the repair of mitochondrial DNA in the moss, Physcomitrella patens. Genes Genet Syst 82, 43-51.

Ogawa, T., Ueda, Y., Yoshimura, K., and Shigeoka, S. (2005). Comprehensive analysis of cytosolic Nudix hydrolases in Arabidopsis thaliana. J Biol Chem 280, 25277-25283.

Ogi, T., Limsirichaikul, S., Overmeer, R.M., Volker, M., Takenaka, K., Cloney, R., Nakazawa, Y., Niimi, A., Miki, Y., Jaspers, N.G., Mullenders, L.H., Yamashita, S., Fousteri, M.I., and Lehmann, A.R. (2010). Three DNA polymerases, recruited by different mechanisms, carry out NER repair synthesis in human cells. Mol Cell 37, 714-727.

Ohtsubo, T., Matsuda, O., Iba, K., Terashima, I., Sekiguchi, M., and Nakabeppu, Y. (1998). Molecular cloning of AtMMH, an Arabidopsis thaliana ortholog of the Escherichia coli mutM gene, and analysis of functional domains of its product. Mol Gen Genet 259, 577-590.

Okafuji, A., Biskup, T., Hitomi, K., Getzoff, E.D., Kaiser, G., Batschauer, A., Bacher, A., Hidema, J., Teranishi, M., Yamamoto, K., Schleicher, E., and Weber, S. (2010). Light-induced activation of class II cyclobutane pyrimidine dimer photolyases. DNA Repair (Amst) 9, 495-505.

Osman, K., Higgins, J.D., Sanchez-Moran, E., Armstrong, S.J., and Franklin, F.C. (2011). Pathways to meiotic recombination in Arabidopsis thaliana. New Phytol.

Ozturk, N., Kao, Y.T., Selby, C.P., Kavakli, I.H., Partch, C.L., Zhong, D., and Sancar, A. (2008). Purification and characterization of a type III photolyase from Caulobacter crescentus. Biochemistry 47, 10255-10261.

Pang, Q., Hays, J.B., and Rajagopal, I. (1992). A plant cDNA that partially complements Escherichia coli recA mutations predicts a polypeptide not strongly homologous to RecA proteins. Proc Natl Acad Sci U S A 89, 8073-8077.

Pang, Q., Hays, J.B., Rajagopal, I., and Schaefer, T.S. (1993). Selection of Arabidopsis cDNAs that partially correct phenotypes of Escherichia coli DNA-damage-sensitive mutants and analysis of two plant cDNAs that appear to express UV-specific dark repair activities. Plant Mol Biol 22, 411-426.

Parsons, J.L., Zharkov, D.O., and Dianov, G.L. (2005). NEIL1 excises 3' end proximal oxidative DNA lesions resistant to cleavage by NTH1 and OGG1. Nucleic Acids Res 33, 4849-4856.

Pascucci, B., Maga, G., Hubscher, U., Bjoras, M., Seeberg, E., Hickson, I.D., Villani, G., Giordano, C., Cellai, L., and Dogliotti, E. (2002). Reconstitution of the base excision repair pathway for 7,8-dihydro-8-oxoguanine with purified human proteins. Nucleic Acids Res 30, 2124-2130.

Perry, J.J., and Tainer, J.A. (2011). All Stressed Out Without ATM Kinase. Sci Signal 4, pe18.

Petersen, J.L., Lang, D.W., and Small, G.D. (1999). Cloning and characterization of a class II DNA photolyase from Chlamydomonas. Plant Mol Biol 40, 1063-1071.

Petrucco, S., Volpi, G., Bolchi, A., Rivetti, C., and Ottonello, S. (2002). A nick-sensing DNA 3'-repair enzyme from Arabidopsis. J Biol Chem 277, 23675-23683.

Phadnis, N., Mehta, R., Meednu, N., and Sia, E.A. (2006). Ntg1p, the base excision repair protein, generates mutagenic intermediates in yeast mitochondrial DNA. DNA Repair (Amst) 5, 829-839.

Pleschke, J.M., Kleczkowska, H.E., Strohm, M., and Althaus, F.R. (2000). Poly(ADP-ribose) binds to specific domains in DNA damage checkpoint proteins. J Biol Chem 275, 40974-40980.

Poirier, G.G., de Murcia, G., Jongstra-Bilen, J., Niedergang, C., and Mandel, P. (1982). Poly(ADP-ribosyl)ation of polynucleosomes causes relaxation of chromatin structure. Proc Natl Acad Sci U S A 79, 3423-3427.

Preuss, S.B., and Britt, A.B. (2003). A DNA-damage-induced cell cycle checkpoint in Arabidopsis. Genetics 164, 323-334.

Puchta, H. (2005). The repair of double-strand breaks in plants: mechanisms and consequences for genome evolution. J Exp Bot 56, 1-14.

Puchta, H., Swoboda, P., Gal, S., Blot, M., and Hohn, B. (1995). Somatic intrachromosomal homologous recombination events in populations of plant siblings. Plant Mol Biol 28, 281-292.

Rapic-Otrin, V., McLenigan, M.P., Bisi, D.C., Gonzalez, M., and Levine, A.S. (2002). Sequential binding of UV DNA damage binding factor and degradation of the p48 subunit as early events after UV irradiation. Nucleic Acids Res 30, 2588-2598.

Reardon, J.T., and Sancar, A. (2003). Recognition and repair of the cyclobutane thymine dimer, a major cause of skin cancers, by the human excision nuclease. Genes Dev 17, 2539-2551.

Ricaud, L., Proux, C., Renou, J.P., Pichon, O., Fochesato, S., Ortet, P., and Montane, M.H. (2007). ATM-mediated transcriptional and developmental responses to gamma-rays in Arabidopsis. PLoS One 2, e430.

Riha, K., Watson, J.M., Parkey, J., and Shippen, D.E. (2002). Telomere length deregulation and enhanced sensitivity to genotoxic stress in Arabidopsis mutants deficient in Ku70. EMBO J 21, 2819-2826.

Roldan-Arjona, T., and Ariza, R.R. (2009). Repair and tolerance of oxidative DNA damage in plants. Mutat Res 681, 169-179.

Roldan-Arjona, T., Garcia-Ortiz, M.V., Ruiz-Rubio, M., and Ariza, R.R. (2000). cDNA cloning, expression and functional characterization of an Arabidopsis thaliana homologue of the Escherichia coli DNA repair enzyme endonuclease III. Plant Mol Biol 44, 43-52.

Ronceret, A., Doutriaux, M.P., Golubovskaya, I.N., and Pawlowski, W.P. (2009). PHS1 regulates meiotic recombination and homologous chromosome pairing by controlling the transport of RAD50 to the nucleus. Proc Natl Acad Sci U S A 106, 20121-20126.

Rowan, B.A., Oldenburg, D.J., and Bendich, A.J. (2010). RecA maintains the integrity of chloroplast DNA molecules in Arabidopsis. J Exp Bot 61, 2575-2588.

Roy, N., Stoyanova, T., Dominguez-Brauer, C., Park, H.J., Bagchi, S., and Raychaudhuri, P. (2010). DDB2, an essential mediator of premature senescence. Mol Cell Biol 30, 2681-2692.

Schaefer, D.G., Delacote, F., Charlot, F., Vrielynck, N., Guyon-Debast, A., Le Guin, S., Neuhaus, J.M., Doutriaux, M.P., and Nogue, F. (2010). RAD51 loss of function abolishes gene targeting and de-represses illegitimate integration in the moss Physcomitrella patens. DNA Repair (Amst) 9, 526-533.

Scrima, A., Konickova, R., Czyzewski, B.K., Kawasaki, Y., Jeffrey, P.D., Groisman, R., Nakatani, Y., Iwai, S., Pavletich, N.P., and Thoma, N.H. (2008). Structural basis of UV DNA-damage recognition by the DDB1-DDB2 complex. Cell 135, 1213-1223.

Selby, C.P., and Sancar, A. (1997). Cockayne syndrome group B protein enhances elongation by RNA polymerase II. Proc Natl Acad Sci U S A 94, 11205-11209.

Shaked, H., Avivi-Ragolsky, N., and Levy, A.A. (2006). Involvement of the Arabidopsis SWI2/SNF2 chromatin remodeling gene family in DNA damage response and recombination. Genetics 173, 985-994.

Shedge, V., Arrieta-Montiel, M., Christensen, A.C., and Mackenzie, S.A. (2007). Plant mitochondrial recombination surveillance requires unusual RecA and MutS homologs. Plant Cell 19, 1251-1264.

Shivji, K.K., Kenny, M.K., and Wood, R.D. (1992). Proliferating cell nuclear antigen is required for DNA excision repair. Cell 69, 367-374.

Siaud, N., Dray, E., Gy, I., Gerard, E., Takvorian, N., and Doutriaux, M.P. (2004). Brca2 is involved in meiosis in Arabidopsis thaliana as suggested by its interaction with Dmc1. EMBO J 23, 1392-1401.

Singh, S.K., Roy, S., Choudhury, S.R., and Sengupta, D.N. (2010). DNA repair and recombination in higher plants: insights from comparative genomics of Arabidopsis and rice. BMC Genomics 11, 443.

Strzalka, W., Oyama, T., Tori, K., and Morikawa, K. (2009). Crystal structures of the Arabidopsis thaliana proliferating cell nuclear antigen 1 and 2 proteins complexed with the human p21 C-terminal segment. Protein Sci 18, 1072-1080.

Subramanian, D., and Griffith, J.D. (2005). Modulation of p53 binding to Holliday junctions and 3-cytosine bulges by phosphorylation events. Biochemistry 44, 2536-2544.

Sugasawa, K., Okuda, Y., Saijo, M., Nishi, R., Matsuda, N., Chu, G., Mori, T., Iwai, S., Tanaka, K., and Hanaoka, F. (2005). UV-induced ubiquitylation of XPC protein mediated by UV-DDB-ubiquitin ligase complex. Cell 121, 387-400.

Takahashi, M., Teranishi, M., Ishida, H., Kawasaki, J., Takeuchi, A., Yamaya, T., Watanabe, M., Makino, A., and Hidema, J. (2011). Cyclobutane pyrimidine dimer (CPD) photolyase repairs ultraviolet-B-induced CPDs in rice chloroplast and mitochondrial DNA. Plant J.

Takeda, J., and Abe, S. (1992). Light-induced synthesis of anthocyanin in carrot cells in suspension. IV. The action spectrum. Photochem Photobiol 56, 69-74.

Tamura, K., Adachi, Y., Chiba, K., Oguchi, K., and Takahashi, H. (2002). Identification of Ku70 and Ku80 homologues in Arabidopsis thaliana: evidence for a role in the repair of DNA double-strand breaks. Plant J 29, 771-781.

Taylor, R.M., Thistlethwaite, A., and Caldecott, K.W. (2002). Central role for the XRCC1 BRCT I domain in mammalian DNA single-strand break repair. Mol Cell Biol 22, 2556-2563.

Taylor, R.M., Hamer, M.J., Rosamond, J., and Bray, C.M. (1998). Molecular cloning and functional analysis of the Arabidopsis thaliana DNA ligase I homologue. Plant J 14, 75-81.

Tchou, J., Michaels, M.L., Miller, J.H., and Grollman, A.P. (1993). Function of the zinc finger in Escherichia coli Fpg protein. J Biol Chem 268, 26738-26744.

Tchou, J., Kasai, H., Shibutani, S., Chung, M.H., Laval, J., Grollman, A.P., and Nishimura, S. (1991). 8-oxoguanine (8-hydroxyguanine) DNA glycosylase and its substrate specificity. Proc Natl Acad Sci U S A 88, 4690-4694.

Teranishi, M., Iwamatsu, Y., Hidema, J., and Kumagai, T. (2004). Ultraviolet-B sensitivities in Japanese lowland rice cultivars: cyclobutane pyrimidine dimer photolyase activity and gene mutation. Plant Cell Physiol 45, 1848-1856.

Teranishi, M., Nakamura, K., Morioka, H., Yamamoto, K., and Hidema, J. (2008). The native cyclobutane pyrimidine dimer photolyase of rice is phosphorylated. Plant Physiol 146, 1941-1951.

Thoma, B.S., and Vasquez, K.M. (2003). Critical DNA damage recognition functions of XPC-hHR23B and XPA-RPA in nucleotide excision repair. Mol Carcinog 38, 1-13.

Tibbetts, R.S., Brumbaugh, K.M., Williams, J.M., Sarkaria, J.N., Cliby, W.A., Shieh, S.Y., Taya, Y., Prives, C., and Abraham, R.T. (1999). A role for ATR in the DNA damage-induced phosphorylation of p53. Genes Dev 13, 152-157.

Tissier, A.F., Lopez, M.F., and Signer, E.R. (1995). Purification and characterization of a DNA strand transferase from broccoli. Plant Physiol 108, 379-386.

Tornaletti, S., and Hanawalt, P.C. (1999). Effect of DNA lesions on transcription elongation. Biochimie 81, 139-146.

Triantaphylides, C., and Havaux, M. (2009). Singlet oxygen in plants: production, detoxification and signaling. Trends Plant Sci 14, 219-228.

Tuteja, N., and Tuteja, R. (2001). Unraveling DNA repair in human: molecular mechanisms and consequences of repair defect. Crit Rev Biochem Mol Biol 36, 261-290.

Tuteja, N., Singh, M.B., Misra, M.K., Bhalla, P.L., and Tuteja, R. (2001). Molecular mechanisms of DNA damage and repair: progress in plants. Crit Rev Biochem Mol Biol 36, 337-397.

Uchiyama, Y., Kimura, S., Yamamoto, T., Ishibashi, T., and Sakaguchi, K. (2004). Plant DNA polymerase lambda, a DNA repair enzyme that functions in plant meristematic and meiotic tissues. Eur J Biochem 271, 2799-2807.

van Gool, A.J., Citterio, E., Rademakers, S., van Os, R., Vermeulen, W., Constantinou, A., Egly, J.M., Bootsma, D., and Hoeijmakers, J.H. (1997). The Cockayne syndrome B protein, involved in transcription-coupled DNA repair, resides in an RNA polymerase II-containing complex. EMBO J 16, 5955-5965.

Vidal, A.E., Boiteux, S., Hickson, I.D., and Radicella, J.P. (2001). XRCC1 coordinates the initial and late stages of DNA abasic site repair through protein-protein interactions. EMBO J 20, 6530-6539.

Vignard, J., Siwiec, T., Chelysheva, L., Vrielynck, N., Gonord, F., Armstrong, S.J., Schlogelhofer, P., and Mercier, R. (2007). The interplay of RecA-related proteins and the MND1-HOP2 complex during meiosis in Arabidopsis thaliana. PLoS Genet 3, 1894-1906.

Vigneron, A., and Vousden, K.H. (2010). p53, ROS and senescence in the control of aging. Aging (Albany NY) 2, 471-474.

Vinocur, B., and Altman, A. (2005). Recent advances in engineering plant tolerance to abiotic stress: achievements and limitations. Curr Opin Biotechnol 16, 123-132.

Virag, L., and Szabo, C. (2002). The therapeutic potential of poly(ADP-ribose) polymerase inhibitors. Pharmacol Rev 54, 375-429.

Wang, H., Zhai, L., Xu, J., Joo, H.Y., Jackson, S., Erdjument-Bromage, H., Tempst, P., Xiong, Y., and Zhang, Y. (2006). Histone H3 and H4 ubiquitylation by the CUL4-DDB-

ROC1 ubiquitin ligase facilitates cellular response to DNA damage. Mol Cell 22, 383-394.

Wang, S., Durrant, W.E., Song, J., Spivey, N.W., and Dong, X. (2010). Arabidopsis BRCA2 and RAD51 proteins are specifically involved in defense gene transcription during plant immune responses. Proc Natl Acad Sci U S A 107, 22716-22721.

Warmerdam, D.O., Kanaar, R., and Smits, V.A. (2010). Differential Dynamics of ATR-Mediated Checkpoint Regulators. J Nucleic Acids 2010.

Waterworth, W.M., Jiang, Q., West, C.E., Nikaido, M., and Bray, C.M. (2002). Characterization of Arabidopsis photolyase enzymes and analysis of their role in protection from ultraviolet-B radiation. J Exp Bot 53, 1005-1015.

Waterworth, W.M., Masnavi, G., Bhardwaj, R.M., Jiang, Q., Bray, C.M., and West, C.E. (2010). A plant DNA ligase is an important determinant of seed longevity. Plant J 63, 848-860.

Waterworth, W.M., Altun, C., Armstrong, S.J., Roberts, N., Dean, P.J., Young, K., Weil, C.F., Bray, C.M., and West, C.E. (2007). NBS1 is involved in DNA repair and plays a synergistic role with ATM in mediating meiotic homologous recombination in plants. Plant J 52, 41-52.

West, C.E., Waterworth, W.M., Jiang, Q., and Bray, C.M. (2000). Arabidopsis DNA ligase IV is induced by gamma-irradiation and interacts with an Arabidopsis homologue of the double strand break repair protein XRCC4. Plant J 24, 67-78.

Wiseman, H., and Halliwell, B. (1996). Damage to DNA by reactive oxygen and nitrogen species: role in inflammatory disease and progression to cancer. Biochem J 313 (Pt 1), 17-29.

Wright, J.A., Keegan, K.S., Herendeen, D.R., Bentley, N.J., Carr, A.M., Hoekstra, M.F., and Concannon, P. (1998). Protein kinase mutants of human ATR increase sensitivity to UV and ionizing radiation and abrogate cell cycle checkpoint control. Proc Natl Acad Sci U S A 95, 7445-7450.

Yamamoto, F., Nishimura, S., and Kasai, H. (1992). Photosensitized formation of 8-hydroxydeoxyguanosine in cellular DNA by riboflavin. Biochem Biophys Res Commun 187, 809-813.

Yang, Z., Roginskaya, M., Colis, L.C., Basu, A.K., Shell, S.M., Liu, Y., Musich, P.R., Harris, C.M., Harris, T.M., and Zou, Y. (2006). Specific and efficient binding of xeroderma pigmentosum complementation group A to double-strand/single-strand DNA junctions with 3'- and/or 5'-ssDNA branches. Biochemistry 45, 15921-15930.

Yatsuhashi, H., Hashimoto, T., and Shimizu, S. (1982). Ultraviolet action spectrum for anthocyanin formation in broom sorghum first internodes. Plant Physiol 70, 735-741.

Ye, J., Meng, X., Yan, C., and Wang, C. (2010). Effect of purple sweet potato anthocyanins on beta-amyloid-mediated PC-12 cells death by inhibition of oxidative stress. Neurochem Res 35, 357-365.

Yoshiyama, K., Conklin, P.A., Huefner, N.D., and Britt, A.B. (2009). Suppressor of gamma response 1 (SOG1) encodes a putative transcription factor governing multiple responses to DNA damage. Proc Natl Acad Sci U S A 106, 12843-12848.

Zhang, C., Guo, H., Zhang, J., Guo, G., Schumaker, K.S., and Guo, Y. (2010). Arabidopsis cóckayne syndrome A-like proteins 1A and 1B form a complex with CULLIN4 and damage DNA binding protein 1A and regulate the response to UV irradiation. Plant Cell 22, 2353-2369.

Zhang, Y., and Schroeder, D.F. (2010). Effect of overexpression of Arabidopsis damaged DNA-binding protein 1A on de-etiolated 1. Planta 231, 337-348.

2

Role of RPA Proteins in Radiation Repair and Recovery

Patrick E. Gygli, J. Scott Lockhart and Linda C. DeVeaux
Idaho State University,
USA

1. Introduction

Repair of radiation-induced DNA damage requires a complex series of protein interactions. Single-stranded DNA (ssDNA) binding proteins (RPA/SSB) have long been known to play a passive, protective role in DNA replication and repair, by coating ssDNA. Recent evidence, however, suggests a much more active function for these ubiquitous proteins. In this review, we provide a summary of the background of ssDNA binding proteins, and incorporate recent experimental observations into current models of dynamic interactions between these proteins and cellular DNA repair enzymes. These results point to a highly choreographed, interactive mechanism, with RPA/SSB at the center of the coordination.

2. Structure

There are two primary classes of ssDNA binding proteins, which share secondary and tertiary structural features, but are distinct in their quaternary structures. The eukaryotic Replication Protein A class (RPAs) consists of heterotrimeric proteins while the bacterial class (SSBs) consists of a range of homo-multimers. Members of the archaeal domain may possess either the RPA or SSB types, or combinations unique to this domain, illustrated in Figure 1 (Kerr, et al., 2003; Lin, et al., 2008; Richard, et al., 2009; Shereda, et al., 2008; Wold, 1997).

SSBs/RPAs are primarily identified by the presence of a structurally conserved oligonucleotide/oligosaccharide binding motif (OB-fold) (Kerr, et al., 2003; Richard, et al., 2009; Shereda, et al., 2008; Theobald, et al., 2003; Wold, 1997). The canonical OB-fold consists of five structurally conserved β-strands, forming two β-sheets, and their inter-spaced variable loops, which form a tertiary flattened β-barrel. The non-specific binding of ssDNA occurs on the surface of the β-barrel in a cleft between the variable loops. The binding of nucleotides is mediated through stacking interactions with aromatic residues and packing interactions with hydrophobic residues. Binding to the phosphodiester backbone also occurs through electrostatic interactions. The OB-folds have a binding polarity that specifies the orientation on the bound ssDNA (Shereda, et al., 2008; Theobald, et al., 2003).

The majority of bacterial and mitochondrial SSBs function as homotetramers, with a single OB-fold per monomer and thus four OB-folds per complex. For members of the *Deinococcus/Thermus* branch, the SSB functions as a homodimer and maintains the theme of four OB-folds per complex by having two non-identical OB-folds per monomer (Bernstein, et al., 2004; Eggington, et al., 2004; Filipkowski, et al., 2006; Filipkowski & Kur, 2007;

Shereda, et al., 2008). These SSB complexes occlude up to 65 and 35 nucleotides of ssDNA, respectively (Filipkowski & Kur, 2007; Meyer & Laine, 1990; Shereda, et al., 2008). Other, less common SSB configurations have also been identified, including an alternative homopentameric Deinococcal SSB (Norais, et al., 2009; Sugiman-Marangos & Junop, 2010). In general, the N-terminal region of the SSB contains the oligomerization domain while the C-terminal region is implicated in heterologous protein interactions (Shereda, et al., 2008).

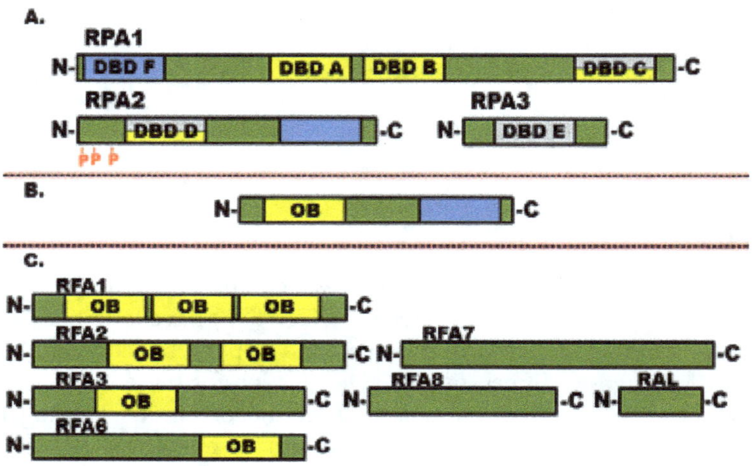

Fig. 1. RPA and SSB structures from eukaryotes, bacteria, and archaea. (A) The canonical eukaryotic RPA comprises three protein subunits, each containing OB-folds designated DBD A-F. Yellow OB-folds are DNA interacting domains, blue domains are involved in heterologous protein interactions, and gray domains are involved in maintenance of RPA structure. The N-terminus of RPA2 is the primary phosphorylation domain, denoted by red Ps. (B) The canonical bacterial SSB functions as a homotetramer and contains a single OB-fold (yellow) and a C-terminal heterologous protein interacting domain (blue) per monomer. (C) Archaeal RPAs are diverse and display characteristics of both eukaryotic RPA and bacterial SSB. Examples from *H. salinarum* are shown. RFA6 resembles bacterial SSB, whereas RFA1 is uniquely archaeal. The genes encoding RFA2 and RFA7, which are found in an operon, likely function as a multimeric protein, as do RFA3, RFA8, and RAL.

The eukaryotic RPA is a heterotrimer composed of a large RPA1 (~72 kDa), medium RPA2 (~32 kDa), and small RPA3 (~14 kDa) subunit. RPA1 and RPA2 tend to be conserved subunits with a variable RPA3, though considerable variation can occur throughout domains (Lin, et al., 2008; Wold, 1997). RPA1 contains four OB-folds referred to as DNA binding domains (DBD). DBD A and B are centrally located, DBD C is in the C-terminal region, and DBD F is in the N-terminal region. RPA2 contains a single centrally located OB-fold, DBD D, and RPA3 a single centrally located OB-fold, DBD E (Binz, et al., 2004; Oakley, et al., 2009; Pretto, et al., 2010). ssDNA binding occurs primarily through interaction with DBD A-D, which together are capable of occluding approximately 30 nucleotides (Blackwell & Borowiec, 1994; Iftode, et al., 1999; C. Kim, et al., 1992; Theobald, et al., 2003). A binding polarity of the complex is achieved through decreased ssDNA affinity from DBD A to D (Oakley, et al., 2009; Pretto, et al., 2010). The N-terminal domain of RPA1 is implicated in heterologous protein interactions and regulation, particularly through DBD F, while the C-terminal domain is involved in heterotrimer structure interactions (Broderick, et al., 2010;

Fanning, et al., 2006; Oakley, et al., 2009; Wold, 1997). The N-terminus of RPA2 contains a regulatory phosphorylation domain that affects interactions of RPA with other proteins, as well as its DNA binding kinetics (Machwe, et al., 2011; Nuss, et al., 2005; Oakley, et al., 2009; Patrick, et al., 2005; Vassin, et al., 2009). The C-terminal region of RPA2 is also involved in heterologous protein interactions and regulation. RPA3 consists almost entirely of DBD E and is thought to be involved primarily in heterotrimer formation, but potential roles in heterologous protein interactions have been identified (Cavero, et al., 2010; Wold, 1997).

3. Multiplicity of homologs

The highly conserved nature of the OB-fold has allowed identification of potential RPA/SSB homologs in the ever-expanding genome sequence database. To our knowledge, there have been no reports of genomes lacking an RPA/SSB homolog, with the possible exception of the crenarchaea *Pyrobaculum aerophilum* and *Aeropyrum pernix* (Luo, et al., 2007).

There are numerous excellent and extensive reviews covering the history, genetics and biochemical characterization of *E. coli* SSB and its encoding gene (Lohman & Ferrari, 1994; Meyer & Laine, 1990; Shereda, et al., 2008). The single gene, *ssb*, is located adjacent to, but divergently transcribed from, the *uvrA* gene (Brandsma, et al., 1985). In *Bacillus subtilis*, there are two SSB genes, *ssb* and *ywpH* (Lindner, et al., 2004). Although the amino acid sequences of the two proteins are similar, YwpH lacks the C-terminal region found in both the *E. coli* and *B. subtilis* SSBs. *B. subtilis ssb* is essential, but unlike in *E. coli*, is found between ribosomal protein genes. Of 87 bacterial genomes analyzed, all contained at least one SSB gene (Lindner, et al., 2004). Based on gene organization, four groupings were proposed: Group I organisms display *B. subtilis*-type gene organization and more than one SSB. Group II organisms contain only one gene for SSB. *E. coli* represents the type organism for Group III bacteria, where the single *ssb* gene is divergently transcribed from the adjacent *uvrA* gene. Group IV consists of organisms whose SSB organization does not resemble either *B. subtilis* or *E. coli*. *Thermotoga maritima* and *T. neopolitana* likely fall into Group IV, whereas *Thermoanaerobacter tengcongensis* is in Group I (Olszewski, et al., 2010; Olszewski, et al., 2008).

Recently, a novel homopentameric SSB, DdrB, was identified in *Deinococcus radiodurans*, which may challenge previous notions regarding canonical SSB structure (Norais, et al., 2009; Sugiman-Marangos & Junop, 2010). Restricted to the Deinococcal lineage, it may represent an adaptation related to the unusually high DNA repair capacity of this organism. However, it should be kept in mind that other SSB proteins that deviate from the traditional consensus may yet be identified (Norais, et al., 2009; G. Xu, et al., 2010).

Three separate genes encode the canonical eukaryotic RPA, which is the subject of several recent review articles (Binz, et al., 2004; Broderick, et al., 2010; Richard, et al., 2009; Wold, 1997). However, in higher plants each subunit of RPA may be represented by multiple genes whose proteins function in distinct processes (Sakaguchi, et al., 2009).

Both *Saccharomyces cerevisiae* and *Schizosaccharomyces pombe* contain a single gene for each of the three RPA subunits. All three are essential in *S. cerevisiae*, but RPA3 appears to be non-essential in *S. pombe* (Brill & Stillman, 1991; Cavero, et al., 2010; Dickson, et al., 2009; Maniar, et al., 1997). Given that RPA3 is the most variable, and the essential role that the intact protein plays in replication, an additional RPA3 gene may yet be identified that carries out this role in *S. pombe*. In addition to heterotrimeric RPA, a protein complex, Stn1/Ten1, resembling an RPA2/RPA3 dimer has been found to be necessary for telomere maintenance and protection in *S. cerevisiae, S. pombe* and *Candida albicans* (Sun, et al., 2009). Together with Cdc13, the Stn1/Ten1 complex may represent a highly conserved telomere binding RPA.

Mammals are thought to have only one nuclear RPA protein, which functions in both replication and repair (Fanning, et al., 2006; Iftode, et al., 1999; Wold, 1997). However, an alternative RPA2 homolog (RPA4) found only in mammals has been identified (Keshav, et al., 1995). RPA4 binds with the single RPA1 and RPA3 subunits to form an alternative RPA that does not interact with DNA polymerase α, and consequently, does not support replication (Haring, et al., 2010; Mason, et al., 2009; Mason, et al., 2010). Rather, its role is restricted to repair, particularly in quiescent cells. A mitochondrial SSB has also been identified in many eukaryotes, which has sequence and structural similarities to *E. coli* SSB (Curth, et al., 1994). In addition, two human proteins, hSSB1 and hSSB2, which structurally resemble bacterial SSB, have been reported. hSSB1 has been characterized, and appears not to be involved in replication, but is required for genome stability and DNA repair processes (Richard, Cubeddu, et al., 2011; Richard, Savage, et al., 2011).

Although much less is known about RPA genes in plants, the recent sequencing of higher plant genomes has revealed a large diversity of homologs (Sakaguchi, et al., 2009). Rice contains three genes each for RPA1 and RPA2, but only a single gene for RPA3 (Ishibashi, et al., 2006; Shultz, et al., 2007). Each RPA1 associates with a particular RPA2, and RPA3 is common among the different complexes. One complex is unique to chloroplasts, whereas the other two are nuclear. Like rice, *Arabidopsis* contains multiple homologs for the RPA1 and RPA2 subunits, but also has two RPA3 genes (Shultz, et al., 2007). In both plants, one of the large subunits has been shown to be non-essential for vegetative growth, but is required for meiosis, demonstrating specialization of function among the multiple species of protein (Chang, et al., 2009; Osman, et al., 2009). This homolog is involved in response to DNA damage as well as maintenance of telomeres (Takashi, et al., 2009). The degree of similarity among the multiple homologs suggests that they arose through duplication of ancestral genes after the establishment of the plant lineage.

By far the most diversity in RPA/SSB homologs is found in the archaea. Although many hypothetical RPA proteins have been identified in the numerous genomes analyzed, there is no quaternary structure that is common to all. In the crenarchaea, the RPA from *Sulfolobus solfataricus* is encoded by a single gene and exists as a monomer or a homotetramer (Haseltine & Kowalczykowski, 2002; Kerr, et al., 2001; Kerr, et al., 2003; Wadsworth & White, 2001). The different quaternary structures confer distinct binding capabilities (Rolfsmeier & Haseltine, 2010). Despite the similarity to bacterial SSB, and the ability of the gene to complement the lethality of an *E. coli ssb* mutation, the DNA-binding domain of this protein more closely resembles those of eukaryotic RPA1 (Haseltine & Kowalczykowski, 2002; Kerr, et al., 2003). Although the genomes of two related crenarchaea, *P. aerophilum* and *A. pernix*, have been reported to contain no obvious RPA or SSB homolog (Luo, et al., 2007), a previous study found a *Sulfolobus*-like SSB in *A. pernix* (Haseltine & Kowalczykowski, 2002). Given the recent identification of a novel SSB in *D. radiodurans*, and the fundamental role that ssDNA binding proteins play in replication and repair, it is likely that a protein carrying out these essential functions will be found in all organisms.

RPAs in euryarchaea present a multitude of OB-fold conformations that presumably provide unique functions (Lin, et al., 2005; Robbins, et al., 2005). Genomes of several euryarchaea, including *Thermoplasma acidophilum, Archaeoglobus fulgidus, Ferroplasma acidarmanus*, and *Halobacterium salinarum*, contain genes with similar organization to the crenarchaeal SSB/RPA gene, with one OB-fold; however, in each case, there is also at least one additional homolog that shows different domain structure, as seen in Figure 1 (Komori & Ishino, 2001; Pugh, et al., 2008; Robbins, et al., 2005). Other euryarchaea, such as *Methanococcus jannaschii, Methanobacter thermoautotrophicus,* and the Methanosarcinae, have proteins with four OB-folds, which may act as monomers, or in a complex with an adjacently encoded RPA2 homolog (Chedin, et al., 1998; Kelly, et al., 1998; Komori & Ishino, 2001; Lin, et al., 2008; Robbins, et al., 2004). In addition, *M. jannaschii* contains a two-OB-fold homolog which appears to function as a homotrimer (Robbins, et al., 2005). The *Pyrococcus furiosis* RPA more closely resembles eukaryotic RPA, with three distinct subunits that function as a heterotrimer and whose genes compose an operon (Komori & Ishino, 2001). In *H. salinarum*, Rfa3, Rfa8, and Ral, and Rfa2 and Rfa7 resemble the *P. furiosis* RPA with respect to operon structure and sequence homology to eukaryotic RPA (Figure 1). Rfa6 resembles the crenarchaeal SSB/RPA in gene and OB-fold structure, while Rfa1 appears more uniquely archaeal, with three OB-folds (DeVeaux, et al., 2007; Robbins, et al., 2005). The roles of the RPA-like homologs in *H. salinarum* will be discussed further below.

4. Characterized mutations of RPA and SSB

E. coli SSB mutants were first isolated in a screen for DNA replication mutants (Meyer & Laine, 1990). Although the two best-characterized of these temperature-sensitive (ts) mutations, *ssb-1* and *ssb-113*, fail to grow at 42° C due to inability of the labile SSB to participate in DNA replication, *ssb-1* mutants have essentially normal phenotypes at the permissive temperature. The mutation (H55Y) resides in the OB-fold and affects the ability of the protein to form homotetramers (Shereda, et al., 2008). In contrast, even at the permissive growth temperature, *ssb-113* mutants are severely compromised in their ability to survive numerous DNA damaging agents, and display recombination deficiencies (Chase, et al., 1984). The extremely pleiotropic phenotype conferred by the amino acid change (P176S of 177) in *ssb-113* suggests that the protein interaction capabilities of the C-terminal region are necessary for more than just replication. A protein lacking only 10 amino acids from the C-terminus is non-functional (Curth, et al., 1996). Indeed, mutation of the terminal phenylalanine is lethal, and disrupts protein-protein interactions (Genschel, et al., 2000). These phenotypes provided support not only for the commonality of protein function in recombination, repair, and replication, but also early evidence that these roles were separable within an individual protein. In contrast, a *B. subtilis* mutant in which SSB lacks the C-terminal 35 amino acids, involved in interaction with the helicase PriA, is viable, demonstrating that this conserved region is not essential in all bacteria (Lecointe, et al., 2007). In the budding yeast *S. cerevisiae*, all three subunits of RPA are essential (Brill & Stillman, 1991; Maniar, et al., 1997). Like *E. coli ssb-113* mutants, ts-mutants of RPA1 are profoundly UV- and ionizing radiation (IR)-sensitive at the permissive temperature (Parker, et al., 1997). Several ts-mutants display a mutator phenotype, which is likely related to defects in replication rather than repair (Chen, et al., 1998). Small insertions in either the RPA1 DNA-binding domain or the N-terminal protein-interaction domain result in a marked decrease in survival after UV exposure; however, only the latter is defective in the cell-cycle response to such damage. In addition, only the DNA-binding mutant is defective in repair of UV-induced lesions (Longhese, et al., 1996; Teng, et al., 1998). The N-terminal domain is required for interactions with the clamp loader. This binding is abolished in the *rfa1-t11* mutation, which contains a single change (K45E) (H. S. Kim & Brill, 2001; Majka, et al., 2006; Umezu, et al., 1998). This same allele is deficient in many pathways requiring interactions with DNA processing proteins, including repair of DNA breaks incurred during meiotic recombination, and interaction with Rad51 and its mediator Rad52 (Soustelle, et al., 2002; Sugiyama & Kantake, 2009). Deletion of either the N-terminal 20 amino acids or any deletion at the C-terminus is lethal (Philipova, et al., 1996). In the fission yeast *S. pombe,* as in *S. cerevisiae,* mutations in the large subunit gene confer sensitivity to DNA damaging agents such as UV; in addition, these mutations confer a deficiency in telomere maintenance that is seen in *S. cerevisiae* only in combination with a Ku mutation (Ono, et al., 2003).

In *S. cerevisiae,* mutations in RPA2 also confer sensitivity to various DNA-damaging agents and display defects in replication fidelity (Maniar, et al., 1997; Santocanale, et al., 1995). Ts-mutants arrest in S phase at the nonpermissive temperature. Although the protein is essential, the DNA-binding domain is not; only the central protein-interaction domain is required (Dickson, et al., 2009; Philipova, et al., 1996). Temperature-sensitive mutations in RPA3 confer a replication defect in *S. cerevisiae.* Whereas replication ceases immediately in ts-mutants of RPA2, RPA3 mutations allow one round of replication before cessation (Maniar, et al., 1997). As in RPA1, deletions of the RPA3 N-terminus are viable, but C-terminal deletions are not tolerated (Philipova, et al., 1996). Interestingly, RPA3 is not essential in *S. pombe,* and is dispensible in meiosis (Cavero, et al., 2010). However, cells containing a gene deletion show marked sensitivity to DNA damaging agents, particularly those interfering with replication, but not to IR. This suggests that RPA3 in *S. pombe* is involved in repair of replication damage, but not homologous recombination. It is possible that an additional RPA3 homolog will be discovered in *S. pombe* that carries out the essential role in replication performed by a single RPA3 in other organisms.

In human cells, depletion of RPA results not only in increased spontaneous DNA damage and decreased cell viability, but also in asynchrony, arrest at the G1/S boundary, a slowing of progression through S phase, and arrest at the G2/M checkpoint (Dodson, et al., 2004; Haring, et al., 2008). The G2/M arrest was found to be the result of constitutive activation of ATM (ataxia telangiectasia mutated) kinase resulting from lack of RPA. Cells harboring mutations in DBD A, B or C are able to replicate DNA, and traverse S phase, but arrest at the G2/M checkpoint. In contrast to yeast, the N-terminal 168 amino acids of RPA1 are not essential for replication or cell-cycle progression. RPA1 mutants defective in ssDNA binding are still able to support replication; however, some mutants with very modest defects in DNA binding are severely compromised in cell-cycle progression (Haring, et al., 2008). One mutation, L221P, in which a highly conserved leucine in DBD A is changed to proline, has been characterized in yeast (Chen & Kolodner, 1999; Chen, et al., 1998), in mice (Wang, et al., 2005), and in humans (Hass, et al., 2010), and has been shown to promote chromosomal instability. This mutation is lethal in mice; heterozygosity leads to shortened life spans and increased cancer incidence. The conservation of this residue and the drastic phenotype associated with its replacement indicates a critical role of this DNA binding domain in the fundamental role of RPA in replication. A mutation changing another conserved residue in the same domain, D227Y, causes telomere shortening in human cancer cells (Kobayashi, et al., 2010), as does the analogous change in yeast (Ono, et al., 2003). Much less is known about mutations of the two smaller subunits in mammalian systems. However, as in yeast, human RPA2 is required for replication, and the only essential region is the central protein-interacting domain (Fanning, et al., 2006; Haring, et al., 2010).

Higher plants contain multiple homologs of at least the large and medium subunits. In rice, one homolog of RPA1 is not essential during vegetative growth, but mutants are sterile, indicating a meiotic defect (Chang, et al., 2009). Also, mutants are sensitive to DNA-damaging agents, indicating a role in repair but not replication. Likewise, in *Arabidopsis thaliana*, deletion of one RPA1 homolog results in meiotic defects; although DNA breaks appear to be repaired normally, there is a deficiency in meiotic crossover (Osman, et al., 2009). During vegetative growth, plants containing this mutation are sensitive to DNA-damaging agents (Takashi, et al., 2009). The presence of multiple homologs, some of which are not essential and appear not to be involved with replication, suggests that RPAs in plants have duplicated and diverged, resulting in specialization and separation of function.

5. Interactive roles of RPA and SSB in DNA metabolism

While RPAs and SSBs are indispensible for normal replication, they are also central to nearly all DNA repair pathways. The overarching theme for RPA/SSB in these repair pathways is their function as directors of key enzymatic proteins without themselves being enzymatic. The following sections will pertain to the canonical RPA and SSB unless otherwise noted.

5.1 Interactive role of RPA and SSB in the unstressed cell cycle

RPA plays a critical role in replication of DNA and was first identified as a factor for replication of the Simian Virus 40 (SV40). Several reviews provide great detail about the role of RPA in replication; however, most current work examines its function in DNA repair (Fanning, et al., 2006; Iftode, et al., 1999; Wold, 1997). Nevertheless, it is important to understand the role of RPA in normal DNA replication as the switch between its replication role and its repair role is of great interest.

During replication, RPA functions to protect ssDNA and direct the assembly of the replication machinery. In SV40 replication, RPA interacts with T-antigen to facilitate unwinding of the replication origin, through ssDNA stabilization as well as DNA-duplex melting (Georgaki & Hubscher, 1993; Georgaki, et al., 1992; Iftode, et al., 1999; Wold, 1997). Interestingly, nearly all RPAs and SSBs are able to replace human RPA in this role, indicating that stability of the ssDNA intermediate is critical for progression of replication (Wold, 1997). In addition, RPA and SSB serve to direct the formation of the replication complex through direct protein-protein interactions (Binz, et al., 2006; Naue, et al., 2011; Shereda, et al., 2008; Witte, et al., 2003; Wold, 1997; Yuzhakov, Kelman, Hurwitz, et al., 1999).

RPA spatially and temporally directs the addition of key proteins of the replication complex at the site of replication. Temporal control is obtained through competitive binding of the replication components to RPA. Initially, the primase complex is directed to the ssDNA template. Following primer synthesis, Replication Factor C (RFC) binds RPA and loads the replicative clamp PCNA. DNA polymerase δ then binds RPA and is loaded at the DNA-primer junction, allowing DNA replication to begin (Yuzhakov, et al., 1999). These protein-protein interactions are RPA-specific; SSB cannot substitute, underscoring the important dual role of RPA in both ssDNA binding and protein interactions (Wold, 1997).

Though RPA and SSB cannot always substitute for each other, they play similar roles in the systems in which they reside. Like RPA, SSB serves not only to stabilize ssDNA but also to direct assembly of the replication complex proteins. Through interactions with the C-terminus of SSB, the primase is loaded and retained at the priming site. This interaction may be facilitated through further interactions of SSB with DnaB. This binding is disrupted by the χ subunit of the replicative DNA polymerase III through a multi-step handoff mechanism (Sharma, et al., 2009; Shereda, et al., 2008; Witte, et al., 2003; Yuzhakov, Kelman, & O'Donnell, 1999). Loss of these protein-protein interactions results in cellular demise.

Integral to the role of RPA in DNA replication is its cell-cycle dependent phosphorylation/ dephosphorylation (Figure 2). Specifically, RPA2 is phosphorylated at two consensus sites for Cdc2/Cdk2, resulting in three forms of RPA: unphosphorylated, and two distinct phosphorylated forms (Iftode, et al., 1999; J. S. Liu, et al., 2006; Oakley, et al., 2003; Patrick, et al., 2005; Wold, 1997; Zernik-Kobak, et al., 1997). The majority of RPA is unphosphorylated during G1 phase, and is phosphorylated at either S23 or S29 of RPA2 at the G1/S phase boundary, which is maintained through S phase and into G2 (Anantha, et al., 2007; Oakley, et al., 2003; Stephan, et al., 2009). Near the G2/M phase boundary, a mitotic phosphorylation form becomes abundant (Oakley, et al., 2003; Zernik-Kobak, et al., 1997). This is presumably due to further phosphorylation of RPA2 at the remaining Cdc2/Cdk2 consensus site, which may regulate the ability of RPA to interact with and bind other proteins, thereby modulating its functional role through the cell-cycle (Oakley, et al., 2003; Stephan, et al., 2009). However, the effects of S phase phosphorylation of RPA have not yet been determined, as its ability to support replication and repair are unchanged (Henricksen, et al., 1996; Oakley, et al., 2003; Pan, et al., 1995). In contrast, M phase phosphorylation of RPA abrogates binding to DNA polymerase α, as well as to the checkpoint proteins ATM and DNA-PK (DNA-dependent protein kinase). In addition, its ability to bind duplex DNA is significantly reduced. These modifications may serve to switch RPA away from its replicative role after S phase (Oakley, et al., 2003; Stephan, et al., 2009). It has also been demonstrated that SSB is phosphorylated on tyrosine residues, but the consequences of this phosphorylation remain to be elucidated (Mijakovic, et al., 2006). As such, phosphorylation will be discussed only in relation to RPA for the remainder of this review. Nevertheless, it is reasonable to hypothesize that phosphorylation of SSB plays a similar regulatory role.

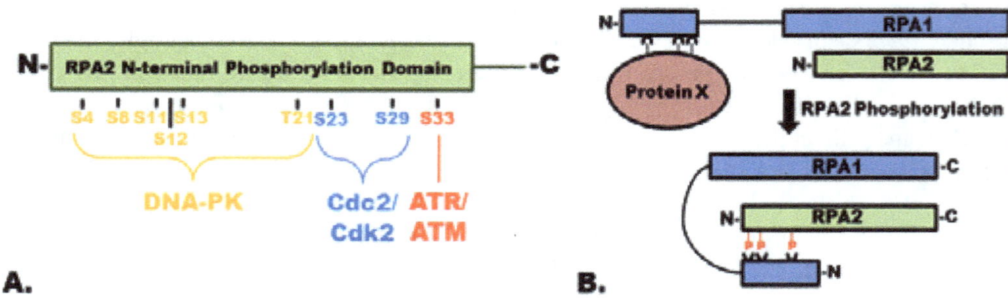

Fig. 2. (A) Phosphorylation sites on the N-terminus of RPA2. DNA-PK, Cdc2/Cdk2 and ATR/ATM phosphorylate different sites, which depends on the type of damage and point in the cell-cycle. (B) Proposed mechanism for phosphoregulation of RPA1 N-terminal heterologous protein interactions. Upon phosphorylation of RPA2, the basic N-terminus of RPA1 binds phosphorylated RPA2 and abrogates heterologous protein binding. Protein X represents any of a number of RPA1-interacting proteins.

5.2 Interactive role of RPA and SSB in NER, BER and MMR

Cellular DNA is under a constant barrage of damaging agents, which may cause crosslinking, base modification or base loss. In general, these types of damage may be repaired by excising the offending lesion and re-synthesizing DNA. RPA and SSB play critical roles in the coordination of these processes. Base excision repair (BER) processes remove damaged bases, forming apurinic/apyrimidinic sites, which are removed and replaced with undamaged DNA (Krokan, et al., 2000). RPA physically interacts with and regulates multiple BER glycosylases, including NEIL1 and Ung2, to facilitate correct repair of lesions, in part by inhibiting excisions on ssDNA and promoting incisions on duplex DNA (Mer, et al., 2000; Theriot, et al., 2010). Similarly, SSB interacts with the glycosylase UDG, stimulating or inhibiting its excision activity, depending on the DNA structure at the lesion (Kumar & Varshney, 1997). Nucleotide excision repair (NER) processes remove helix-distorting lesions by excising a patch of DNA, followed by re-synthesis. In this case, RPA physically interacts with the NER mediator XPA to direct incision to the damaged strand, and to help prevent excessive incision events, which could lead to further degradation of the genome (Krasikova, et al., 2010; Overmeer, et al., 2011; Saijo, et al., 2011). In mismatch repair (MMR), RPA and SSB interact with the exonuclease EXO1 to stimulate excision processes, as well as ensure correct excision termination (Genschel & Modrich, 2009; Lu & Keck, 2008).

5.3 Interactive role of RPA and SSB in the recovery of stalled replication forks

An advancing replication fork must traverse a myriad of DNA lesions through a normal replicative cycle, and the abundance of these lesions increases dramatically under DNA-damaging conditions. Depletion of the nucleotide pool or a single-strand lesion blocks progression of the polymerase complex, while the replicative helicase uncouples from the replisome and continues to unwind template DNA. Such uncoupling results in long segments of ssDNA to which RPA or SSB may bind and actively participate in restart of the stalled fork (Atkinson & McGlynn, 2009; Byun, et al., 2005; McInerney & O'Donnell, 2007; Pages & Fuchs, 2003). Additionally, lesions such as inter-strand crosslinks or covalently linked proteins block advancement of the entire replisome. Such stalls may be repaired and restarted through a fork regression pathway. Several competing fork regression models exist, but all of them require protein elements that closely function and interact with RPA and SSB (Atkinson & McGlynn, 2009; Dronkert & Kanaar, 2001; Machwe, et al., 2011; Shereda, et al., 2007; Shereda, et al., 2008; Sowd, et al., 2009; Sugiyama & Kantake, 2009; Suhasini, et al., 2009; Woodman, et al., 2010; Yuan, et al., 2009; Yusufzai, et al., 2009).

When the replicative helicase is uncoupled from the replisome, large tracts of ssDNA are formed. In eukaryotes this lengthy ssDNA is rapidly coated with RPA, which serves as a signal of replication stress to activate the S phase checkpoint kinase ATR (ATM and Rad3-related), a member of the phosphatidylinositol 3-kinase-like kinase (PIKK) family (Byun, et al., 2005; J. S. Liu, et al., 2006; Zou & Elledge, 2003). In bacteria, the ssDNA is similarly coated with SSB, but a strict cell-cycle control response is absent. ATR is found in a complex with its activator ATRIP (ATR interacting protein) and recruitment of ATR/ATRIP to sites of replication stress is mediated by direct interaction between the N-terminus of RPA1 (DBD F) and ATRIP. This interaction is sufficient for localization of ATR/ATRIP to the stalled replication fork, but activation of ATR requires further protein interactions, also mediated by RPA (X. Xu, et al., 2008; Zou & Elledge, 2003). The Rad17 complex, which comprises Rad17 and RFC subunits 2-5, loads the Rad9-Rad1-Hus1 (9-1-1) DNA damage checkpoint clamp at damage sites. To facilitate loading of the 9-1-1 complex, the Rad17 complex is recruited to damage sites in an RPA-dependent manner (Majka, et al., 2006; Zou, et al., 2003). Rad9 of the 9-1-1 complex binds topoisomerase 2 binding protein 1 (TopBP1), another factor for ATR activation. Simultaneously, Rad9 binds the N-terminus of RPA1 which correctly orients TopBP1 for activation of ATR. Rad9 and ATRIP compete for binding of the N-terminus of RPA1, but each must be bound for efficient activation of ATR. This suggests a model in which two adjacent RPAs are required to be bound to ssDNA at a damage site (X. Xu, et al., 2008). This model is further supported by studies describing a ssDNA length-dependent activation of ATR via RPA (J. S. Liu, et al., 2006; Zou & Elledge, 2003).

Activated ATR initiates the intra-S phase checkpoint signal cascade resulting in cell-cycle arrest, stabilization of replication forks, and initiation of damage repair through phosphorylation of effector molecules, including the checkpoint kinase Chk1 (Cimprich & Cortez, 2008; Kastan & Bartek, 2004; Yang, et al., 2003). Activation also leads ATR to phosphorylate S33, a PIKK consensus site, of the RPA2 subunit of ssDNA-bound RPA, which stimulates the Cdc2/Cdk2 kinases to phosphorylate their consensus sites on RPA2 if not already phosphorylated. This, in turn, stimulates phosphorylation of T21 by DNA-PK, which leads to further phosphorylation of RPA2 at residues S4, S8, S11, S12, and S13 by DNA-PK (Anantha, et al., 2007; Vassin, et al., 2009; Zernik-Kobak, et al., 1997). Such hyperphosphorylation of RPA is the major switch from its role in normal uninterrupted replication to an activator and director of DNA damage repair.

Hyperphosphorylation inhibits replicative functions of RPA while stimulating repair and fork stabilization, likely by modifying its protein interaction and duplex DNA binding and destabilizing capabilities. In a rather elegant regulatory mechanism, the phosphorylated RPA2 competitively binds the basic N-terminal region of RPA1, displacing proteins from one of the primary binding surfaces and modulating its interaction capability (Figure 2) (Oakley, et al., 2009). Competitive binding and conformational changes such as this may be responsible for many of the protein interactions that are altered upon phosphorylation of RPA2. Hyperphosphorylation abolishes interaction of RPA with DNA polymerase α, as well as decreases its duplex unwinding ability, which is critical for replication (Oakley, et al., 2003; Patrick, et al., 2005; Wold, 1997). Additionally, in an SV40 *in vitro* system, hyperphosphorylation of RPA leads to a 50% reduction in replication, which can be rescued by unphosphorylated RPA (Patrick, et al., 2005). Hyperphosphorylation, coupled with other aspects of the intra-S phase checkpoint, effectively halts chromosomal replication. However, other RPA-dependent processes, such as damage-dependent DNA synthesis, are unchanged or stimulated. Hyperphosphorylated RPA stimulates *in vivo* synthesis of DNA on RPA-coated ssDNA via a currently unidentified repair polymerase, minimizing ssDNA accumulation during replication stress (Vassin, et al., 2009). Additionally, essential interactions between RPA and NER proteins are unaffected by hyperphosphorylation of RPA (see above) (Oakley, et al., 2003; Patrick, et al., 2005). Many of these repair proteins are capable of interacting with the unphosphorylated C-terminus of RPA2 rather than the N-terminus of RPA1, which may explain the separation of functions between unphosphorylated and hyperphosphorylated RPA (Ali, et al., 2010; Saijo, et al., 2011). Regardless of the mechanism, this demonstrates the versatility of RPA in DNA metabolism.

The previous discussion has focused on a restart and repair pathway for replication fork stalls in which the replicative helicase uncouples from the replisome. A replisome may also encounter double-strand lesions, such as interstrand crosslinks, that prevent progression of the entire complex. These lesions, as well as some ssDNA lesions, result in stalled forks that may be repaired and restarted though fork regression. Among the most important proteins in fork regression are repair helicases including those in the RecQ, RecG, HARP, and FANC families. These helicases may perform the complex winding and unwinding of nascent and template strands necessary to form a Holliday junction-like structure referred to as a "chicken foot." Additionally, proteins of the Fanconi anemia pathway may be important for

RPA focus formation in regression of forks stalled by interstrand crosslinks (Huang, et al., 2010). For a review of fork regression models, see Atkinson and McGlynn, 2009.

Many studies support the hypothesis that RPA directs activity of helicases in fork regression. In eukaryotes, RPA interacts with the RecQ-like helicases WRN and BLM, which have been implicated in the regression of stalled replication forks *in vitro*. RecQ helicases are important for maintenance of chromosome stability; it is therefore not unexpected that they would be involved in fork regression. The interaction of RPA with these proteins may also recruit them to stalled forks; regardless, it stimulates their helicase activity (Brosh, et al., 2000; Brosh, et al., 1999; Doherty, et al., 2005; Machwe, et al., 2011; Machwe, et al., 2006; Machwe, et al., 2007; Ralf, et al., 2006). RPA also recruits the annealing helicase HARP to stalled forks through direct interaction. HARP has been implicated in stabilization and restart of stalled replication forks and may be well suited to assisting fork regression in which complementary DNA strands must be annealed to form stable structures (Ciccia, et al., 2009; Yuan, et al., 2009; Yusufzai, et al., 2009). Thus, the RecQ-like helicases may work with the HARP helicases in the regression of stalled forks. In addition to the human RecQ-like helicases, the archaeal RecQ-like helicase Hel308 is also recruited by RPA and is capable of fork regression *in vitro* (Li, et al., 2008; Woodman, et al., 2010). Additionally, the FANCM protein, which is involved in fork regression, interacts with RPA at stalled forks to promote formation of RPA foci (Banerjee, et al., 2008; Huang, et al., 2010).

In bacterial fork regression, similar interactions between SSB and helicases have been observed. SSB binds RecQ through its C-terminus *in vitro* and stimulates RecQ helicase activity (Lecointe, et al., 2007; Shereda, et al., 2007; Shereda, et al., 2008). RecG helicase not only interacts with SSB through the C-terminus but is stabilized by this interaction and supports fork regression (Buss, et al., 2008; Lecointe, et al., 2007; Shereda, et al., 2008). The replication restart helicase PriA also interacts with SSB, which would complete the fork regression process and initiate restart of replication (Cadman & McGlynn, 2004; Kozlov, et al., 2010; Lecointe, et al., 2007; Shereda, et al., 2008). In addition to helicases, SSB interacts with and actively directs the activity of several recombination proteins necessary for the repair of regressed forks before they may be restarted. These processes are essential to other aspects of DNA repair as well, including double-strand break (DSB) repair, discussed below.

5.4 Interactive role of RPA and SSB in DNA double-strand break repair

The types of DNA damage discussed previously may be repaired directly through NER or in response to replication fork stall. A far more grave form of DNA damage is the DSB, arising from either exogenous or endogenous stresses. A well-known exogenous physical stress that causes DSBs is IR, which is the major reason that it is so detrimental to living systems. A variety of chemical agents, such as bleomycin, phleomycin, and mitomycin C, also act by inducing DSBs. Additionally, a stalled replication fork that is unrepaired may collapse into a special type of DSB with a single double-strand end (Allen, et al., 2011). Regardless, these DSBs are all repaired via similar pathways, which rely on RPA and SSB.

Until recently, models of eukaryotic DSB repair indicated that the conserved DNA repair protein complex MRN (Mre11-Rad50-Nbs1) was the first responder and signaler at the site of a DSB. However, recent evidence implicates the novel ssDNA binding protein hSSB1 as the DSB-recognition protein in humans. At the site of damage this protein may bind short ssDNA overhangs and provide protection from incorrect end-processing by nucleases. Additionally, hSSB1 is found complexed with MRN independent of damage, through an interaction between the C-terminal tail of hSSB1 and the N-terminal region of Nbs1. This direct interaction, along with the ssDNA-bound hSSB1, stimulates the recruitment of the MRN complex to DSB sites. RPA cannot replace hSSB1 in this function (Richard, Cubeddu, et al., 2011; Richard, Savage, et al., 2011). hSSB1 may also have duplex melting capabilities similar to that seen in other SSBs, which would further help to provide a substrate for MRN binding (Cubeddu & White, 2005; Eggington, et al., 2006; Richard, Cubeddu, et al., 2011).

Once recruited to a DSB, the MRN complex tethers the broken DNA ends; its endonuclease activity is stimulated through hSSB1 association. MRN then activates the ATM kinase, which in turn initiates a phosphorylation signal cascade similar to ATR. Among the many phosphorylation targets of ATM are the cell-cycle checkpoint kinase Chk2, histone variant H2AX, and hSSB1 (Czornak, et al., 2008; Richard, et al., 2008; Richard, Cubeddu, et al., 2011; Richard, Savage, et al., 2011; Williams, et al., 2010). Phosphorylation of Chk2 results in cell-cycle arrest, while phosphorylated H2AX serves as a local binding point for repair proteins (Kastan & Bartek, 2004; J. E. Kim, et al., 2006). hSSB1 phosphorylation has unknown consequences, but it is likely to alter its repair role in a manner similar to the phospho-regulation of RPA (Richard, et al., 2008; Richard, Savage, et al., 2011). The nuclease activity of MRN results in limited end-resection at the DSB providing a substrate to which RPA may then bind (Richard, Cubeddu, et al., 2011; Richard, Savage, et al., 2011). ssDNA-bound RPA activates the ATR response and may also be phosphorylated by either activated ATM or ATR, switching it to a repair-process director (Jazayeri, et al., 2006; Oakley, et al., 2001).

In both eukaryotic and bacterial systems, DSB repair and fork regression may proceed via homologous recombination when a homologous template is present. Not surprisingly, RPA and SSB play central roles in this process as well. The RPA or SSB coating ssDNA at the site of damage is replaced with recombinase Rad51 or RecA, respectively, through direct interaction with mediators of homologous recombination. Specifically, the replacement of RPA by Rad51 is facilitated by interactions between the N-terminus of RPA1 and the homologous recombination mediator Rad52 (Plate, et al., 2008; Sugiyama & Kantake, 2009). Akin to requirements for ATR activation, multiple RPAs are necessary to promote this exchange. Similarly, bacterial SSB interacts through its C-terminal tail with the recombination mediator RecO to facilitate loading of RecA onto ssDNA by RecFOR (Costes, et al., 2010; Inoue, et al., 2011). Another interesting interaction of SSB is its apparent competition with the RecA inhibitor RecX for the common ssDNA ligand. By outcompeting RecX for access to ssDNA, SSB prevents RecX from inhibiting RecA loading onto the ssDNA (Baitin, et al., 2008). Interactions between archaeal SSB and a RadA-mediator Rad55 have also been demonstrated *in vitro*. This interaction promotes loading of RadA onto ssDNA suggesting a similar function to that seen in eukaryotes and bacteria (Sheng, et al., 2008).

6. Transcriptional regulation

The post-translational modifications of RPA/SSB provide virtually instantaneous response to conditions within the cell. Less well-documented, but potentially as important to survival, is transcriptional regulation of the genes in response to more global DNA damage. There is evidence of such regulation in all three domains of life. In general, where damage-induced transcriptional regulation has been reported, the organism contains multiple homologs, and the damage-regulated RPA is generally not required for replication.

In bacteria, the well-studied *E. coli ssb* gene contains multiple promoters, one of which has been shown to be damage-inducible (Brandsma, et al., 1985). Despite this, the level of *E. coli*

SSB protein does not appear to respond to DNA damage, suggesting that any regulation on this promoter is compensated by opposite regulation on the others (Meyer & Laine, 1990). One of the two homologs in *B. subtilis* functions in natural competence, whereas the gene for the replication SSB is not damage-inducible (Lindner, et al., 2004). The promoters for both the canonical SSB and the newly identified DdrB in *D. radiodurans* contain a recognizable "radiation-desiccation response motif"; both genes are up-regulated in response to IR, but *ssb* is not induced by desiccation or UV (Ujaoney, et al., 2010). The SSB protein is present in *D. radiodurans* at ten-fold higher levels than in *E. coli*, and, unlike in *E. coli*, levels increase 4-fold after irradiation (Bernstein, et al., 2004; Y. Liu, et al., 2003). In contrast, the transcript for the *ddrB* gene is normally almost absent, but is induced 40-fold within minutes after exposure to IR (Tanaka, et al., 2004). The IR-sensitivity, and viability, of *ddrB* knockouts underscores its specific role in DNA repair, and not replication.

In yeast and humans, the presence of a single RPA makes transcriptional regulation in response to damage less likely. In yeast, expression of RPA is cell-cycle dependent, with maximal expression prior to S phase (Brill & Stillman, 1991). Human RPA levels remain constant throughout the cell cycle (Wold, 1997). However, the alternative RPA2 subunit, RPA4, is more highly expressed in quiescent cells, and, since it competes with RPA2 for binding to RPA1 and RPA3, must be down-regulated in dividing cells (Haring, et al., 2010). This long-term regulation, however, is presumably not readily reversible, and is not a damage response. Interestingly, RPA1 and RPA2 levels are higher in colon cancer cells but it is not clear how this increase is achieved (Givalos, et al., 2007). Plants have multiple homologs, which are differentially expressed in tissues. There is evidence for regulation of certain homologs in response to DNA damage, as well as in response to certain hormones (Marwedel, et al., 2003; Sakaguchi, et al., 2009).

The single crenarchaeal RPA homolog would not be expected to be transcriptionally regulated to any significant extent, given its essential role in replication. In the euryarchaea, however, where multiple homologs are common, regulation has been reported. The transcriptome of *H. salinarum* during recovery from exposure to IR or UV has been analyzed and only one of the five RPA homologs showed any any increase in expression (Baliga, et al., 2004; Kottemann, et al., 2005; McCready, et al., 2005). This homolog, encoded by the *rfa3* operon, is one of two eukaryotic-like RPAs present in *H. salinarum*. Constitutive up-regulation of this operon was found as the only transcriptomic difference among multiple radiation-resistant mutants of *H. salinarum* (DeVeaux, et al., 2007). This homolog is significantly up-regulated following IR-treatment of wild type *H. salinarum*, but not in the radiation-resistant mutants, presumably because the protein is being constitutively expressed at the induced level. In addition, both wild-type and mutant strains show induced expression of the second RPA-like homolog, encoded by the *rfa2* operon. Neither of the crenarchaeal nor the euryarchaeal-like SSB/RPA homologs shows significant transcriptional differences after irradiation (Gygli and DeVeaux, unpublished observations). These results suggest that the eukaryotic RPA-like homologs present in this organism may be more directly involved in repair of radiation damage.

7. Conclusion

The highly conserved and essential nature of the RPA/SSB family underscores the fundamental role that these proteins play in basic DNA metabolic processes. The interactions that these proteins are involved in illustrate an intricate network and temporal sequence of events that are only beginning to be understood. The multiplicity of homologs present in some lineages suggests that ancestral duplications have resulted in specialization of function. These organisms provide models for study of individual activities, such as DNA repair, which are not essential for viability.

8. Acknowledgment

We thank all of the researchers whose hard work provided us with material for this review. We thank Dr. Dring Crowell and the members of the DeVeaux lab for support and helpful comments. The following agencies provided support for P.E.G. and J.S.L.: The Henry M. Jackson Foundation, NASA ISGC, and The United States Department of Defense.

9. References

Ali, S. I., Shin, J. S., Bae, S. H., et al. (2010). Replication Protein A 32 interacts through a similar binding interface with TIPIN, XPA, and UNG2. *Int J Biochem Cell Biol*, Vol. 42, No. 7 (pp. 1210-1215), 1878-5875 (Electronic) 1357-2725 (Linking)

Allen, C., Ashley, A. K., Hromas, R., et al. (2011). More forks on the road to replication stress recovery. *J Mol Cell Biol*, Vol. 3, No. 1 (pp. 4-12), 1759-4685 (Electronic)

Anantha, R. W., Vassin, V. M., & Borowiec, J. A. (2007). Sequential and synergistic modification of human RPA stimulates chromosomal DNA repair. *J Biol Chem*, Vol. 282, No. 49 (pp. 35910-35923), 0021-9258 (Print) 0021-9258 (Linking)

Atkinson, J., & McGlynn, P. (2009). Replication fork reversal and the maintenance of genome stability. *Nucleic Acids Res*, Vol. 37, No. 11 (pp. 3475-3492), 1362-4962 (Electronic) 0305-1048 (Linking)

Baitin, D. M., Gruenig, M. C., & Cox, M. M. (2008). SSB antagonizes RecX-RecA interaction. *J Biol Chem*, Vol. 283, No. 21 (pp. 14198-14204), 0021-9258 (Print) 0021-9258 (Linking)

Baliga, N. S., Bjork, S. J., Bonneau, R., et al. (2004). Systems level insights into the stress response to UV radiation in the halophilic archaeon *Halobacterium* NRC-1. *Genome Res*, Vol. 14, No. 6 (pp. 1025-1035), 1088-9051 (Print) 1088-9051 (Linking)

Banerjee, S., Smith, S., Oum, J. H., et al. (2008). Mph1p promotes gross chromosomal rearrangement through partial inhibition of homologous recombination. *J Cell Biol*, Vol. 181, No. 7 (pp. 1083-1093), 1540-8140 (Electronic) 0021-9525 (Linking)

Bernstein, D. A., Eggington, J. M., Killoran, M. P., et al. (2004). Crystal structure of the *Deinococcus radiodurans* single-stranded DNA-binding protein suggests a mechanism for coping with DNA damage. *Proc Natl Acad Sci U S A*, Vol. 101, No. 23 (pp. 8575-8580), 0027-8424 (Print) 0027-8424 (Linking)

Binz, S. K., Dickson, A. M., Haring, S. J., et al. (2006). Functional assays for Replication Protein A (RPA). *Methods Enzymol*, Vol. 409, (pp. 11-38), 0076-6879 (Print) 0076-6879 (Linking)

Binz, S. K., Sheehan, A. M., & Wold, M. S. (2004). Replication Protein A phosphorylation and the cellular response to DNA damage. *DNA Repair (Amst)*, Vol. 3, No. 8-9 (pp. 1015-1024), 1568-7864 (Print) 1568-7856 (Linking)

Blackwell, L. J., & Borowiec, J. A. (1994). Human Replication Protein A binds single-stranded DNA in two distinct complexes. *Mol Cell Biol*, Vol. 14, No. 6 (pp. 3993-4001), 0270-7306 (Print) 0270-7306 (Linking)

Brandsma, J. A., Bosch, D., de Ruyter, M., et al. (1985). Analysis of the regulatory region of the *ssb* gene of *Escherichia coli*. *Nucleic Acids Res*, Vol. 13, No. 14 (pp. 5095-5109), 0305-1048 (Print) 0305-1048 (Linking)

Brill, S. J., & Stillman, B. (1991). Replication factor-A from *Saccharomyces cerevisiae* is encoded by three essential genes coordinately expressed at S phase. *Genes Dev*, Vol. 5, No. 9 (pp. 1589-1600), 0890-9369 (Print) 0890-9369 (Linking)

Broderick, S., Rehmet, K., Concannon, C., et al. (2010). Eukaryotic single-stranded DNA binding proteins: central factors in genome stability. *Subcell Biochem*, Vol. 50, (pp. 143-163), 0306-0225 (Print) 0306-0225 (Linking)

Brosh, R. M., Jr., Li, J. L., Kenny, M. K., et al. (2000). Replication Protein A physically interacts with the Bloom's syndrome protein and stimulates its helicase activity. *J Biol Chem*, Vol. 275, No. 31 (pp. 23500-23508), 0021-9258 (Print) 0021-9258 (Linking)

Brosh, R. M., Jr., Orren, D. K., Nehlin, J. O., et al. (1999). Functional and physical interaction between WRN helicase and human Replication Protein A. *J Biol Chem*, Vol. 274, No. 26 (pp. 18341-18350), 0021-9258 (Print) 0021-9258 (Linking)

Buss, J. A., Kimura, Y., & Bianco, P. R. (2008). RecG interacts directly with SSB: implications for stalled replication fork regression. *Nucleic Acids Res*, Vol. 36, No. 22 (pp. 7029-7042), 1362-4962 (Electronic) 0305-1048 (Linking)

Byun, T. S., Pacek, M., Yee, M. C., et al. (2005). Functional uncoupling of MCM helicase and DNA polymerase activities activates the ATR-dependent checkpoint. *Genes Dev*, Vol. 19, No. 9 (pp. 1040-1052), 0890-9369 (Print) 0890-9369 (Linking)

Cadman, C. J., & McGlynn, P. (2004). PriA helicase and SSB interact physically and functionally. *Nucleic Acids Res*, Vol. 32, No. 21 (pp. 6378-6387), 1362-4962 (Electronic) 0305-1048 (Linking)

Cavero, S., Limbo, O., & Russell, P. (2010). Critical functions of Rpa3/Ssb3 in S-phase DNA damage responses in fission yeast. *PLoS Genet*, Vol. 6, No. 9, 1553-7404 (Electronic) 1553-7390 (Linking)

Chang, Y., Gong, L., Yuan, W., et al. (2009). Replication Protein A (RPA1a) is required for meiotic and somatic DNA repair but is dispensable for DNA replication and homologous recombination in rice. *Plant Physiol*, Vol. 151, No. 4 (pp. 2162-2173), 1532-2548 (Electronic) 0032-0889 (Linking)

Chase, J. W., L'Italien, J. J., Murphy, J. B., et al. (1984). Characterization of the *Escherichia coli* SSB-113 mutant single-stranded DNA-binding protein. Cloning of the gene, DNA and protein sequence analysis, high pressure liquid chromatography peptide mapping, and DNA-binding studies. *J Biol Chem*, Vol. 259, No. 2 (pp. 805-814), 0021-9258 (Print) 0021-9258 (Linking)

Chedin, F., Seitz, E. M., & Kowalczykowski, S. C. (1998). Novel homologs of Replication Protein A in archaea: implications for the evolution of ssDNA-binding proteins. *Trends Biochem Sci*, Vol. 23, No. 8 (pp. 273-277), 0968-0004 (Print) 0968-0004 (Linking)

Chen, C., & Kolodner, R. D. (1999). Gross chromosomal rearrangements in *Saccharomyces cerevisiae* replication and recombination defective mutants. *Nat Genet*, Vol. 23, No. 1 (pp. 81-85), 1061-4036 (Print) 1061-4036 (Linking)

Chen, C., Umezu, K., & Kolodner, R. D. (1998). Chromosomal rearrangements occur in *S. cerevisiae rfa1* mutator mutants due to mutagenic lesions processed by double-strand-break repair. *Mol Cell*, Vol. 2, No. 1 (pp. 9-22), 1097-2765 (Print) 1097-2765 (Linking)

Ciccia, A., Bredemeyer, A. L., Sowa, M. E., et al. (2009). The SIOD disorder protein SMARCAL1 is an RPA-interacting protein involved in replication fork restart. *Genes Dev*, Vol. 23, No. 20 (pp. 2415-2425), 1549-5477 (Electronic) 0890-9369 (Linking)

Cimprich, K. A., & Cortez, D. (2008). ATR: an essential regulator of genome integrity. *Nat Rev Mol Cell Biol*, Vol. 9, No. 8 (pp. 616-627), 1471-0080 (Electronic) 1471-0072 (Linking)

Costes, A., Lecointe, F., McGovern, S., et al. (2010). The C-terminal domain of the bacterial SSB protein acts as a DNA maintenance hub at active chromosome replication forks. *PLoS Genet*, Vol. 6, No. 12 (pp. e1001238), 1553-7404 (Electronic) 1553-7390 (Linking)

Cubeddu, L., & White, M. F. (2005). DNA damage detection by an archaeal single-stranded DNA-binding protein. *J Mol Biol*, Vol. 353, No. 3 (pp. 507-516), 0022-2836 (Print) 0022-2836 (Linking)

Curth, U., Genschel, J., Urbanke, C., et al. (1996). *In vitro* and *in vivo* function of the C-terminus of *Escherichia coli* single-stranded DNA binding protein. *Nucleic Acids Res*, Vol. 24, No. 14 (pp. 2706-2711), 0305-1048 (Print) 0305-1048 (Linking)

Curth, U., Urbanke, C., Greipel, J., et al. (1994). Single-stranded-DNA-binding proteins from human mitochondria and *Escherichia coli* have analogous physicochemical properties. *Eur J Biochem*, Vol. 221, No. 1 (pp. 435-443), 0014-2956 (Print) 0014-2956 (Linking)

Czornak, K., Chughtai, S., & Chrzanowska, K. H. (2008). Mystery of DNA repair: the role of the MRN complex and ATM kinase in DNA damage repair. *J Appl Genet*, Vol. 49, No. 4 (pp. 383-396), 1234-1983 (Print) 1234-1283 (Linking)

DeVeaux, L. C., Muller, J. A., Smith, J., et al. (2007). Extremely Radiation-Resistant Mutants of a Halophilic Archaeon with Increased Single-Stranded DNA-Binding Protein (RPA) Gene Expression. *Radiat Res*, Vol. 168, No. 4 (pp. 507-514), 0033-7587 (Print) 0033-7587 (Linking)

Dickson, A. M., Krasikova, Y., Pestryakov, P., et al. (2009). Essential functions of the 32 kDa subunit of yeast Replication Protein A. *Nucleic Acids Res*, Vol. 37, No. 7 (pp. 2313-2326), 1362-4962 (Electronic) 0305-1048 (Linking)

Dodson, G. E., Shi, Y., & Tibbetts, R. S. (2004). DNA replication defects, spontaneous DNA damage, and ATM-dependent checkpoint activation in Replication Protein A-deficient cells. *J Biol Chem*, Vol. 279, No. 32 (pp. 34010-34014), 0021-9258 (Print) 0021-9258 (Linking)

Doherty, K. M., Sommers, J. A., Gray, M. D., et al. (2005). Physical and functional mapping of the Replication Protein A interaction domain of the Werner and Bloom syndrome helicases. *J Biol Chem*, Vol. 280, No. 33 (pp. 29494-29505), 0021-9258 (Print) 0021-9258 (Linking)

Dronkert, M. L., & Kanaar, R. (2001). Repair of DNA interstrand cross-links. *Mutat Res*, Vol. 486, No. 4 (pp. 217-247), 0027-5107 (Print) 0027-5107 (Linking)

Eggington, J. M., Haruta, N., Wood, E. A., et al. (2004). The single-stranded DNA-binding protein of *Deinococcus radiodurans*. *BMC Microbiol*, Vol. 4, (pp. 2), 1471-2180 (Electronic) 1471-2180 (Linking)

Eggington, J. M., Kozlov, A. G., Cox, M. M., et al. (2006). Polar destabilization of DNA duplexes with single-stranded overhangs by the *Deinococcus radiodurans* SSB protein. *Biochemistry,* Vol. 45, No. 48 (pp. 14490-14502), 0006-2960 (Print) 0006-2960 (Linking)

Fanning, E., Klimovich, V., & Nager, A. R. (2006). A dynamic model for Replication Protein A (RPA) function in DNA processing pathways. *Nucleic Acids Res,* Vol. 34, No. 15 (pp. 4126-4137), 1362-4962 (Electronic) 0305-1048 (Linking)

Filipkowski, P., Duraj-Thatte, A., & Kur, J. (2006). Novel thermostable single-stranded DNA-binding protein (SSB) from *Deinococcus geothermalis. Arch Microbiol,* Vol. 186, No. 2 (pp. 129-137), 0302-8933 (Print) 0302-8933 (Linking)

Filipkowski, P., & Kur, J. (2007). Identification and properties of the *Deinococcus grandis* and *Deinococcus proteolyticus* single-stranded DNA binding proteins (SSB). *Acta Biochim Pol,* Vol. 54, No. 1 (pp. 79-87), 0001-527X (Print) 0001-527X (Linking)

Genschel, J., Curth, U., & Urbanke, C. (2000). Interaction of *E. coli* single-stranded DNA binding protein (SSB) with exonuclease I. The carboxy-terminus of SSB is the recognition site for the nuclease. *Biol Chem,* Vol. 381, No. 3 (pp. 183-192), 1431-6730 (Print) 1431-6730 (Linking)

Genschel, J., & Modrich, P. (2009). Functions of MutLα, Replication Protein A (RPA), and HMGB1 in 5'-directed mismatch repair. *J Biol Chem,* Vol. 284, No. 32 (pp. 21536-21544), 0021-9258 (Print) 0021-9258 (Linking)

Georgaki, A., & Hubscher, U. (1993). DNA unwinding by Replication Protein A is a property of the 70 kDa subunit and is facilitated by phosphorylation of the 32 kDa subunit. *Nucleic Acids Res,* Vol. 21, No. 16 (pp. 3659-3665), 0305-1048 (Print) 0305-1048 (Linking)

Georgaki, A., Strack, B., Podust, V., et al. (1992). DNA unwinding activity of Replication Protein A. *FEBS Lett,* Vol. 308, No. 3 (pp. 240-244), 0014-5793 (Print) 0014-5793 (Linking)

Givalos, N., Gakiopoulou, H., Skliri, M., et al. (2007). Replication Protein A is an independent prognostic indicator with potential therapeutic implications in colon cancer. *Mod Pathol,* Vol. 20, No. 2 (pp. 159-166), 0893-3952 (Print) 0893-3952 (Linking)

Haring, S. J., Humphreys, T. D., & Wold, M. S. (2010). A naturally occurring human RPA subunit homolog does not support DNA replication or cell-cycle progression. *Nucleic Acids Res,* Vol. 38, No. 3 (pp. 846-858), 1362-4962 (Electronic) 0305-1048 (Linking)

Haring, S. J., Mason, A. C., Binz, S. K., et al. (2008). Cellular functions of human RPA1. Multiple roles of domains in replication, repair, and checkpoints. *J Biol Chem,* Vol. 283, No. 27 (pp. 19095-19111), 0021-9258 (Print) 0021-9258 (Linking)

Haseltine, C. A., & Kowalczykowski, S. C. (2002). A distinctive single-strand DNA-binding protein from the Archaeon *Sulfolobus solfataricus. Mol Microbiol,* Vol. 43, No. 6 (pp. 1505-1515), 0950-382X (Print) 0950-382X (Linking)

Hass, C. S., Gakhar, L., & Wold, M. S. (2010). Functional characterization of a cancer causing mutation in human Replication Protein A. *Mol Cancer Res,* Vol. 8, No. 7 (pp. 1017-1026), 1557-3125 (Electronic) 1541-7786 (Linking)

Henricksen, L. A., Carter, T., Dutta, A., et al. (1996). Phosphorylation of human Replication Protein A by the DNA-dependent protein kinase is involved in the modulation of

DNA replication. *Nucleic Acids Res*, Vol. 24, No. 15 (pp. 3107-3112), 0305-1048 (Print) 0305-1048 (Linking)

Huang, M., Kim, J. M., Shiotani, B., et al. (2010). The FANCM/FAAP24 complex is required for the DNA interstrand crosslink-induced checkpoint response. *Mol Cell*, Vol. 39, No. 2 (pp. 259-268), 1097-4164 (Electronic) 1097-2765 (Linking)

Iftode, C., Daniely, Y., & Borowiec, J. A. (1999). Replication Protein A (RPA): the eukaryotic SSB. *Crit Rev Biochem Mol Biol*, Vol. 34, No. 3 (pp. 141-180), 1040-9238 (Print) 1040-9238 (Linking)

Inoue, J., Nagae, T., Mishima, M., et al. (2011). A Mechanism for Single-stranded DNA-binding Protein (SSB) Displacement from Single-stranded DNA upon SSB-RecO Interaction. *J Biol Chem*, Vol. 286, No. 8 (pp. 6720-6732), 1083-351X (Electronic) 0021-9258 (Linking)

Ishibashi, T., Kimura, S., & Sakaguchi, K. (2006). A higher plant has three different types of RPA heterotrimeric complex. *J Biochem*, Vol. 139, No. 1 (pp. 99-104), 0021-924X (Print) 0021-924X (Linking)

Jazayeri, A., Falck, J., Lukas, C., et al. (2006). ATM- and cell cycle-dependent regulation of ATR in response to DNA double-strand breaks. *Nat Cell Biol*, Vol. 8, No. 1 (pp. 37-45), 1465-7392 (Print) 1465-7392 (Linking)

Kastan, M. B., & Bartek, J. (2004). Cell-cycle checkpoints and cancer. *Nature*, Vol. 432, No. 7015 (pp. 316-323), 1476-4687 (Electronic) 0028-0836 (Linking)

Kelly, T. J., Simancek, P., & Brush, G. S. (1998). Identification and characterization of a single-stranded DNA-binding protein from the archaeon *Methanococcus jannaschii*. *Proc Natl Acad Sci U S A*, Vol. 95, No. 25 (pp. 14634-14639), 0027-8424 (Print) 0027-8424 (Linking)

Kerr, I. D., Wadsworth, R. I., Blankenfeldt, W., et al. (2001). Overexpression, purification, crystallization and data collection of a single-stranded DNA-binding protein from *Sulfolobus solfataricus*. *Acta Crystallogr D Biol Crystallogr*, Vol. 57, No. Pt 9 (pp. 1290-1292), 0907-4449 (Print) 0907-4449 (Linking)

Kerr, I. D., Wadsworth, R. I., Cubeddu, L., et al. (2003). Insights into ssDNA recognition by the OB fold from a structural and thermodynamic study of *Sulfolobus* SSB protein. *EMBO J*, Vol. 22, No. 11 (pp. 2561-2570), 0261-4189 (Print) 0261-4189 (Linking)

Keshav, K. F., Chen, C., & Dutta, A. (1995). Rpa4, a homolog of the 34-kilodalton subunit of the Replication Protein A complex. *Mol Cell Biol*, Vol. 15, No. 6 (pp. 3119-3128), 0270-7306 (Print) 0270-7306 (Linking)

Kim, C., Snyder, R. O., & Wold, M. S. (1992). Binding properties of Replication Protein A from human and yeast cells. *Mol Cell Biol*, Vol. 12, No. 7 (pp. 3050-3059), 0270-7306 (Print) 0270-7306 (Linking)

Kim, H. S., & Brill, S. J. (2001). Rfc4 interacts with Rpa1 and is required for both DNA replication and DNA damage checkpoints in *Saccharomyces cerevisiae*. *Mol Cell Biol*, Vol. 21, No. 11 (pp. 3725-3737), 0270-7306 (Print) 0270-7306 (Linking)

Kim, J. E., Minter-Dykhouse, K., & Chen, J. (2006). Signaling networks controlled by the MRN complex and MDC1 during early DNA damage responses. *Mol Carcinog*, Vol. 45, No. 6 (pp. 403-408), 0899-1987 (Print) 0899-1987 (Linking)

Kobayashi, Y., Sato, K., Kibe, T., et al. (2010). Expression of mutant RPA in human cancer cells causes telomere shortening. *Biosci Biotechnol Biochem*, Vol. 74, No. 2 (pp. 382-385), 1347-6947 (Electronic) 0916-8451 (Linking)

Komori, K., & Ishino, Y. (2001). Replication Protein A in *Pyrococcus furiosus* is involved in homologous DNA recombination. *J Biol Chem*, Vol. 276, No. 28 (pp. 25654-25660), 0021-9258 (Print) 0021-9258 (Linking)

Kottemann, M., Kish, A., Iloanusi, C., et al. (2005). Physiological responses of the halophilic archaeon *Halobacterium* sp. strain NRC1 to desiccation and gamma irradiation. *Extremophiles*, Vol. 9, No. 3 (pp. 219-227), 1431-0651 (Print) 1431-0651 (Linking)

Kozlov, A. G., Jezewska, M. J., Bujalowski, W., et al. (2010). Binding specificity of *Escherichia coli* single-stranded DNA binding protein for the chi subunit of DNA pol III holoenzyme and PriA helicase. *Biochemistry*, Vol. 49, No. 17 (pp. 3555-3566), 1520-4995 (Electronic) 0006-2960 (Linking)

Krasikova, Y. S., Rechkunova, N. I., Maltseva, E. A., et al. (2010). Localization of xeroderma pigmentosum group A protein and Replication Protein A on damaged DNA in nucleotide excision repair. *Nucleic Acids Res*, Vol. 38, No. 22 (pp. 8083-8094), 1362-4962 (Electronic) 0305-1048 (Linking)

Krokan, H. E., Nilsen, H., Skorpen, F., et al. (2000). Base excision repair of DNA in mammalian cells. *FEBS Lett*, Vol. 476, No. 1-2 (pp. 73-77), 0014-5793 (Print) 0014-5793 (Linking)

Kumar, N. V., & Varshney, U. (1997). Contrasting effects of single stranded DNA binding protein on the activity of uracil DNA glycosylase from *Escherichia coli* towards different DNA substrates. *Nucleic Acids Res*, Vol. 25, No. 12 (pp. 2336-2343), 0305-1048 (Print) 0305-1048 (Linking)

Lecointe, F., Serena, C., Velten, M., et al. (2007). Anticipating chromosomal replication fork arrest: SSB targets repair DNA helicases to active forks. *EMBO J*, Vol. 26, No. 19 (pp. 4239-4251), 0261-4189 (Print) 0261-4189 (Linking)

Li, Z., Lu, S., Hou, G., et al. (2008). Hjm/Hel308A DNA helicase from *Sulfolobus tokodaii* promotes replication fork regression and interacts with Hjc endonuclease *in vitro*. *J Bacteriol*, Vol. 190, No. 8 (pp. 3006-3017), 1098-5530 (Electronic) 0021-9193 (Linking)

Lin, Y., Lin, L. J., Sriratana, P., et al. (2008). Engineering of functional Replication Protein A homologs based on insights into the evolution of oligonucleotide/oligosaccharide-binding folds. *J Bacteriol*, Vol. 190, No. 17 (pp. 5766-5780), 1098-5530 (Electronic) 0021-9193 (Linking)

Lin, Y., Robbins, J. B., Nyannor, E. K., et al. (2005). A CCCH zinc finger conserved in a Replication Protein A homolog found in diverse Euryarchaeotes. *J Bacteriol*, Vol. 187, No. 23 (pp. 7881-7889), 0021-9193 (Print) 0021-9193 (Linking)

Lindner, C., Nijland, R., van Hartskamp, M., et al. (2004). Differential expression of two paralogous genes of *Bacillus subtilis* encoding single-stranded DNA binding protein. *J Bacteriol*, Vol. 186, No. 4 (pp. 1097-1105), 0021-9193 (Print) 0021-9193 (Linking)

Liu, J. S., Kuo, S. R., & Melendy, T. (2006). Phosphorylation of Replication Protein A by S-phase checkpoint kinases. *DNA Repair (Amst)*, Vol. 5, No. 3 (pp. 369-380), 1568-7864 (Print) 1568-7856 (Linking)

Liu, Y., Zhou, J., Omelchenko, M. V., et al. (2003). Transcriptome dynamics of *Deinococcus radiodurans* recovering from ionizing radiation. *Proc Natl Acad Sci U S A*, Vol. 100, No. 7 (pp. 4191-4196), 0027-8424 (Print) 0027-8424 (Linking)

Lohman, T. M., & Ferrari, M. E. (1994). *Escherichia coli* single-stranded DNA-binding protein: multiple DNA-binding modes and cooperativities. *Annu Rev Biochem*, Vol. 63, (pp. 527-570), 0066-4154 (Print) 0066-4154 (Linking)

Longhese, M. P., Neecke, H., Paciotti, V., et al. (1996). The 70 kDa subunit of Replication Protein A is required for the G1/S and intra-S DNA damage checkpoints in budding yeast. *Nucleic Acids Res*, Vol. 24, No. 18 (pp. 3533-3537), 0305-1048 (Print) 0305-1048 (Linking)

Lu, D., & Keck, J. L. (2008). Structural basis of *Escherichia coli* single-stranded DNA-binding protein stimulation of exonuclease I. *Proc Natl Acad Sci U S A*, Vol. 105, No. 27 (pp. 9169-9174), 1091-6490 (Electronic) 0027-8424 (Linking)

Luo, X., Schwarz-Linek, U., Botting, C. H., et al. (2007). CC1, a novel crenarchaeal DNA binding protein. *J Bacteriol*, Vol. 189, No. 2 (pp. 403-409), 0021-9193 (Print) 0021-9193 (Linking)

Machwe, A., Lozada, E., Wold, M. S., et al. (2011). Molecular cooperation between the Werner syndrome protein and Replication Protein A in relation to replication fork blockage. *J Biol Chem*, Vol. 286, No. 5 (pp. 3497-3508), 1083-351X (Electronic) 021-9258 (Linking)

Machwe, A., Xiao, L., Groden, J., et al. (2006). The Werner and Bloom syndrome proteins catalyze regression of a model replication fork. *Biochemistry*, Vol. 45, No. 47 (pp. 13939-13946), 0006-2960 (Print) 0006-2960 (Linking)

Machwe, A., Xiao, L., Lloyd, R. G., et al. (2007). Replication fork regression *in vitro* by the Werner syndrome protein (WRN): holliday junction formation, the effect of leading arm structure and a potential role for WRN exonuclease activity. *Nucleic Acids Res*, Vol. 35, No. 17 (pp. 5729-5747), 1362-4962 (Electronic) 0305-1048 (Linking)

Majka, J., Binz, S. K., Wold, M. S., et al. (2006). Replication Protein A directs loading of the DNA damage checkpoint clamp to 5'-DNA junctions. *J Biol Chem*, Vol. 281, No. 38 (pp. 27855-27861), 0021-9258 (Print) 0021-9258 (Linking)

Maniar, H. S., Wilson, R., & Brill, S. J. (1997). Roles of Replication Protein-A subunits 2 and 3 in DNA replication fork movement in *Saccharomyces cerevisiae*. *Genetics*, Vol. 145, No. 4 (pp. 891-902), 0016-6731 (Print) 0016-6731 (Linking)

Marwedel, T., Ishibashi, T., Lorbiecke, R., et al. (2003). Plant-specific regulation of Replication Protein A2 (OsRPA2) from rice during the cell cycle and in response to ultraviolet light exposure. *Planta*, Vol. 217, No. 3 (pp. 457-465), 0032-0935 (Print) 0032-0935 (Linking)

Mason, A. C., Haring, S. J., Pryor, J. M., et al. (2009). An alternative form of Replication Protein A prevents viral replication *in vitro*. *J Biol Chem*, Vol. 284, No. 8 (pp. 5324-5331), 0021-9258 (Print) 0021-9258 (Linking)

Mason, A. C., Roy, R., Simmons, D. T., et al. (2010). Functions of alternative Replication Protein A in initiation and elongation. *Biochemistry*, Vol. 49, No. 28 (pp. 5919-5928), 1520-4995 (Electronic) 0006-2960 (Linking)

McCready, S., Muller, J. A., Boubriak, I., et al. (2005). UV irradiation induces homologous recombination genes in the model archaeon, *Halobacterium* sp. NRC-1. *Saline Systems*, Vol. 1, (pp. 3)

McInerney, P., & O'Donnell, M. (2007). Replisome fate upon encountering a leading strand block and clearance from DNA by recombination proteins. *J Biol Chem*, Vol. 282, No. 35 (pp. 25903-25916), 0021-9258 (Print) 0021-9258 (Linking)

Mer, G., Bochkarev, A., Gupta, R., et al. (2000). Structural basis for the recognition of DNA repair proteins UNG2, XPA, and RAD52 by replication factor RPA. *Cell*, Vol. 103, No. 3 (pp. 449-456), 0092-8674 (Print) 0092-8674 (Linking)

Meyer, R. R., & Laine, P. S. (1990). The single-stranded DNA-binding protein of *Escherichia coli*. *Microbiol Rev*, Vol. 54, No. 4 (pp. 342-380), 0146-0749 (Print) 0146-0749 (Linking)

Mijakovic, I., Petranovic, D., Macek, B., et al. (2006). Bacterial single-stranded DNA-binding proteins are phosphorylated on tyrosine. *Nucleic Acids Res*, Vol. 34, No. 5 (pp. 1588-1596), 1362-4962 (Electronic) 0305-1048 (Linking)

Naue, N., Fedorov, R., Pich, A., et al. (2011). Site-directed mutagenesis of the χ subunit of DNA polymerase III and single-stranded DNA-binding protein of *E. coli* reveals key residues for their interaction. *Nucleic Acids Res*, Vol. 39, No. 4 (pp. 1398-1407), 1362-4962 (Electronic) 0305-1048 (Linking)

Norais, C. A., Chitteni-Pattu, S., Wood, E. A., et al. (2009). DdrB protein, an alternative *Deinococcus radiodurans* SSB induced by ionizing radiation. *J Biol Chem*, Vol. 284, No. 32 (pp. 21402-21411), 0021-9258 (Print) 0021-9258 (Linking)

Nuss, J. E., Patrick, S. M., Oakley, G. G., et al. (2005). DNA damage induced hyperphosphorylation of Replication Protein A. 1. Identification of novel sites of phosphorylation in response to DNA damage. *Biochemistry*, Vol. 44, No. 23 (pp. 8428-8437), 0006-2960 (Print) 0006-2960 (Linking)

Oakley, G. G., Loberg, L. I., Yao, J., et al. (2001). UV-induced hyperphosphorylation of Replication Protein A depends on DNA replication and expression of ATM protein. *Mol Biol Cell*, Vol. 12, No. 5 (pp. 1199-1213), 1059-1524 (Print) 1059-1524 (Linking)

Oakley, G. G., Patrick, S. M., Yao, J., et al. (2003). RPA phosphorylation in mitosis alters DNA binding and protein-protein interactions. *Biochemistry*, Vol. 42, No. 11 (pp. 3255-3264), 0006-2960 (Print) 0006-2960 (Linking)

Oakley, G. G., Tillison, K., Opiyo, S. A., et al. (2009). Physical interaction between Replication Protein A (RPA) and MRN: involvement of RPA2 phosphorylation and the N-terminus of RPA1. *Biochemistry*, Vol. 48, No. 31 (pp. 7473-7481), 1520-4995 (Electronic) 0006-2960 (Linking)

Olszewski, M., Grot, A., Wojciechowski, M., et al. (2010). Characterization of exceptionally thermostable single-stranded DNA-binding proteins from *Thermotoga maritima* and *Thermotoga neapolitana*. *BMC Microbiol*, Vol. 10, (pp. 260), 1471-2180 (Electronic) 1471-2180 (Linking)

Olszewski, M., Mickiewicz, M., & Kur, J. (2008). Two highly thermostable paralogous single-stranded DNA-binding proteins from *Thermoanaerobacter tengcongensis*. *Arch Microbiol*, Vol. 190, No. 1 (pp. 79-87), 0302-8933 (Print) 0302-8933 (Linking)

Ono, Y., Tomita, K., Matsuura, A., et al. (2003). A novel allele of fission yeast *rad11* that causes defects in DNA repair and telomere length regulation. *Nucleic Acids Res*, Vol. 31, No. 24 (pp. 7141-7149), 1362-4962 (Electronic) 0305-1048 (Linking)

Osman, K., Sanchez-Moran, E., Mann, S. C., et al. (2009). Replication protein A (AtRPA1a) is required for class I crossover formation but is dispensable for meiotic DNA break repair. *EMBO J*, Vol. 28, No. 4 (pp. 394-404), 1460-2075 (Electronic) 0261-4189 (Linking)

Overmeer, R. M., Moser, J., Volker, M., et al. (2011). Replication Protein A safeguards genome integrity by controlling NER incision events. *J Cell Biol*, Vol. 192, No. 3 (pp. 401-415), 1540-8140 (Electronic) 0021-9525 (Linking)

Pages, V., & Fuchs, R. P. (2003). Uncoupling of leading- and lagging-strand DNA replication during lesion bypass *in vivo*. *Science*, Vol. 300, No. 5623 (pp. 1300-1303), 1095-9203 (Electronic) 0036-8075 (Linking)

Pan, Z. Q., Park, C. H., Amin, A. A., et al. (1995). Phosphorylated and unphosphorylated forms of human single-stranded DNA-binding protein are equally active in simian virus 40 DNA replication and in nucleotide excision repair. *Proc Natl Acad Sci U S A*, Vol. 92, No. 10 (pp. 4636-4640), 0027-8424 (Print) 0027-8424 (Linking)

Parker, A. E., Clyne, R. K., Carr, A. M., et al. (1997). The *Schizosaccharomyces pombe rad11+* gene encodes the large subunit of Replication Protein A. *Mol Cell Biol*, Vol. 17, No. 5 (pp. 2381-514), 0270-7306 (Print) 0270-7306 (Linking)

Patrick, S. M., Oakley, G. G., Dixon, K., et al. (2005). DNA damage induced hyperphosphorylation of Replication Protein A. 2. Characterization of DNA binding activity, protein interactions, and activity in DNA replication and repair. *Biochemistry*, Vol. 44, No. 23 (pp. 8438-8448), 0006-2960 (Print) 0006-2960 (Linking)

Philipova, D., Mullen, J. R., Maniar, H. S., et al. (1996). A hierarchy of SSB protomers in Replication Protein A. *Genes Dev*, Vol. 10, No. 17 (pp. 2222-2233), 0890-9369 (Print) 0890-9369 (Linking)

Plate, I., Hallwyl, S. C., Shi, I., et al. (2008). Interaction with RPA is necessary for Rad52 repair center formation and for its mediator activity. *J Biol Chem*, Vol. 283, No. 43 (pp. 29077-29085), 0021-9258 (Print) 0021-9258 (Linking)

Pretto, D. I., Tsutakawa, S., Brosey, C. A., et al. (2010). Structural dynamics and single-stranded DNA binding activity of the three N-terminal domains of the large subunit of Replication Protein A from small angle X-ray scattering. *Biochemistry*, Vol. 49, No. 13 (pp. 2880-2889), 1520-4995 (Electronic) 0006-2960 (Linking)

Pugh, R. A., Lin, Y., Eller, C., et al. (2008). *Ferroplasma acidarmanus* RPA2 facilitates efficient unwinding of forked DNA substrates by monomers of FacXPD helicase. *J Mol Biol*, Vol. 383, No. 5 (pp. 982-998), 1089-8638 (Electronic) 0022-2836 (Linking)

Ralf, C., Hickson, I. D., & Wu, L. (2006). The Bloom's syndrome helicase can promote the regression of a model replication fork. *J Biol Chem*, Vol. 281, No. 32 (pp. 22839-22846), 0021-9258 (Print) 0021-9258 (Linking)

Richard, D. J., Bolderson, E., Cubeddu, L., et al. (2008). Single-stranded DNA-binding protein hSSB1 is critical for genomic stability. *Nature*, Vol. 453, No. 7195 (pp. 677-681), 1476-4687 (Electronic) 0028-0836 (Linking)

Richard, D. J., Bolderson, E., & Khanna, K. K. (2009). Multiple human single-stranded DNA binding proteins function in genome maintenance: structural, biochemical and functional analysis. *Crit Rev Biochem Mol Biol*, Vol. 44, No. 2-3 (pp. 98-116), 1549-7798 (Electronic) 1040-9238 (Linking)

Richard, D. J., Cubeddu, L., Urquhart, A. J., et al. (2011). hSSB1 interacts directly with the MRN complex stimulating its recruitment to DNA double-strand breaks and its endo-nuclease activity. *Nucleic Acids Res*, 1362-4962 (Electronic) 0305-1048 (Linking)

Richard, D. J., Savage, K., Bolderson, E., et al. (2011). hSSB1 rapidly binds at the sites of DNA double-strand breaks and is required for the efficient recruitment of the MRN complex. *Nucleic Acids Res*, Vol. 39, No. 5 (pp. 1692-1702), 1362-4962 (Electronic) 0305-1048 (Linking)

Robbins, J. B., McKinney, M. C., Guzman, C. E., et al. (2005). The euryarchaeota, nature's medium for engineering of single-stranded DNA-binding proteins. *J Biol Chem*, Vol. 280, No. 15 (pp. 15325-15339), 0021-9258 (Print) 0021-9258 (Linking)

Robbins, J. B., Murphy, M. C., White, B. A., et al. (2004). Functional analysis of multiple single-stranded DNA-binding proteins from *Methanosarcina acetivorans* and their effects on DNA synthesis by DNA polymerase BI. *J Biol Chem*, Vol. 279, No. 8 (pp. 6315-6326), 0021-9258 (Print) 0021-9258 (Linking)

Rolfsmeier, M. L., & Haseltine, C. A. (2010). The single-stranded DNA binding protein of *Sulfolobus solfataricus* acts in the presynaptic step of homologous recombination. *J Mol Biol*, Vol. 397, No. 1 (pp. 31-45), 1089-8638 (Electronic) 0022-2836 (Linking)

Saijo, M., Takedachi, A., & Tanaka, K. (2011). Nucleotide Excision Repair by Mutant Xeroderma Pigmentosum Group A (XPA) Proteins with Deficiency in Interaction with RPA. *J Biol Chem*, Vol. 286, No. 7 (pp. 5476-5483), 1083-351X (Electronic) 0021-9258 (Linking)

Sakaguchi, K., Ishibashi, T., Uchiyama, Y., et al. (2009). The multi-Replication Protein A (RPA) system--a new perspective. *FEBS J*, Vol. 276, No. 4 (pp. 943-963), 1742-4658 (Electronic) 1742-464X (Linking)

Santocanale, C., Neecke, H., Longhese, M. P., et al. (1995). Mutations in the gene encoding the 34 kDa subunit of yeast Replication Protein A cause defective S phase progression. *J Mol Biol*, Vol. 254, No. 4 (pp. 595-607), 0022-2836 (Print) 0022-2836 (Linking)

Sharma, A., Nitharwal, R. G., Singh, B., et al. (2009). *Helicobacter pylori* single-stranded DNA binding protein--functional characterization and modulation of *H. pylori* DnaB helicase activity. *FEBS J*, Vol. 276, No. 2 (pp. 519-531), 1742-4658 (Electronic) 1742-464X (Linking)

Sheng, D., Zhu, S., Wei, T., et al. (2008). The *in vitro* activity of a Rad55 homologue from *Sulfolobus tokodaii*, a candidate mediator in RadA-catalyzed homologous recombination. *Extremophiles*, Vol. 12, No. 1 (pp. 147-157), 1431-0651 (Print) 1431-0651 (Linking)

Shereda, R. D., Bernstein, D. A., & Keck, J. L. (2007). A central role for SSB in *Escherichia coli* RecQ DNA helicase function. *J Biol Chem*, Vol. 282, No. 26 (pp. 19247-19258), 0021-9258 (Print) 0021-9258 (Linking)

Shereda, R. D., Kozlov, A. G., Lohman, T. M., et al. (2008). SSB as an organizer/mobilizer of genome maintenance complexes. *Crit Rev Biochem Mol Biol*, Vol. 43, No. 5 (pp. 289-318), 1549-7798 (Electronic) 1040-9238 (Linking)

Shultz, R. W., Tatineni, V. M., Hanley-Bowdoin, L., et al. (2007). Genome-wide analysis of the core DNA replication machinery in the higher plants *Arabidopsis* and rice. *Plant Physiol*, Vol. 144, No. 4 (pp. 1697-1714), 0032-0889 (Print) 0032-0889 (Linking)

Soustelle, C., Vedel, M., Kolodner, R., et al. (2002). Replication Protein A is required for meiotic recombination in *Saccharomyces cerevisiae*. *Genetics*, Vol. 161, No. 2 (pp. 535-547), 0016-6731 (Print) 0016-6731 (Linking)

Sowd, G., Wang, H., Pretto, D., et al. (2009). Replication Protein A stimulates the Werner syndrome protein branch migration activity. *J Biol Chem*, Vol. 284, No. 50 (pp. 34682-34691), 1083-351X (Electronic) 0021-9258 (Linking)

Stephan, H., Concannon, C., Kremmer, E., et al. (2009). Ionizing radiation-dependent and independent phosphorylation of the 32-kDa subunit of Replication Protein A during mitosis. *Nucleic Acids Res*, Vol. 37, No. 18 (pp. 6028-6041), 1362-4962 (Electronic) 0305-1048 (Linking)

Sugiman-Marangos, S., & Junop, M. S. (2010). The structure of DdrB from *Deinococcus*: a new fold for single-stranded DNA binding proteins. *Nucleic Acids Res*, Vol. 38, No. 10 (pp. 3432-3440), 1362-4962 (Electronic) 0305-1048 (Linking)

Sugiyama, T., & Kantake, N. (2009). Dynamic regulatory interactions of rad51, rad52, and Replication Protein-A in recombination intermediates. *J Mol Biol*, Vol. 390, No. 1 (pp. 45-55), 1089-8638 (Electronic) 0022-2836 (Linking)

Suhasini, A. N., Sommers, J. A., Mason, A. C., et al. (2009). FANCJ helicase uniquely senses oxidative base damage in either strand of duplex DNA and is stimulated by Replication Protein A to unwind the damaged DNA substrate in a strand-specific manner. *J Biol Chem*, Vol. 284, No. 27 (pp. 18458-18470), 1083-351X (Electronic) 0021-9258 (Linking)

Sun, J., Yu, E. Y., Yang, Y., et al. (2009). Stn1-Ten1 is an Rpa2-Rpa3-like complex at telomeres. *Genes Dev*, Vol. 23, No. 24 (pp. 2900-2914), 1549-5477 (Electronic) 0890-9369 (Linking)

Takashi, Y., Kobayashi, Y., Tanaka, K., et al. (2009). *Arabidopsis* Replication Protein A 70a is required for DNA damage response and telomere length homeostasis. *Plant Cell Physiol*, Vol. 50, No. 11 (pp. 1965-1976), 1471-9053 (Electronic) 0032-0781 (Linking)

Tanaka, M., Earl, A. M., Howell, H. A., et al. (2004). Analysis of *Deinococcus radiodurans*'s transcriptional response to ionizing radiation and desiccation reveals novel proteins that contribute to extreme radioresistance. *Genetics*, Vol. 168, No. 1 (pp. 21-3), 0016-6731 (Print) 0016-6731 (Linking)

Teng, Y., Longhese, M., McDonough, G., et al. (1998). Mutants with changes in different domains of yeast Replication Protein A exhibit differences in repairing the control region, the transcribed strand and the non-transcribed strand of the *Saccharomyces cerevisiae* MFA2 gene. *J Mol Biol*, Vol. 280, No. 3 (pp. 355-363), 0022-2836 (Print) 0022-2836 (Linking)

Theobald, D. L., Mitton-Fry, R. M., & Wuttke, D. S. (2003). Nucleic acid recognition by OB-fold proteins. *Annu Rev Biophys Biomol Struct*, Vol. 32, (pp. 115-133), 1056-8700 (Print) 1056-8700 (Linking)

Theriot, C. A., Hegde, M. L., Hazra, T. K., et al. (2010). RPA physically interacts with the human DNA glycosylase NEIL1 to regulate excision of oxidative DNA base damage in primer-template structures. *DNA Repair (Amst)*, Vol. 9, No. 6 (pp. 643-652), 1568-7856 (Electronic) 1568-7856 (Linking)

Ujaoney, A. K., Potnis, A. A., Kane, P., et al. (2010). Radiation desiccation response motif-like sequences are involved in transcriptional activation of the Deinococcal *ssb* gene by ionizing radiation but not by desiccation. *J Bacteriol*, Vol. 192, No. 21 (pp. 5637-5644), 1098-5530 (Electronic) 0021-9193 (Linking)

Umezu, K., Sugawara, N., Chen, C., et al. (1998). Genetic analysis of yeast RPA1 reveals its multiple functions in DNA metabolism. *Genetics*, Vol. 148, No. 3 (pp. 989-1005), 0016-6731 (Print) 0016-6731 (Linking)

Vassin, V. M., Anantha, R. W., Sokolova, E., et al. (2009). Human RPA phosphorylation by ATR stimulates DNA synthesis and prevents ssDNA accumulation during DNA-replication stress. *J Cell Sci*, Vol. 122, No. Pt 22 (pp. 4070-4080), 1477-9137 (Electronic) 0021-9533 (Linking)

Wadsworth, R. I., & White, M. F. (2001). Identification and properties of the crenarchaeal single-stranded DNA binding protein from *Sulfolobus solfataricus*. *Nucleic Acids Res*, Vol. 29, No. 4 (pp. 914-920), 1362-4962 (Electronic) 0305-1048 (Linking)

Wang, Y., Putnam, C. D., Kane, M. F., et al. (2005). Mutation in Rpa1 results in defective DNA double-strand break repair, chromosomal instability and cancer in mice. *Nat Genet*, Vol. 37, No. 7 (pp. 750-755), 1061-4036 (Print) 1061-4036 (Linking)

Williams, G. J., Lees-Miller, S. P., & Tainer, J. A. (2010). Mre11-Rad50-Nbs1 conformations and the control of sensing, signaling, and effector responses at DNA double-strand breaks. *DNA Repair (Amst)*, Vol. 9, No. 12 (pp. 1299-1306), 1568-7856 (Electronic) 1568-7856 (Linking)

Witte, G., Urbanke, C., & Curth, U. (2003). DNA polymerase III chi subunit ties single-stranded DNA binding protein to the bacterial replication machinery. *Nucleic Acids Res*, Vol. 31, No. 15 (pp. 4434-4440), 1362-4962 (Electronic) 0305-1048 (Linking)

Wold, M. S. (1997). Replication Protein A: a heterotrimeric, single-stranded DNA-binding protein required for eukaryotic DNA metabolism. *Annu Rev Biochem*, Vol. 66, (pp. 61-92), 0066-4154 (Print) 0066-4154 (Linking)

Woodman, I. L., Brammer, K., & Bolt, E. L. (2010). Physical interaction between archaeal DNA repair helicase Hel308 and Replication Protein A (RPA). *DNA Repair (Amst)*, 1568-7856 (Electronic) 1568-7856 (Linking)

Xu, G., Lu, H., Wang, L., et al. (2010). DdrB stimulates single-stranded DNA annealing and facilitates RecA-independent DNA repair in *Deinococcus radiodurans*. *DNA Repair (Amst)*, Vol. 9, No. 7 (pp. 805-812), 1568-7856 (Electronic) 1568-7856 (Linking)

Xu, X., Vaithiyalingam, S., Glick, G. G., et al. (2008). The basic cleft of RPA70N binds multiple checkpoint proteins, including RAD9, to regulate ATR signaling. *Mol Cell Biol*, Vol. 28, No. 24 (pp. 7345-7353), 1098-5549 (Electronic) 0270-7306 (Linking)

Yang, J., Yu, Y., Hamrick, H. E., et al. (2003). ATM, ATR and DNA-PK: initiators of the cellular genotoxic stress responses. *Carcinogenesis*, Vol. 24, No. 10 (pp. 1571-1580), 0143-3334 (Print) 0143-3334 (Linking)

Yuan, J., Ghosal, G., & Chen, J. (2009). The annealing helicase HARP protects stalled replication forks. *Genes Dev*, Vol. 23, No. 20 (pp. 2394-2399), 1549-5477 (Electronic) 0890-9369 (Linking)

Yusufzai, T., Kong, X., Yokomori, K., et al. (2009). The annealing helicase HARP is recruited to DNA repair sites via an interaction with RPA. *Genes Dev*, Vol. 23, No. 20 (pp. 2400-2404), 1549-5477 (Electronic) 0890-9369 (Linking)

Yuzhakov, A., Kelman, Z., Hurwitz, J., et al. (1999). Multiple competition reactions for RPA order the assembly of the DNA polymerase delta holoenzyme. *EMBO J*, Vol. 18, No. 21 (pp. 6189-6199), 0261-4189 (Print) 0261-4189 (Linking)

Yuzhakov, A., Kelman, Z., & O'Donnell, M. (1999). Trading places on DNA--a three-point switch underlies primer handoff from primase to the replicative DNA polymerase. *Cell*, Vol. 96, No. 1 (pp. 153-163), 0092-8674 (Print) 0092-8674 (Linking)

Zernik-Kobak, M., Vasunia, K., Connelly, M., et al. (1997). Sites of UV-induced phosphorylation of the p34 subunit of Replication Protein A from HeLa cells. *J Biol Chem*, Vol. 272, No. 38 (pp. 23896-23904), 0021-9258 (Print) 0021-9258 (Linking)

Zou, L., & Elledge, S. J. (2003). Sensing DNA damage through ATRIP recognition of RPA-ssDNA complexes. *Science*, Vol. 300, No. 5625 (pp. 1542-1548), 1095-9203 (Electronic) 0036-8075 (Linking)

3

Interactions by Carcinogenic Metal Compounds with DNA Repair Processes

Simona Catalani and Pietro Apostoli
Department of Experimental and Applied Medicine,
Section of Occupational Health and Industrial Hygiene,
University of Brescia,
Italy

1. Introduction

Some metal compounds, including arsenic, beryllium, cadmium, chromium and nickel have long been recognized as human and animal carcinogens, while for other as antimony, cobalt, lead and vanadium their carcinogenic action are probable or possible. Except chromium (VI), carcinogenic metals are only weak mutagens in mammalian cells and often inactive in bacterial assays. Since the mutagenicity in bacterial assays indicates reactivity with DNA, metals are thought to exert genotoxicity mainly by indirect mechanisms. The four main, partly overlapping, DNA repair pathways operating in mammalian cells are base excision, mismatch, nucleotide excision and recombinational repair; each of repair pathways is involved in the removal of the specific DNA lesions. In addition, many carcinogenic metal compounds at low concentrations have been identified as inhibitors of the repair of DNA damage caused by other xenobiotics or endogenous factor. Furthermore, DNA is not only damaged by environmental mutagens including UV-light and polycyclic aromatic hydrocarbons, but also by reactive oxygen species generated from the same metallic elements. Failure to repair DNA damage can result in the accumulation of damaged DNA, mutation and carcinogenesis.

2. Mechanism of action

The potential target of metallic elements on DNA repair proteins are the zinc finger structures in their DNA binding motifs. Within these structures, zinc is complexed to four cysteines and/or histidines, folding different structural domains mediating DNA-protein as well as protein-protein interactions. It is estimated that about 1% of all mammalian genes encode zinc finger proteins, which are involved in many processes maintaining genomic integrity (Mackay & Crossley, 1998). The zinc ions do not participate in interactions conveyed by zinc finger domains, but are necessary for their function since they maintain their three-dimensional structures. In the case of transcription factors and DNA repair proteins, the absence of metal ions lead to loss in DNA-binding capacity. The functions of individual zinc finger include recognition of structures and sequences of nucleic acids and proteins. The majority of identified zinc finger may be classified as transcription factors. Another well known function of various zinc finger motifs, is the assembly of multiprotein complexes having structural or enzymatic functions. The main zinc finger proteins involved are the bacterial formamidopyrimidine-DNA glicosylase (fpg), the xeroderma pigmentosum A (XPA) protein, the poly(ADP-ribose) polymerase (PARP) and tumor suppression protein p53. The studies about of metal ions interaction indicated that apparently similar zinc finger domains may have different reactivity and suggested to draw a sort of list of possible mechanisms of zinc finger damage (Hartwig, 2001). Among these mechanisms, the most important are isostructural substitution, substitution with altered geometry, mixed complex formation, and catalysis of thiol oxidation. Many studies showed that different concentrations are needed to observe an inhibition and wide differences were observed for example when comparing the results obtained with Fpg and XPA (Witkiewicz-Kucharczyk & Bal., 2006). Regarding XPA, arsenic and lead did not decrease its binding to a UV-irradiated oligoucleotide, whereas cadmium, cobalt and nickel interfere with its DNA binding ability. A simultaneous treatment with zinc largely prevented this inhibition (Asmuß et al., 2000). Structural investigations by different spectroscopic methods revealed a tetrahedrally co-ordination of all three metal ions with no major distortion of XPA while for cadmium an increased Cd-S bond length was observed. Poly(ADP-ribosyl)ation of various proteins is one of the earliest nuclear events following DNA strand break induction. Yager & Wiencke (1997) and Hartwig et al., (2002) demonstrated an inhibition of H_2O_2-induced PARP activity in intact cells by nickel, cobalt, cadmium and very low concentration of arsenic in HeLa cells, while no effect was observed with lead. One other zinc-dependent protein with great impact on the processing of DNA damage and genomic stability is the p53 suppressor protein. Zinc has been shown to be required for proper folding in wild type conformation, and exposure to either isolate p53 protein or human breast cancer cells to cadmium resulted in disruption of native p53 conformation and inhibition of DNA binding (Meplan et al., 1999). Witkiewicz-Kucharczyk & Bal (2006) assessed the different metal binding properties of zinc finger and reported that cobalt is practically isostructural with zinc in zinc finger peptides and proteins, regardless of the number of cysteine residues involved. However, there is a strong, although quantitative variable thermodynamic preference for zinc over cobalt in tetrahedral environments provided by zinc finger. This effect is due to the ligand field stabilization effect, modulated by entropic contributions (Lachenmann et al., 2004). The substitution of nickel into zinc finger can also be achieved, but it results in distortions of the binding geometry and alterations of the peptide fold. A distorted tetrahedral coordination was found for cysteine$_2$-Histidine$_2$ zinc fingers (Posewitz & Wilcox, 1995), while a nearly square planar arrangement of donors was demonstrated in a cysteine$_4$ environment (Bal et al., 2003). Also the efficacy of cadmium binding is related to the number of coordinated thiolates (Krizek et al., 1993). Zinc seems to be preferred in the cysteine$_2$-histidine$_2$ environment, the affinities of zinc and cadmium may be comparable for cysteine$_3$-histidine, and cadmium is strongly preferred in cysteine$_4$ zinc finger peptides (Kopera et al., 2004). This preference is due to the high enthalpy of the cadmium-S bond. The cadmium ion fits into tetrahedral environments with little strain, however, it is significantly larger than zinc and cobalt ions, which results in local distortions of zinc finger geometries (Buchko et al., 2000). Finally lead, element with high affinities to thiolates, can replace zinc in zinc finger domains and disrupt their fold. Arsenic too is known to have a high affinity to -SH groups and it is demonstrated by arsenic-mediated repair inhibition not related with a direct mechanism of one or more specific repair proteins, but rather with changes in gene expression and/or signal transduction (Asmuß et al., 2000). Finally redox regulation has been *in vitro* and *in vivo* demonstrated in several DNA-binding zinc finger proteins. The metal ions can oxidize the essential cysteines and/or other residues in zinc finger structures interfering in metal binding domain. Taken together, the above mentioned mechanisms indicate that DNA repair, zinc homeostasis, oxidative assault and the redox status of the cell are all interconnected (Fig 1). The toxic/carcinogenic metals with sufficiently high affinities to thiols may interfere at all stages of zinc homeostasis and signaling, but specific ways of their actions can only be understood in appropriately complicated experimental designs. Yet each zinc finger protein exerts its own structural function toward metallic compounds but no general prediction about this phenomenon appear to be possible.

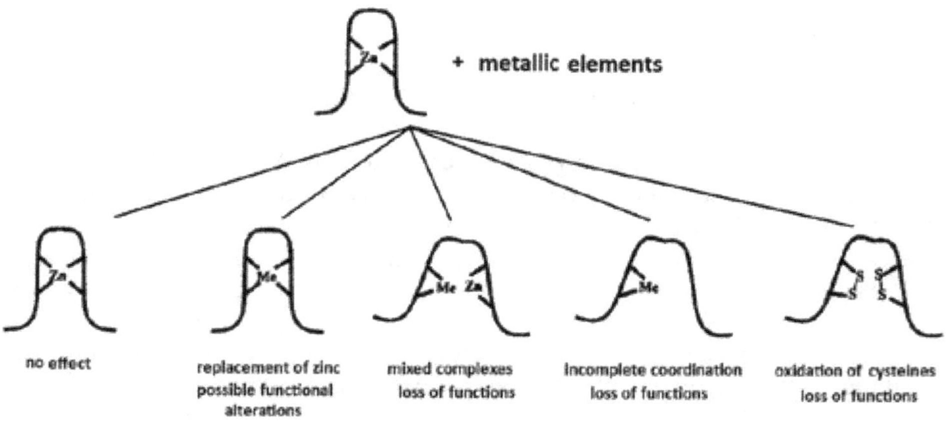

Fig. 1. Schematic representation of potential interactions of metallic elements with zinc-binding structures in transcription factors and DNA repair protein (modified from Hartwig et al.,2001).

3. Arsenic

Different mechanism of action have been suggested for arsenic carcinogenicity including the induction of oxidative stress, induction of genetic damage, altered DNA methylation patterns, enhanced cell proliferation, inhibition of the tumor suppressor protein p53, DNA repair alteration and recently biomethylation (Aposhian & Aposhian 2006). A possible molecular mechanism for arsenic toxicity may lie in its ability to react with thiols, for example, in zinc binding structures of transcription factors, cell cycle control and DNA repair proteins (Kitchin & Wallace, 2008). Nucleotide excision repair (NER) in particular is strongly inhibited by arsenic. NER is capable of removing a wide variety of bulky, DNA helix distorting lesions, caused, e.g., by UV-irradiation or environmental mutagens. Arsenic is known to enhance the persistence of bulky DNA lesions and consequently the mutagenicity induced by UV and benzo[a]pyrene (Hartmann & Speit 1996; Gebel, 2001). Since bulky lesion formation is the possible responsible for their carcinogenicity, genetic integrity depends largely on NER efficiency. Many studies have shown that inorganic arsenic inhibits repair of bulky DNA adducts induced by UV-irradiation (Hartwig et al., 1997; Danaee et al., 2004) or benzo[a]pyrene in cultured cells and laboratory animals (Schwerdtle et al., 2003; Shen et al., 2008); additionally arsenite has been shown to down-regulate expression of some NER genes in cultured human cells (Hamadeh et al., 2005). In humans, arsenic exposure via drinking water was correlated with a dose relationship dependent to decreased expression of some NER genes and reduced repair of lesions in lymphocytes (Andrew et al., 2006). Human lymphoblastoid cells were pre-exposed to arsenite (As(III)) alone and in combination with UV, the pre-treatment with As(III) specifically inhibited the repair of UV-induced pyrimidine dimer-related DNA damage and leads to enhanced UV mutagenesis. Hartwig et al (1997) investigated the effects of arsenite in removal of benzo[a]pyrene-induced DNA damage. When damaged DNA is replicated prior to repair, these adducts can lead to mutations and cancer. This study was carried out in A549 human lung cancer cells; in absence of arsenite, about 45% of benzo[a]pyrene diolepoxide–DNA adducts were repaired within 6–8 h, in presence of arsenite, there was a significant increase of adduct formation. Additionally, the repair capacity towards the stable lesions was decreased in a concentration-dependent shape reaching about 25% of the control at 75 μM, a still slightly cytotoxic effect for this cell line (Schwerdtle et al., 2003b). Similar results have been obtained *in vivo*. Thus, in rats the frequency of benzo[a]pyrene-induced DNA adducts quantified by ^{32}P post-labeling was drastically reduced in the presence of arsenite (Tran et al., 2002). Interesting was the evidence in the human study, arsenic exposure was associated with decreased expression of excision repair cross-complement 1 (ERCC1) in isolated human lymphocytes at the mRNA and protein levels. The mRNA levels of ERCC1 expression were positively associated with water arsenic concentration and nail arsenic concentration and significantly correlated with the amount of OGG1, a base pair excision repair gene (Mo et al., 2009). More detailed studies have been undertaken to assess the potential effects of the trivalent and pentavalent methylated metabolites on DNA repair processes. In humans and many other mammals, inorganic arsenic is converted into trivalent and pentavalent methylated metabolites, monomethylarsonous (MMA(III)) and dimethylarsinous (DMA(III)) acid, monomethylarsonic (MMA(V)) and dimethylarsinic (DMA(V)) acid. Biomethylation has long been thought to be a sort of detoxification process, yet nowadays it is reasonable to conclude that some adverse health effects seen in humans chronically exposed to inorganic arsenic are in fact caused by these metabolites. When considering MMA(III) and DMA(III) been demonstrated in some investigations as toxic, or even more toxic, compared to inorganic arsenic with an increase in benzo[a]pyrene diolepoxide–DNA adducts formation and repair inhibition for MMA(III), at much lower concentrations than arsenite (Schwerdtle et al., 2003). Repair inhibition was also observed at 5 μM DMA(III), but no effect on adduct generation was evident. Nevertheless, the cytotoxicity of the trivalent metabolites was also higher as compared to arsenite (Hartwig et al., 2003). Moreover, significant but less repair inhibition was mediated by 250 and 500μM of DMA(V) or MMA(V). Altogether, the results demonstrate that arsenite as well as the methylated metabolites interfere with cellular repair systems; the strongest effects with respect to inhibitory concentration were found for the trivalent metabolites (Schwerdtle et al., 2003b). Shen et al. (2009) investigated the difference manifested by DMA(III) compared to other trivalent arsenic species on the formation of benzo[a]pyrene diolepoxide–DNA adducts. At concentrations comparable to those used in the study by Schwerdtle et al. (2003) they found that each of the three trivalent arsenic species were able to enhance the formation of benzo[a]pyrene diolepoxide–DNA adducts with the potency in a decreasing order of MMA(III) > DMA(III) > As(III), well related with their cytotoxicity. Similar to As(III), DMA(III) the modulation of reduced glutathione (GSH) or total glutathione S-transferase (GST) activity could not account for its enhanced effect on DNA adduct formation. Additionally, similar effects elicited by the trivalent arsenic species were demonstrated to be highly time-dependent. Nollen et al. (2009) investigated the gene expression, total protein level and localization of proteins during NER and comparing inorganic arsenite and MMA(III). Arsenite and MMA(III) strongly decreased expression and protein level of the main initiator of global genome NER, i.e. Xeroderma pigmentosum complementation group C (XPC). This led to diminished association of XPC to sites of local UVC damage, resulting in decreased recruitment of further NER proteins. These data demonstrate that in human skin fibroblasts arsenite and MMA(III) more interacts with XPC expression, resulting in decreased XPC protein level and diminished assembly of the NER. The observed stronger impact on XPC by MMA(III) may explain the more potent NER inhibition by MMA(III) as compared to arsenite (Schwerdtle et al., 2003; Shen et al., 2008). Finally, these data provide further evidence that in the case of DNA repair inhibition the biomethylation of arsenic increases inorganic arsenic induced genotoxicity and probably contributes to its carcinogenicity. With respect to DNA repair inhibition, several studies point to an interaction of arsenic with various DNA repair pathways, which may in turn decrease genomic integrity. The effect of arsenic on the extent of poly(ADP-ribosyl)ation has been investigated previously in two studies with controversial conclusion. Yager & Wiencke (1997) observed a decreased amount of poly(ADP-ribose) in human T-cell lymphoma-derived at arsenite concentrations above 5 μM. In contrast, an increase of poly(ADP-ribosyl)ation reaction was reported at higher concentrations in CHO-K1 cells (Lynn et al., 1998). Hartwig et al., 2003b investigated the effects of arsenite on poly(ADP-ribosyl)ation stimulated by H_2O_2 in intact cells by applying an anti-poly(ADP-ribose) monoclonal antibody. The experiments demonstrated a clear reduction of poly(ADP-ribosyl)ation level just evident at the extremely low and non-cytotoxic concentration of 10nM arsenite and reaching about 40% of residual activity at 0.5 μM arsenite. There was an increase in induced DNA single strand break formation by arsenite in agreement with the assumed role of poly(ADP-ribosyl)ation in DNA strand break repair (Hartwig et al., 2003b). Also the effect of the arsenicals on the activity of the isolated formamidopyrimidine glycosylase (Fpg) was examined. Fpg is a glycosylase initiating base excision repair in Escherichia coli: it recognizes and removes a lot of DNA base modification including 7,8-dihydro-8-oxoguanine (8-oxoguanine). Even though Fpg is a bacterial repair protein, the recent discovery of human homologues suggests its relevance for mammalian cells too (Hazra et al., 2003). After 30 min preincubation MMA(III) and DMA(III) inhibited Fpg activity in dose-dependent shape, yielding 48 and 15% of the Fpg activity at 1 mM, respectively. In contrast, arsenite and the pentavalent metabolites did not show any effects on Fpg activity up to 10mM (Schwerdtle et al., 2003b). Finally, we describe the effects of arsenic compounds on the zinc finger structure of XPA. Different arsenicals promote the release of zinc from a peptide consisting of 37 amino acids representing the zinc finger domain of the human XPA protein (XPAzf). All trivalent arsenic compounds induced zinc release from XPAzf, starting at low micromolar concentrations, with MMA(III) and DMA(III) more active than arsenite. In contrast, MMA(V) and DMA(V) showed no or only slight effects up to 10mM (Schwerdtle et al., 2003b). Moreover there are some evidence about the influence of arsenic on BER, the predominant repair pathway for DNA lesions caused by reactive oxygen species (ROS) (Liu et al., 2001). Some studies have shown that low doses of arsenic can also cause an hormetic response in DNA polymerase β (Pol β), as well as telomerase activity (Zhang et al., 2003; Snow et al. 2005). DNA polymerase β is not only responsible for the incorporation of nucleotides in BER, but also excises the 5′-deoxyribose-5-phosphate (dRP) moiety prior to completion of repair (Wilson, 1998). Sykora et al. (2008) investigated the regulation of DNA polymerase β (Pol β) and AP endonuclease (APE1), in response to low but physiologically relevant doses of arsenic. Lung fibroblasts and keratinocytes were exposed to As(III), and mRNA, protein levels and BER activity were assessed. Both Pol β and APE1 mRNA exhibited significant dose-dependent down regulation at doses of As(III) above 1 μM. However, at lower doses Pol β mRNA and protein levels, and consequently, BER activity were significantly increased. In contrast, APE1 protein levels were only marginally increased by low doses of As(III) and there was no correlation between APE1 and overall BER activity. Enzyme supplementation of nuclear extracts confirmed that Pol β was rate limiting. These changes in BER are related to the overall protective against sunlight UV-induced toxicity at low doses of As(III) while at high doses there is a synergistic toxicity action. The results provide evidence that changes in BER due to low doses of arsenic could contribute to a non-linear, threshold dose response for arsenic carcinogenesis. The primary function of APE1 in BER is to act as an endonuclease responsible for the excision of apurinic/apyrimidinic (AP) sites. However, APE1 is also a redox factor responsible for signal transduction in response to oxidative stress (Hsieh et al., 2001). Arsenic has the potential to affect both the endonuclease and the functions of APE1, through its increase in ROS levels and inhibition of DNA repair (Hamadeh et al., 2002).

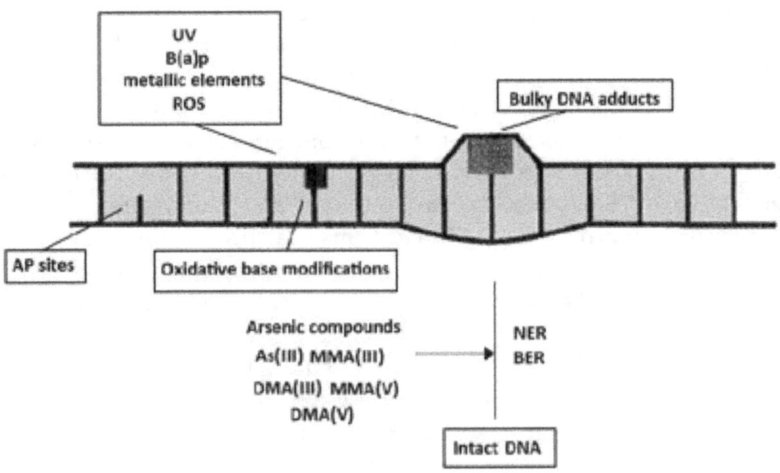

Fig. 2. Schematic outline of DNA repair inhibition by arsenite and its methylated metabolites(modified from Hartwig et al., 2003).

4. Beryllium

Beryllium does not directly damage the DNA but it can lead to morphological cell transformation and inhibition of DNA repair synthesis. However, the effects observed on DNA repair are not specific for beryllium since similar findings are reported for other metallic compounds. A possible hypothesis is that the mechanism of genotoxicity is unlikely to be a non-threshold mechanism. A practical threshold can be postulated for beryllium since both direct DNA repair enzyme inhibition or DNA/protein expression-mediated effects do definitely require more than one ion to inhibit all DNA repair enzyme molecules (Strupp, 2011a). Dylevoĭ (1990), using four strains of E. coli with different DNA repairing capacities, established that beryllium efficacy in the DNA repair test depended on pH of medium and ions concentration. The DNA of rat primary hepatocytes was treated by incubation with 2-acetylaminofluorene, a known DNA damaging agent, and co-incubated with beryllium metal extracts (Strupp, 2011b). They observed that, the DNA repair synthesis were reduced by co-incubation with beryllium metal extract. However, it should be noted that this effect was observed only when the concurrent DNA damage was massive (>80% cells in repair), while no effects were observed in cells with lower DNA damage. These findings deserve however further investigations about their relevance in vivo.

5. Cadmium

Several reports suggested that cadmium genotoxicity is not direct but rather mediated by reactive oxygen free radicals and resulting oxidative stress. In spite of being a weak genotoxic chemical, cadmium exhibits remarkable potential to inhibit DNA damage repair, and this has been identified as a major mechanism for its carcinogenicity (Giaginis et al., 2006). Cadmium is comutagenic and increases the mutagenicity of UV radiaton, alkylation and oxidation in mammalian cells. These effects may be explained by cadmium inhibition on several types of DNA repair: base excision repair, nucleotide excision repair, mismatch repair and the elimination of the premutagenic DNA precursor 8-oxodGTP. Regarding base excision repair, low concentrations of cadmium which did not generate oxidative damage as such, inhibited the repair of oxidative DNA damage in mammalian cells (Dally & Hartwig 1997; Fatur et al. 2003). Exposure of human cells to sub-lethal concentrations of cadmium leads to a time and concentration dependent decrease in hOGG1 activity, i.e. of the main DNA glycosylase activity responsible for the initiation of the base excision repair of 8-oxoguanine, an abundant and mutagenic form of oxidized guanine. The study of Bravard et al. (2010) confirms that part of the inhibitory effect of low dose cadmium on the cellular 8-oxoguanine DNA glycosylase activity can be attributed to an already described reduced hOGG1 transcription (Youn et al., 2005). This moderate inhibitory effect of cadmium on hOGG1 mRNA levels cannot explain the dramatic decrease observed in the levels and activity of hOGG1 protein. Indeed, inhibition of the ectopically expressed hOGG1-GFP in cells exposed to the metal confirmed the post-transcriptional effect of cadmium on hOGG1 protein and activity levels. A different response of the second enzyme in the cellular BER pathway has been described. Bravard et al (2010) found that in vivo treatment of human cells with cadmium has no effect on the APE1 activity, suggesting that in their experimental conditions most cadmium is complexed within the cells and therefore the intracellular concentrations of free cadmium do not reach the levels required for the inhibition of APE1. These results, taken together with the indirect inhibition of hOGG1 by oxidation, support the hypothesis that the effects on the BER pathway are in the consequence of the cellular redox imbalance rather than the direct interaction with proteins. Candelas et al. (2010) showed that cadmium inhibits the repair of uracile (U) in DNA, resulting both from mis-incorporation and cytosine (C) deamination. These lesions, as those on AP sites, are common in any cell, and must constantly be repaired to avoid mutagenic events. The necessity to continuously repair these lesions is underscored by the high levels of expression of UNG2 and APE1 (Cappelli et al., 2001). This genotoxic consequence of cadmium exposure might participate in the deregulation of physiological cellular processes by altering the pattern of gene expression on the one hand (U), and increasing the mutation rate on the other hand (on

AP site), thereby interfering with the normal control of cell growth and division. Moreover cadmium exposure inhibits and modifies some proteins of BER such as formamidopyrimidine glycosylase (Fpg): the substitution of a cysteine in the zinc finger localized in the C terminal of Fpg protein may inhibit the binding of the protein to DNA (O' Connor et al., 1993). With respect to nucleotide excision repair, cadmium interferes with the removal of thymine dimers after UV irradiation by inhibiting the first step of this repair pathway (Hartwig & Schwerdtle 2002; Fatur et al. 2003). Also both association and dissociation of essential NER proteins are disturbed in presence of cadmium. Because of decreased of XPC nuclear protein levels, a reduced XPC localization to UVC-induced DNA damage in cells was observed after incubation with a non cytotoxic concentration of $CdCl_2$. Interestingly, the tumor suppressor protein p53 also contain a zinc binding domain, which is essential for DNA binding and p53 function in transcription mechanism. In this context, Meplan et al. (1999) demonstrated that cadmium chloride alters p53 conformation in MCF7 cells, inhibits its DNA binding and down regulates transcriptional activation of a reporter gene. As p53 has been shown to act as a transcription factor for two important NER genes XPC and P48 and cadmium induced p53 conformational change may also result in altered p53 NER downstream effects (Adimoolam & Ford 2002). Cadmium exposure inhibits the xeroderma pigmentosum A (XPA) protein. XPA contains a typical four-cysteine zinc finger, which is not directly involved in DNA binding of the protein. The DNA binding capacity of XPA is strongly reduced after intoxication with cadmium (Hartmann et al., 1998; Hartwig et al., 2002). Another aspect is that cadmium found in liver and kidney cortex is bound to metallothioneins (MT), small, cystein-rich metal-binding proteins which are considered to be protective from cadmium toxicity (Klaassen et al., 1999; Nordberg 2009; Chang et al., 2009). Nevertheless, Hartwig et al 2002 demonstrated that the inhibitory cadmium effect for fpg proteins were comparable independent of whether CdCl2 or MT-bound Cd(II) was applied. Thus, metal ions complexed to MT may still be available for toxic reactions. In a recent study Schwerdtle et al., (2010) compared genotoxic effects of particulate CdO and soluble $CdCl_2$ in cultured human cells and reported that both cadmium compounds inhibited the nucleotide excision repair of benzo[a]pyrene diol epoxide-induced bulky DNA adducts and UVC-induced photolesions in a dose-dependent shape at non-cytotoxic concentrations. This agreement with the similar carcinogenic effects of both water-soluble and water insoluble cadmium compound indicates that Cd^{2+} is the most common species responsible for indirect genotoxicity of the element (Oldiges et al., 1989).

6. Chromium

Among the carcinogenic metal compounds, only chromium (VI) has been clearly defined mutagenic in bacterial and mammalian test systems and its carcinogenic activity is thought to be due to the induction of DNA damage generated by reactive intermediates arising in its intracellular reduction to chromium (III) (Klein, 1996). Cr(VI)-carcinogenesis may be initiated or promoted through several mechanistic processes including, the intracellular metabolic reduction of Cr(VI) producing chromium species capable of interacting with DNA to yield genotoxic and mutagenic effects, Cr(VI)-induced inflammatory/immunological responses, and alteration of survival signaling pathways. The intracellular reduction of Cr(VI) produces a broad spectrum of DNA lesions including binary DNA adducts, DNA interstrand crosslinks (ICLs), DNA-protein adducts, DNA double-strand breaks and oxidized bases (Nickens et al., 2010). On the contrary the knowledge about the role of DNA repair system in this process is lacking. Several lesions generated by Cr(VI) reduction (i.e. oxidized bases) are substrates for base excision repair (BER). In BER, damaged (alkylated or oxidized) bases are recognized by specific DNA glycosylases and are excised, resulting in the formation of apurinic/ apyrimidinic (AP) sites. Interesting to note that chromium(VI) can be reduced in body fluids, which results in its detoxification, due to the poor ability of chromium(III) to cross cell membranes. Infact chromium(VI), when introduced by the oral route, is efficiently detoxified up reduction by saliva and gastric juice and sequestration by intestinal bacteria (De Flora, 2000). Administration of up to 20 mg chromium (VI), either in drinking water or by gavage, failed to produce any effect in the mouse bone marrow micronucleus assay or in the rat hepatocyte DNA rapair assay (Mirsalis et al., 1996).The results of studies carried out by O'Brien et al (2002; 2005) suggested that NER functions is essential in the protection of cells from Cr(VI) lethality and for the removal of Cr(III)-DNA adducts. Brooks et al., (2008) suggest that NER and BER are required for Cr(VI) genomic instability and postulate that, in the absence of excision repair, DNA damage is directed an error-free system of DNA repair or damage tolerance.

7. Nickel

Epidemiological studies in exposed workers identified some species of nickel as carcinogenic for upper respiratory tract and lung (Polednak 1981; Roberts et al. 1984; Roberts et al. 1989). The carcinogenic potency depends largely on properties such as solubility and kind of salts, which influence its bioavailability. Water soluble nickel salts are taken up only slowly by cells, while particulate of nickel compounds are phagocytosed and, due to the low pH, gradually dissolved in lysosomes, yielding high concentrations of nickel ions in the nucleus (Costa et al., 2005). Using in vitro cells and animal models, nickel compounds have been found to generate various types of adverse effects, including chromosomal aberrations, DNA strand breaks, high reactive oxygen species production, impaired DNA repair, hypoxia-mimic stress, aberrant epigenetic changes, and signaling cascade activation (Lu et al., 2005). Nickel has been shown to interfere with the repair mechanisms involved in removing UV-, platinum-, mitomycin C, g-radiation- and benzo[a]pyrene-induced DNA damage (Dally et al., 1997; Hartmann et al., 1998; Schwerdtle et al., 2002). These comutagenic effects are explained by the inhibition of all major types of DNA repair processes. Potentially sensitive targets for the toxic action of nickel(II) are zinc finger structures present in several DNA repair enzymes, including the bacterial Fpg protein and the mammalian XPA protein, DNA ligase III and poly(ADP-ribose) polymerase (PARP). Some studies investigated the effects of nickel compounds on the repair of DNA and showed that both soluble and particulate nickel can inhibit repair of benzo[a]pyrene DNA adducts in human lung cells (Schwerdtle et al., 2002). Low doses of nickel chloride (1 μmol/L) inhibited repair of UV or N-Methyl-N-nitro-N'-nitrosoguanidine -induced DNA damage as indicated by accumulating strand breaks, and 1-5 μm nickel chloride inhibited the formamidopyrimidine-DNA glycosylase (Fpg), 3-methyladenine-DNA glycosylase II (Alk A) and endonuclease III (Endo III) enzymes involved in DNA excision repair (Wozniak and Blaziak, 2004). The mechanisms of this action may include interactions with a specific structure containing zinc or the –SH groups of repair proteins. Because nickel compounds, such as NiS, Ni_3S_2, NiO (black and green), and soluble $NiCl_2$, have been shown to be active inducers of reactive oxygen species (ROS) in Chinese hamster ovary cells, the involvement of reactive oxygen species has been implicated in the inhibition of DNA repair (Lynn, 1997). Inhibition of glutathione synthesis or catalase activity increased the enhancing effect of nickel on the cytotoxicity of ultraviolet light. Inhibition of catalase and glutathione peroxidase activities also enhanced the retardation effect of nickel on the rejoining of DNA strand breaks accumulated by hydroxyurea plus cytosine-beta-D-arabinofuranoside in UV-irradiated cells. Lynn et al., (1997) showed that nickel, in the presence of H_2O_2, exhibited a synergistic inhibition on both DNA polymerization and ligation and caused protein fragmentation. In addition, glutathione could completely repair the inhibition by nickel or H_2O_2 alone but only partially the inhibition by nickel when associated with H_2O_2. Therefore, nickel may bind to DNA-repair enzymes and generate oxygen-free radicals to cause protein degradation in situ. Schwerdtle et al., (2002) studied the effect of soluble and particulated nickel compounds on the formation and repair of stable benzo(a)pyrene DNA adducts in human lung cells. With respect to adduct formation, NiO, but not $NiCl_2$, reduced the generation of DNA lesions by ~30%. Regarding their repair in the absence of nickel compounds most lesions were removed within 24h; nevertheless, between 20 and 35% of induced adducts remained longer than 48h after treatment; $NiCl_2$ (100μM) led to ~80% residual repair capacity; after 500μM the repair was reduced to ~36%. Also, even at the completely non-cytotoxic concentration of 0.5 μg/cm^2 NiO, lesion removal was reduced to ~35% of control and to 15% at 2.0 μg/cm^2. Nevertheless, under the same experimental conditions, the extent of DNA strand breaks and oxidative DNA base modifications were increased only at highly cytotoxic concentrations of both compounds (Hartwig et al., 2002). Repair inhibition by nickel appears therefore to be independent from metal compounds, and the results do not provide an explanation for the marked differences in carcinogenic potencies between soluble and particulated nickel species. However when considering the carcinogenicity in human or in experimental animals the retentions times in the body have to be taken into account. Thus, analysis of nickel contents in rat lungs after inhalation of different nickel species, especially for NiO, an impaired clearance and up to 1000-fold higher and persistent nickel lung burdens have been shown when compared to water-soluble nickel sulphate (Dunnick et al., 1995). Therefore, exposure to particulate nickel compounds may give rise to continuous DNA repair impairment and thus the biological consequences may be far more severe. The overall data add further evidences that the inhibition of DNA repair processes is an important mechanism in nickel genotoxicity, especially, because these effects are observed at low, non-cytotoxic concentrations. Since oxidative DNA damage is continuously induced during aerobic metabolism, an impaired repair of these lesions might explain the carcinogenic action of nickel(II).

8. Interaction on DNA repair processes of metallic elements classified as a possible or probable human carcinogen

8.1 Antimony

Trivalent antimony is a known genotoxic agent and it is classified as a possible human carcinogen by the International Agency for Research on Cancer (1989) and as an animal carcinogen by the Deutsche Research Foundation (DFG 2008). The chemico-toxicological characteristics of antimony are similar to those of arsenic: their trivalent species are responsible for toxicological properties, and they have carcinogenic potential. In contrast to arsenic, however, informations about the toxicity of antimony and its possible mechanisms are limited. Tkahashi et al., (2002) investigated the effects of antimony trichloride ($SbCl_3$) and antimony potassium tartrate ($C_4H_4KO_7Sb$) on the repair of DNA double strand breaks induced by γ-radiation. Antimony compounds inhibited repair of DNA double strand breaks in a dose dependent manner. Both in trichloride, 0.2 mM antimony significantly inhibited the rejoining of double strand breaks, while 0.4 mM was necessary in potassium antimony tartrate. The mean lethal doses (D_0) for the treatment with antimony trichloride and antimony potassium tartrate, were approximately 0.21 and 0.12 mM, respectively. This indicates that the repair inhibition by antimony trichloride occurred in the dose range near D_0, but the antimony potassium tartrate inhibited the repair mechanism at doses where most cells lost their proliferating ability. This relationship is consistent with the general tendency of their respective toxicity: trivalent antimony compounds are less toxic than trivalent arsenic compounds, but more toxic than bismuth compounds (Leonard & Gerber, 1996; Huang et al., 1998). Grosskopf et al., (2010) show that trivalent antimony interferes with proteins involved in nucleotide excision repair and partly impairs this pathway, pointing to an indirect mechanism in the genotoxicity of trivalent antimony. After irradiation of human lung carcinoma cells with UVC, a higher number of cyclobutane pyrimidine dimers (CPD) remained in the presence of $SbCl_3$, whereas processing of the 6−4 photoproducts and benzo[a]pyrene diol epoxide (BPDE)-induced DNA adducts were not impaired. Nevertheless, cell viability was reduced more than in additive mode after combined treatment of $SbCl_3$ with UVC as well as with BPDE. A decrease in gene expression and protein level of XPE was found and moreover, trivalent antimony was shown to interact with the zinc finger domain of XPA with concentration dependent release of zinc from peptide of this domain. Compared to the data on arsenite, antimony is more effective in zinc releasing from XPA, yielding 50% zinc release at 10 times lower concentration (Schwerdtle et al., 2003). Antimony might be able to interact with proteins involved in DNA repair, via their cysteine or histidine side chains. Complexes between antimony(III) and glutathione via sulphur binding site of the tripeptide have already been confirmed (Burford et al., 2005).

8.2 Cobalt

The carcinogenic potential of cobalt and its compounds was evaluated in 1991 by the International Agency for Research on Cancer (1991, 2006), the Commision concluded that cobalt and its compounds are possibly carcinogenic to humans (group 2B). Also the Deutsche Research Foundation (DFG 2008) has classified cobalt among the carcinogens of Category 2. Production of active oxygen species and inhibition of DNA repair appear to be the predominant mechanism of action in cobalt genotoxicity (Lison et al., 2001). Specifically by nucleotide excise repair pathway, in fact cobalt inhibits the removal of UV-induced cyclobutane pyrimidine dimers in mammalian cells but did not inhibit DNA strand rejoining after X-irradiation (Hartwig et al., 1991). Furthermore, by applying the nucleoid sedimentation assay in HeLa cells, Snyder et al (1989) demonstrated that cobalt causes an accumulation of DNA strand breaks after UV irradiation, indicating an impairment of the polymerization and/or the ligation step of nucleotide excision repair. Kasten et al. (1992) provided further evidence that cobalt at low non-cytotoxic concentration, inhibits both the incision and polymerization step of nucleotide excision repair in human fibroblasts. De Boeck et al., (1998) assessed the interference of cobalt compounds with the repair of primarily-induced DNA damage and showed that cobalt was able to cause persistence of methylmethanesulphonate-induced DNA lesions by interference its repair. In particular, cobalt inhibited the Xeroderma pigmentosum group A (XPA) protein, a zinc finger protein involved in nucleotide excision repair (Asmuß et al. 2000) where it substituted for the zinc ion (Kopera et al. 2004). Cobalt at low, non-cytotoxic concentrations interferes with the incision step of UV-induced DNA repair, but the removal of lesions may not be uniformly affected (Kasten et al., 1997). This effect may be related to differences in processing these lesions. Regarding the effect of cobalt on the incision frequency, a potentially preferential inhibition of incisions at 6-4-photoproducts could be due to either the disruption of the highly effective damage recognition at the site of this lesion or to a enhanced inhibition of the global genome repair system, while the transcription-coupled repair is unaffected at low doses. In addition to the incision step, the polymerization is inhibited by cobalt as well, while the ligation of repair patches is not affected by this element. A possible mechanism of the interference of cobalt with DNA polymerases could be the competition with magnesium; in fact the inhibition of the polymerization step was completely reversed in the presence of magnesium ions (Kasten et al. 1992, 1997). Sirover and Loeb (1976) demonstrated a dose-dependent reduction of the catalytic activity as well as the fidelity of isolated DNA polymerases from different organisms after substitution of magnesium ions by cobalt. Taken together, the data indicate that cobalt belongs to a group of metal compounds which enhance the genotoxicity of direct mutagens.

8.3 Lead

The toxicity of lead and its compounds is well known for many centuries for anaemia, effects on nervous system and developmental disorders above all. Nevertheless, during the last years potential carcinogenic effects have been focused, leading to the classification of inorganic lead compounds as "Probably carcinogenic to humans" (Group 2A) by IARC (1987; 2006) and in the Group 2 by the Deutsche Research Foundation (DFG 2008). Although inorganic lead compounds exhibit only a weak mutagenic potential, they show more pronounced co-mutagenic activities in combination with DNA alkylating and oxidizing agents (Roy & Rossman, 1992; Hartwig et al., 1994). These effects were due to an interference with DNA repair processes, following an accumulation of DNA strand breaks, as shown in human HeLa cells after UV irradiation. Lead enhanced the frequencies of UV-induced mutations and sister chromatid exchanges at very low, nontoxic concentrations. Mutations as well as DNA strand breaks occurred only after long-term treatment at doses much higher than cytotoxic ones (Roy & Rossman, 1992). Considering the base excision repair, lead has been shown to inhibit the apurinic/apyrimidinic endonuclease (APE1) in micromolar concentration range both in an isolated enzymic test and in cells leading to an accumulation of apurinic sites in DNA and to an increase in methyl methansulfonate-induced mutagenicity (McNeill et al. 2007). Current evidences suggest that inactivation of APE1 is mediated by an unique and specific interaction of metal with active site residues then disrupting the in magnesium-dependent catalytic reaction. Furthermore, lead interferes with the repair of DNA double strand breaks via interaction with the stress response pathway induced by a phosphoinositol-3-kinase (PIKK) related kinase (Gastaldo et al. 2007). Due to its high affinity for sulfhydryl groups, a mechanism for lead interaction with proteins could be the displacement of zinc from zinc binding structures. In support of this assumption, in cell-free systems lead has been shown to reduce DNA binding of transcription factors (TFIIIA) and Sp1 (Huang et al. 2004). No impact was however described on the zinc-containing DNA repair proteins Fpg or XPA (Asmuß et al. 2000).

8.4 Vanadium

The International Agency for Research on Cancer has classified vanadium pentoxide (V_2O_5) as a possible carcinogen (Group 2B) (2006) while the Deutsche Research Foundation included vanadium among the carcinogens of Category 2 (DFG, 2008). The genotoxicity of vanadium compounds is explained by mechanisms of induction of oxidative stress, inhibition of DNA repair and interference with the activity of protein phosphatases and kinases. Only few studies have been carried out about the genotoxic action of vanadium compounds; Ivancsits et al. (2002) tested the impact of vanadate(V) on DNA repair kinetics of UV and bleomycin treated human fibroblasts. They observed a significant increase of DNA migration in the alkaline comet assay accompanied by persistent double-stranded breaks after exposure to vanadate in combination with UV-light or bleomycin, as compared to vanadate treatment alone. This indicates that vanadate may act as an indirect genotoxic agent by converting repairable single-stranded breaks into non-repairable double-stranded breaks. This effect was confirmed by the strong differences between lymphocytes of workers exposed to vanadium pentoxide after bleomycin treatment and controls. Bleomycin-induced DNA migration was higher in the exposed group (25%), whereas the repair of bleomycin-induced lesions was reduced (Erlich et al., 2008).

9. Conclusion

The carcinogenic action of some metallic elements includes different mechanism such as induction of oxidative stress, inhibition of DNA repair, activation of mitogenic signalling, and epigenetic modification of gene expression. Nevertheless, each metallic elements and also each metal species exert characteristic interactions, and even though similar cellular pathways are affected, the underlying mechanisms are quite different. A relevant factor in metal carcinogenesis is the bioavailability of different metal species and the capacity to penetrate the cell barrier. The DNA does not appear to be the primary binding site for carcinogenic metal ions. This suggests that an inhibition of DNA repair processes may be a predominant mechanism in metal-induced genotoxicity. In addition, most carcinogenic metal compounds have been shown to increase the cytotoxicity, mutagenicity, and clastogenicity in mammalian cells when combined with different types of DNA-damaging agents (UV-light and/or alkylating agents). For most metal compounds, interactions with proteins appear to be more relevant for carcinogenicity as compared to direct DNA damage, and several targets have been identified, such as DNA repair, tumor suppressor and signal transduction proteins. Since metal ions can bind in principle to many electron rich centers in proteins the existence of particularly metal-sensitive protein structures may be suggested. The zinc finger proteins have been identified as potential molecular targets for toxic metal compounds and are involved not only in DNA binding but also in protein-protein interactions. Thus, there is an increasing evidence for zinc binding as structures very sensitive for toxic metal compounds. Significant factors appear to be not only the physicochemical properties but also accessibility and the protein microenvironment. The efficient repair of DNA lesions induced by endogenous processes and by environmental factors are an important prerequisite to maintain DNA integrity; if repair is not efficient, cells may accumulate DNA damage, leading to increased probabilities of genes instability and alteration in cellular cycle control and thus to tumor formation. The study and elaboration of metallic elements carcinogenicity should be conducted in parallel with dose-response studies in order to have a real idea of exposures especially when considering the possibility of co-exposures to other carcinogenic organic.

10. Abbreviations

APE1: Apurinic/apyrimidinic endonuclease
As(III): Arsenite
BER: Base excision rapair
BPDE: Benzo[a]pyrene diol epoxide
CPD: Cyclobutane pyrimidine dimers
DFG: Deutsche Forschungsgemeinschaft, German Research Foundation
DMA(III): Dimethylarsinous acid
DMA(V): Dimethylarsinic acid
dRP: 5′-deoxyribose-5-phosphate
ERCC1: Excision repair cross-complement 1
Fpg: Formamidopyrimidine-DNA glicosylase
GSH: Reduced glutathione
GST: Total glutathione S-transferase
IARC: International Agency for Research on Cancer
MMA(III): Monomethylarsonous acid
MMA(V): Monomethylarsonic acid
MMR: Mismatch repair
MT: Metallothioneins
NER: Nucleotide excision repair
PARP: Poly(ADP-ribose) polymerase
Pol β: Polymerase β
ROS: Reactive oxygen species
XPA: Xeroderma pigmentosum A
XPAzf: Zinc finger domain of the human XPA protein
XPC: Xeroderma pigmentosum complementation group C

11. References

Adimoolam, S. & Ford, J.M. (2002). p53 and DNA damage-inducible expression of the xeroderma pigmentosum group C gene. *Proceedings of the National Academy of Sciences of the U.S.A.* Vol. 99, pp. 12985-12990

Andrew, A. S., Burgess, J. L., Meza, M. M., Demidenko, E., Waugh, M.G., Hamilton, J.W. & Karagas, MR. (2006). Arsenic exposure is associated with decreased DNA repair in vitro and in individuals exposed to drinking water arsenic. Environ Health Perspectives.Vol.114, pp.1193-1198

Aposhian, H. V. & Aposhian, M. M. (2006). Arsenic toxicology: Five questions. *Chemical Research in Toxicology.* Vol. 19, pp. 1–15

Asmuß, M., Mullenders, L.H. & Hartwig, A. (2000). Interference by toxic metal compounds with isolated zinc finger DNA repair proteins. *Toxicology Letters.* Vol. 112-113, pp. 227-231

Bravard, A., Campalans, A., Vacher, M., Gouget, B., Levalois, C., Chevillard, S. & Radicella JP. (2009). Inactivation by oxidation and recruitment into stress granules of hOGG1 but not APE1 in human cells exposed to sub-lethal concentrations of cadmium. *Mutation Research.* Vol. 685, pp. 61–69

Brooks, B., O'Brien, T.J., Ceryak, S., Wise, J.P. Sr, Wise, S.S., Wise, J.P. Jr, Defabo, E. & Patierno SR. (2008). Excision repair is required for genotoxin-induced mutagenesis in mammalian cells. *Carcinogenesis*. Vol.29, pp. 1064-1069

Buchko, G.W., Hess, N.J. & Kennedy, M.A. (2000). Cadmium mutagenicity and human nucleotide excision repair proteinXPA: CD,EXAFS and (1)H/(15)N-NMR spectroscopic studies on the zinc(II)- and cadmium(II)-associated minimal DNA-binding domain (M98- F219). *Carcinogenesis*. Vol. 21, pp. 1051–1057

Burford, N., Eelman, M.D. & Groom, K. (2005). Identification of complexes containing glutathione with As(III), Sb(III), Cd(II), Hg(II), Tl(I), Pb(II) or Bi(III) by electrospray ionization mass spectrometry. Journal of Inorganic Biochemistry. Vol. 99, pp. 1992-1997

Candéias, S., Pons, B., Viau, M., Caillat, S. & Sauvaigo, S. (2010). Direct inhibition of excision/synthesis DNA repair activities by cadmium: analysis on dedicated biochips. *Mutation Research*. Vol.694, pp. 53-59

Cappelli, E., Hazra, T., Hill, J.W., Slupphaug, G., Bogliolo, M. & Frosina G. (2001). Rates of base excision repair are not solely dependent on levels of initiating enzymes. *Carcinogenesis*. Vol. 22, pp. 387–393

Chang, X., Jin, T., Chen, L., Nordberg, M. & Lei, L. (2009). Metallothionein I isoform mRNA expression in peripheral lymphocytes as a biomarker for occupational cadmium exposure. *Experimental and Biological Medicine (Maywood)*. Vol. 234:666-672

Commission for the Investigation of Health hazards of Chemical Compounds in the Work Area, DFG (2008) *List of MAK and BAT values 2008, report no. 44*. Wiley. VCH, Weinheim

Costa, M., Davidson, T.L., Chen, H., Ke, Q., Zhang, P., Yan, Y., Huang, C. & Kluz, T. (2005). Nickel carcinogenesis: epigenetics and hypoxia signaling. *Mutation Research*. Vol.592, No.1-2, pp.79-88

Dally, H. & Hartwig, A. (1997). Induction and repair inhibition of oxidative DNA damage by nickel(II) and cadmium(II) in mammalian cells. *Carcinogenesis*. Vol. 18, pp. 1021-1026

Danaee, H., Nelson, H.H., Liber, H., Little, J.B. & Kelsey, K.T. (2004). Low dose exposure to sodium arsenite synergistically interacts with UV radiation to induce mutations and alter DNA repair in human cells. *Mutagenesis*. Vol. 19, pp. 143–148

De Boeck, M., Lison, D. & Kirsch-Volders, M. (1998). Evaluation of the in vitro direct and indirect genotoxic effects of cobalt compounds using the alkaline comet assay. Influence of interdonor and interexperimental variability. *Carcinogenesis*. Vol.19, pp. 2021-2029

De Flora, S. (2000). Threshold mechanisms and site specificity in chromium(VI) carcinogenesis. *Carcinogenesis*. Vol.21: 533-541

Dunnick, J.K., Elwell, M.R., Radovsky, A.E., Benson, J.M., Hahn, F.F., Nikula, K.J., Barr, E.B. & Hobbs, C.H. (1995). Comparative carcinogenic effects of nickel subsulfide, nickel oxide, or nickel sulfate hexahydrate chronic exposures in the lung. *Cancer Research*. Vol. 55, No. 22, pp. 5251-5256

Dylevoĭ, MV. (1990). An evaluation of the DNA-damaging action of the metal carcinogen beryllium using a bacterial repair test. *Mikrobiologicheskiĭ zhurnal*.Vol.52, pp. 34-38

Ehrlich, V.A., Nersesyan, A.K., Atefie, K., Hoelzl, C., Ferk, F., Bichler, J., Valic, E., Schaffer, A., Schulte-Hermann, R., Fenech, M., Wagner, K.H. & Knasmüller, S. (2008).

Inhalative exposure to vanadium pentoxide causes DNA damage in workers: results of a multiple end point study. *Environmental Health Perspective*. Vol.116, pp. 1689-1693

Fatur, T., Tusek, M., Falnoga, I., Scancar, J., Lah, T.T. & Filipic, M. (2003). Cadmium inhibits repair of UV-, methyl methanesulfonate- and Nmethyl- N-nitrosourea-induced DNA damage in Chinese hamster ovary cells. *Mutation Research*. Vol. 529, pp. 109-116

Gastaldo, J., Viau, M., Bencokova, Z., Joubert, A., Charvet, A.M., Balosso, J. & Foray, N. (2007). Lead contamination results in late and slowly repairable DNA double-strand breaks and impacts upon the ATM-dependent signaling pathways. *Toxicology Letters*. Vol. 173, pp. 201-214

Gebel, T. W. (2001). Genotoxicity of arsenical compounds. International Journal of Hygiene and Environmental Health. Vol. 203, pp. 249–262

Giaginis, C., Gatzidou, E. & Theocharis, S. (2006). DNA repair systems as targets of cadmium toxicity. *Toxicology and Applied Pharmacology*. Vol. 213, pp. 282–290

Grosskopf, C., Schwerdtle, T., Mullenders, L.H. & Hartwig, A. (2010). Antimony impairs nucleotide excision repair: XPA and XPE as potential molecular targets. *Chemical Research in Toxicology*. Vol.23, pp. 1175-1183

Hamadeh, H. K., Trouba, K. J., Amin, R. P., Afshari, C. A. & Germolec, D. (2002). Coordination of altered DNA repair and damage pathways in arsenite-exposed keratinocytes. *Toxicology Science*. Vol. 69, pp. 306–316

Hartmann, M. & Hartwig, A. (1998). Disturbance of DNA damage recognition after UV-irradiation by nickel(II) and cadmium(II) in mammalian cells. *Carcinogenesis*. Vol. 19, pp. 617-621

Hartwig, A., Groblinghoff, U.D., Beyersmann, D., Natarajan, A. T., Filon, R. & Mullenders, L.H.(1997). Interaction of arsenic(III) with nucleotide excision repair in UV-irradiated human fibroblasts, *Carcinogenesis*. Vol. 18, pp. 399–405

Hartwig, A., Snyder, R.D., Schlepegrell, R. & Beyersmann, D. (1991). Modulation by Co(II) of UV-induced DNA repair, mutagenesis and sister-chromatid exchanges in mammalian cells. *Mutation Research*. Vol. 248, pp. 177-185

Hartwig, A., Mullenders, L.H., Schlepegrell, R., Kasten, U. & Beyersmann, D. (1994). Nickel(II) interferes with the incision step in nucleotide excision repair in mammalian cells. *Cancer Research*. Vol. 54, pp.4045-4051

Hartwig, A. (2001). Zinc finger proteins as potential targets for toxic metal ions: differential effects on structure and function. *Antioxidant & Redox Signaling*. Vol. 3, pp. 625-634

Hartwig, A. & Schwerdtle, T. (2002). Interactions by carcinogenic metal compounds with DNA repair processes: toxicological implications. *Toxicology Letters*. Vol. 127, pp. 47-54

Hartwig, A., Asmuß, M., Blessing, H., Hoffmann, S. , Jahnkem, G., Khandelwal, S., Pelzer, A. & Bürkle, A. (2002). Interference by toxic metal ions with zinc-dependent proteins involved in maintaining genomic stability. *Food and Chemical Toxicology*. Vol.40, pp. 1179-1184

Hartwig, A., Blessing, H., Schwerdtle, T. & Walter, I. (2003). Modulation of DNA repair processes by arsenic and selenium compounds. Toxicology. Vol. 193, pp. 161–169

Hartwig, A., Pelzer, A., Asmuß, M. & Bürkle, A. (2003b). Very low concentrations of arsenite suppress poly(ADP-ribosyl)ation in mammalian cells. *International Journal of Cancer*. Vol. 104, pp. 1-6

Hazra, T.K., Izumi, T., Kow, Y.W. & Mitra, S. (2003). The discovery of a new family of mammalian enzymes for repair of oxidatively damaged DNA, and its physiological implications. *Carcinogenesis*. Vol. 24, pp. 155-157

Hsieh, M., Hegde, V., Kelley, M. & Deutsch, W. (2001). Activation of APE/Ref-1 redox activity is mediated by reactive oxygen species and PKC phosphorylation. *Nucleic Acids Research*. Vol. 29, pp. 3116-3122

Huang, H., Shu, S.C., Shih, J.H., Kuo, C.J. & Chiu, I.D. (1998). Antimony trichloride induces DNA damage and apoptosis in mammalian cells. *Toxicology*. Vol. 129, pp. 113-123

IARC (1989). Some Organic Solvents, Resin Monomers and Related Compounds, Pigments and Occupational Exposures in Paint Manufacture and Painting. *Monographs on the Evaluation of Carcinogenic Risks to Humans*. Vol. 47

IARC (1991). Chlorinated Drinking-water; Chlorination By-products; Some Other Halogenated Compounds; Cobalt and Cobalt Compounds. *Monographs on the Evaluation of Carcinogenic Risks to Humans*. Vol.52.

IARC (2006). Cobalt in Hard Metals and Cobalt Sulfate, Gallium Arsenide, Indium Phosphide and Vanadium Pentoxide. *Monographs on the Evaluation of Carcinogenic Risks to Humans*. Vol. 86

IARC (2006). Inorganic and Organic Lead Compounds. *Monographs on the Evaluation of Carcinogenic Risks to Humans*. Vol. 87

Ivancsits, S., Pilger, A., Diem, E., Schaffer, A. & Rüdiger, H.W. (2002). Vanadate induces DNA strand breaks in cultured human fibroblasts at doses relevant to occupational exposure. *Mutation Research*. Vol. 519, pp. 25-35

Kasten, U, Hartwig, A. & Beyermann, D. (1992). Mechanisms of cobalt(II) uptake into V79 Chinese hamster cells. *Archives of Toxicology*. Vol. 66, pp. 592-597

Kasten, U., Mullenders, L.H. & Hartwig, A. (1997). Cobalt(II) inhibits the incision and the polymerization step of nucleotide excision repair in human fibroblasts. *Mutation Research*. Vol. 383, pp. 81-89

Kitchin, K. T. & Wallace, K. (2008). The role of protein binding of trivalent arsenicals in arsenic carcinogenesis and toxicity, *Journal of inorganic biochemistry*. Vol. 102, pp. 532-539

Klaassen, C.D., Liu, J. & Choudhuri, S. (1999). Metallothionein: an intracellular protein to protect against cadmium toxicity. *The Annual Review of Pharmacology and Toxicology*. Vol. 39, pp. 267-294

Klein, C.B. (1996). Carcinogenicity and genotoxicity of chromium. In *Toxicology of Metals*, Chang, L.W. pp. 205-219, Ed. Lewis, Boca Raton

Kopera, E., Schwerdtle, T., Hartwig, A. & Bal, W. (2004). Co(II) and Cd(II) substitute for Zn(II) in the zinc finger derived from the DNA repair protein XPA, demonstrating a variety of potential mechanisms of toxicity. *Chemical Research in Toxicology*. Vol.17, pp.1452-1458

Krizek, B.A., Merkle, D.L. & Berg, J.M. (1993). Ligand variation and metal ion binding specificity in zinc finger peptides. *Inorganic Chemistry*. Vol. 32, pp. 937-940

Lachenmann, M.J., Ladbury, J.E., Dong, J., Huang, K., Carey, P. & Weiss, M.A.(2004). Why zinc fingers prefer zinc: ligand-field symmetry and the hidden thermodynamics of metal ion selectivity. *Biochemistry*. Vol. 43, pp. 13910–13925

Leonard, A. & Gerber, G.B. (1996). Mutagenicity, carcinogenicity and teratogenicity of antimony compounds. *Mutation Research*. Vol. 366, pp. 1-8

Lison, D., De Boeck, M., Verougstraete, V. & Kirsch-Volders M. (2001). Update on the genotoxicity and carcinogenicity of cobalt compounds. *Occupational Environmental Medicine*. Vol. 58, No. 10, pp. 619–625

Liu, S.X., Athar, M., Lippai, I., Waldren, C. & Hei, T.K. (2001). Induction of oxyradicals by arsenic: implication for mechanism of genotoxicity. *Proceedings of the National Academy of Sciences of the U.S.A*. Vol. 98, pp. 1643–1648

Lu, H., Shi, X., Costa, M. & Huang, C. (2005) Carcinogenic effect of nickel compounds. *Molecular Cellular Biochemistry*. Vol. 279, pp. 45–67

Lynn, S., Yew, F.H., Chen, K.S. & Jan, K.Y. (1997). Reactive oxygen species are involved in nickel inhibition of DNA repair. *Environmental and Molecular Mutagenesis*. Vol.29, pp. 208-216

Lynn, S., Shiung, J.N., Gurr, J.R. & Jan, K.Y. (1998). Arsenite stimulates poly(ADP-ribosylation) by generation of nitric oxide. *Free Radical Biology & Medicine*. Vol. 24, pp. 442–449

Mackay, J.P. & Crossley, M. (1998). Zinc fingers are sticking together. *Trends in Biochemical Science*. Vol. 23, pp. 1–4

McNeill, D.R., Wong, H.K., Narayana, A. & Wilson, D.M. 3rd. (2007). Lead promotes a basic site accumulation and co-mutagenesis in mammalian cells by inhibiting the major abasic endonuclease Ape1. *Molecular Carcinogenesis*. Vol. 46, pp. 91 - 99

Meplan, C., Richard, M.J. & Hainaut P. (1999). Redox signalling and transition metals in the control of the p53 pathway. *Biochemical Pharmacology*. Vol.59, pp. 25-33

Mirsalis, J.C., Hamilton, C.M., O'Loughlin, K.G., Paustenbach, D.J., Kerger, B.D. & Patierno, S. (1996). Chromium (VI) at plausible drinking water concentrations is not genotoxic in the in vivo bone marrow micronucleus or liver unscheduled DNA synthesis assays. *Environmental and Molecular Mutagenesis*. Vol. 28: 60-63

Mo, J., Xia, Y., Ning, Z., Wade, T.J. & Mumford, J.L. (2009). Elevated ERCC1 gene expression in blood cells associated with exposure to arsenic from drinking water in Inner Mongolia. *Anticancer Research*. Vol. 29, pp. 3253-3259

Nickens, K.P., Patierno, S.R. & Ceryak, S. (2010). Chromium genotoxicity: A double-edged sword. *Chemico Biological Interactions*. Vol.188, pp.276-288

Nordberg, G.F. (2009). Historical perspectives on cadmium toxicology. *Toxicology and Applied Pharmacology*. Vol. 238:192-200.

O'Brien, T.J., Fornsaglio, J.L., Ceryak, S. & Patierno, S.R. (2002). Effects of hexavalent chromium on the survival and cell cycle distribution of DNA repair-deficient S. cerevisiae. *DNA Repair (Amst)*. Vol.1, pp.617-627

O'Brien, T.J., Brooks, B.R. & Patierno, S.R. (2005). Nucleotide excision repair functions in the removal of chromium-induced DNA damage in mammalian cells. *Molecular and Cellular Biochemistry*. Vol.279, pp. 85-95

Oldiges, H., Hochrainera, D. & Glasera, U. (1989). Long-term inhalation study with Wistar rats and four cadmium compounds. *Toxicological & Environmental Chemistry*. Vol. 19, pp. 217-222

Polednak, A.P. (1981). Mortality among welders, including a group exposed to nickel oxides. Archive of Environmental Health. Vol. 36, pp. 235–242

Posewitz, M.C. & Wilcox, D.E. (1995). Properties of the Sp1 zinc finger 3 peptide: coordination chemistry, redox reactions, and metal binding competition with metallothionein. *Chemical Research in Toxicology*. Vol. 8, pp. 1020–1028

Roberts, R.S., Julian, J.A., Muir, D.C. & Shannon, H.S. (1984) Cancer mortality associated with the high-temperature oxidation of nickel subsulfide. *IARC Scientific Publications*. Vol. 53, pp. 23–35

Roberts, R.S., Julian, J.A., Muir, D.C. & Shannon, H.S. (1989) A study of mortality in workers engaged in the mining, smelting, and refining of nickel. II: mortality from cancer of the respiratory tract and kidney. *Toxicology Industrial Health*. Vol. 5, pp. 975–993.

Roy, N.K. & Rossman, T.G. (1992). Mutagenesis and comutagenesis by lead compounds. *Mutation Research*. Vol. 298, pp.97-103

Schwerdtle, T., Ebert, F., Thuy, C., Richter, C., Mullenders, L.H. & Hartwig, A. (2010). Genotoxicity of soluble and particulate cadmium compounds: impact on oxidative DNA damage and nucleotide excision repair. *Chemical Research in Toxicology*. Vol.23, pp. 432-442

Schwerdtle, T., Walter, I. & Hartwig, A. (2003). Arsenite and its biomethylated metabolites interfere with the formation and repair of stable BPDE-induced DNA adducts in human cells and impair XPAzf and Fpg. *DNA Repair (Amst)*. Vol. 2, pp. 1449-1463

Schwerdtle, T., Walter, I., Mackiw, I. & Hartwig, A. (2003b). Induction of oxidative DNA damage by arsenite and its trivalent and pentavalent methylated metabolites in cultured human cells and isolated DNA. *Carcinogenesis*. Vol. 24, pp. 967–974

Shen, S., Lee, J., Weinfeld, M. & Le, X. C. (2008). Attenuation of DNA damage-induced p53 expression by arsenic: A possible mechanism for arsenic co-carcinogenesis. *Molecular Carcinogenesis*. Vol. 47, pp.508–518

Shen, S., Lee, J., Cullen, W.R., Le, X.C. & Weinfeld, M. (2009). Arsenite and its mono- and dimethylated trivalent metabolites enhance the formation of benzo[a]pyrene diol epoxide-DNA adducts in Xeroderma pigmentosum complementation group A cells. *Chemical Research in Toxicology*. Vol. 22, pp.382-390

Sirover A. & Loeb, L.A. (1976). Infidelity of DNA synthesis in vitro: screening for potential metal mutagens or carcinogens. *Science*. Vol. 194, pp. 1434–1436

Snow, E.T., Sykora, P., Durham, T.R. & Klein, C.B. (2005). Arsenic, mode of action at biologically plausible low doses: what are the implications for low dose cancer risk? *Toxicology and Applied Pharmacology*. Vol. 207, pp. S557–S564

Snyder, R.D., G.F. Davis & P.J. Lachmann. (1989) .Inhibition by metals of X-ray and ultraviolet-induced DNA repair in human cells. *Biological Trace Element Research*. Vol. 21, pp. 389–398

Strupp, C. (2011a). Beryllium metal II. a review of the available toxicity data. *The Annals of Occupational Hygiene*. Vol.55, No.1, pp. 43-56

Strupp, C. (2011b). Beryllium metal I. experimental results on acute oral toxicity, local skin and eye effects, and genotoxicity. *The Annals of Occupational Hygiene*. Vol.55, pp.30-42

Sykora, P. & Snow, E.T. (2008). Modulation of DNA polymerase beta-dependent base excision repair in cultured human cells after low dose exposure to arsenite. *Toxicology and Applied Pharmacology*. Vol. 228, pp. 385-394

Takahashi, S., Takeda, E., Kubota, Y. & Okayasu, R. (2000). Inhibition of repair of radiation-induced DNA double-strand breaks by nickel and arsenite. *Radiation Research*.Vol.154, pp. 686-691.

Tran, H.P., Prakash, A.S., Barnard, R., Chiswell, B. & Ng, J.C. (2002). Arsenic inhibits the repair of DNA damage induced by benzo(a)pyrene, *Toxicology Letters*. Vol.133, pp. 59–67

Wilson, S. (1998). Mammalian base excision repair and DNA polymerase beta. *Mutation Research*. Vol. 407, pp. 203–215

Witkiewicz-Kucharczyk, A & Bal, W. (2006). Damage of zinc fingers in DNA repair proteins, a novel molecular mechanism in carcinogenesis. *Toxicology Letters*. Vol.162, pp. 29-42

Yager, J.W. & Wiencke, J.K. (1997). Inhibition of poly(ADP-ribose) polymerase by arsenite. *Mutation Research*. Vol. 386, pp. 345–351

Youn, C.K., Kim, S.H., Lee do, Y., Song, S.H., Chang, I.Y., Hyun, J.W,. Chung, M.H & You H.J. (2005). Cadmium down-regulates human OGG1 through suppression of Sp1 activity. *Journal of Biological Chemistry*. Vol. 280, pp. 25185–25195.

Zhang, T., Schmitt, M. & Mumford, J. (2003). Effects of arsenic on telomerase and telomeres in relation to cell proliferation and apoptosis in human keratinocytes and leukemia cell in vivo. *Carcinogenesis*. Vol. 24, pp. 1811–1817

4

Involvement of Non-Homologous End-Joining in Radiation-Induced Genomic Instability

Keiji Suzuki, Motohiro Yamauchi, Masatoshi Suzuki,
Yasuyoshi Oka and Shunichi Yamashita
*Nagasaki University Graduate School of Biomedical Sciences,
Atomic Bomb Disease Institute, Department of Radiation Medical Sciences,
Japan*

1. Introduction

DNA double-strand breaks are the most detrimental form of DNA damage induced by either endogenous and exogenous sources. DNA double-strand breaks are generated in response to ionizing radiation, radiomimic drugs, and topoisomerase inhibitors. They also created during V(D)J and class switch recombination in lymphocytes, meiotic recombination in germ cells, and by retroviral integrations (Downs et al., 2007, Polo and Jackson, 2011). Since DNA double-strand breaks discontinue chromosome structure, they may result in cell death that are associated with radiosensitivity, immunodeficiency, neurodegeneration, and developmental defects (Jackson and Bartek, 2009, Mahaney et al., 2009, O'Driscoll and Jeggo, 2006, Weterings and Chen, 2007, Wyman and Kanaar, 2006). Thus, cells have evolved sophisticated mechanisms, by which DNA double-strand breaks are repaired. Two major pathways to repair DNA double-strand breaks are non-homologous end-joining and homologous and homologous recombination (Hartlerode and Scully, 2009, Mahaney et al., 2009, Weterings and Chen, 2007, Wyman and Kanaar, 2006). While rejoining of DNA breaks are indispensable for the survival of cells, DNA repair, by itself, may threaten the stability of the genome. (Burma et al., 2006, Pastink et al., 2001, Sonoda et al., 2006, van Gent et al., 2001). In particular, non-homologous end-joining, which is the primary DNA repair pathway functions in G1 phase, is error-prone (Hartlerode and Scully, 2009, Lieber, 2010). It causes loss or rearrangement of the genetic information through mis-rejoining of DNA double strand breaks. Processing of DNA broken ends by exonucleases and endonucleases also provide another chance to alter DNA sequences. Consequently, surviving cells can avoid lethal effects of DNA double-strand breaks but it results in a loss of heterozygosity as well as gross genome rearrangements that are associated with cancer predisposition. Although most genome rearrangements have been thought to be generated directly by the initial radiation exposure (Leonhardt et al., 1999), recent findings have demonstrated that the integrity of the genome is also endangered eventually, if the cells were survived exposure to DNA damaging agents. In this chapter, the results showing that delayed DNA double-strand breaks are induced several generations after the initial insult in the progenies of surviving cells are presented, and a role of non-homologous end-joining on delayed manifestation of radiation effects and the integrity of the genome in the cells surviving radiation exposure will be discussed.

2. Radiation-induced genomic instability

It has been well established that ionizing radiation induces delayed effects in the progeny of surviving cells (Little, 2003, Lorimore et al., 2003, Morgan et al., 1996, Suzuki et al., 2003). This phenomenon is now called radiation-induced genomic instability, which is manifested as the delayed expression of various radiation effects, such as delayed reproductive death, delayed chromosomal instability, and delayed mutagenesis (Figure 1). Radiation-induced genomic instability has been commonly observed in many cell culture systems as well as in various animals (Lorimore et al., 2003, Morgan, 2003). In addition, there are a series of studies showing that radiation-induced genomic instability is attributed to transgenerational effects in mice using hypervariable minisatellite sequences, which have been renamed as expanded simple tandem repeats (Niwa, 2006). Radiation-induced genomic instability results in accumulating gene mutations and chromosomal rearrangements in addition to the direct genome damage caused by the primary radiation exposure. Therefore, it has been thought to play a pivotal role in accelerating the process of radiation-induced carcinogenesis (Huang et al., 2003, Kadhim et al., 1992, Niwa, 2003, Suzuki, 1997).

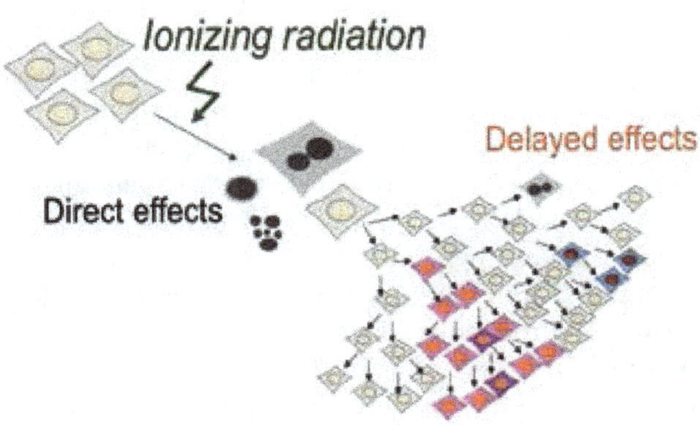

Fig. 1. Radiation-induced genomic instability.

Because radiation-induced genomic instability is induced in a certain fraction of the progenies originated from a single survived cell, not a single gene mutation but some epigenetic changes could be involved in the initiation of radiation-induced genomic instability (Wright, 2010). Persistently elevated levels of oxidative stress was found is association with radiation-induced genomic instability (Azzam et al., 2003, Kim et al., 2006a, Limoli et al., 2003). Further association was confirmed in studies where chronic hydrogen peroxide treatment initiated instability. Administration of free-radical scavengers, antioxidant treatment, and reducing oxygen tension each reduced delayed chromosomal instability, suggesting a role of oxidative stress in perpetuating genomic instability (Roy et al., 2000). Moreover, unstable clones showed mitochondrial dysfunction, which might explain elevated levels of oxidative stress (Kim et al., 2006b). An inflammatory response has also been proposed to be involved in radiation-induced genomic instability particularly in bone marrow (Wright, 2010). Furthermore, possible involvement of bystander effects has also been discussed. Bystander effects are responses observed in unirradiated cells as a result of receiving signals from irradiated cells (Mothersill and Seymour, 2004, Prise and O'Sullivan, 2009). A variety of responses have been described including DNA damage induction, chromosomal instability, and cell death. As bystander effects have been observed in coculture of irradiated and unirradiated cells, and after the transfer of medium from irradiated cells to unirradiated cells, secreted factor(s) may be involved in transducing the bystander signals (Sowa and Morgan, 2004). It has been hypothesized that increased secretion of transforming growth factor beta results in stimulation of production of reactive oxygen species through a membrane NADPH oxidase. In fact, previous study demonstrated that transforming growth factor beta increased oxidative stress through decreased activity of mitochondrial complex IV (Kim et al., 2006b).

Although oxidative stress is surely involved in perpetuation of radiation-induced genomic instability (Azzam et al., 2003, Coates et al., 2008, Miller et al., 2008, Kim et al., 2006a, Limoli et al., 2003, Wright, 2007), alternative mechanisms could be associated with manifestation of radiation-induced genomic instability in non-hematopoietic cells. We have shown that delayed unscheduled induction of DNA double strand breaks is involved in the manifestation of delayed phenotypes (Suzuki et al., 2003). In fact, our study indicated that increased phosphorylated histone H2AX foci, which correspond to DNA double-strand breaks, were frequently detected in the progeny of normal human diploid cells surviving X-rays. Moreover, delayed reactivation of p53 in response to DNA damage was manifested in the surviving clones. Delayed induction of DNA double strand breaks was also confirmed by delayed induction of chromosomal aberrations (Toyokuni et al., 2009). Thus, it is evidenced that induction of DNA double strand breaks is induced indirectly in surviving cells from exposure to radiation, indicating that DNA repair pathways could play roles in amending delayed DNA double-strand breaks in surviving cells.

Previously, Chang and Little reported that radiation-induced genomic instability was absent in xrs5 cells, which are NHEJ-deficient Chinese hamster cells defective in Ku80 protein (Chang and Little, 1992a). Interestingly, delayed reproductive death was not observed in these cells, even though they harbor sufficient amount of DNA double-strand breaks. Since the mechanism of delayed reproductive death has not been fully described yet, we have hypothesized that defective NHEJ in xrs5 cells decreases the chance of mis-rejoining of the broken ends, which result in the formation of dicentric chromosomes involved in division halt. To test this possibility we examined delayed chromosomal instability in two NHEJ-defective cells, xrs-5 and xrs-6 cells, and compared the frequency with the wild-type CHO cells. Furthermore, delayed induction of dicentric chromosomes was examined in cells defective in the catalytic subunit of DNA-dependent protein kinase (DNA-PKcs).

3. Non-homologous end-joining and its mutants

Non-homologous end-joining is one of the two major pathways involved in amending DNA double-strand breaks in multicellular eukaryotes. It primarily plays a critical role during G0-, G1- and early S-phase of cell cycle (Lieber 2010, Polo and Jackson, 2011). Non-homologous end-joining is initiated by binding a heterodimeric protein complex consists of Ku80 and Ku70 to both ends of DNA double-strand breaks (Jackson and Bartek, 2009, Mahaney et al., 2009, O'Driscoll and Jeggo, 2006, Weterings and Chen, 2007, Wyman and Kanaar, 2006). Then, DNA-PKcs, a catalytic subunit of DNA-dependent protein kinase, is recruited to Ku-DNA complex, which results in activation of the protein kinase activity of DNA-PKcs and tethering two broken DNA ends. DNA-PKcs phosphorylates a number of proteins,

including Ku80, Ku70, XRCC4, Artemis, DNA ligase IV and DNA-PKcs itself (Mahaney et al., 2009, Weterings and Chen, 2007). Autophosphorylation alters the conformation of DNA-PKcs, allowing the recruitment of DNA end-processing enzymes, such as MRE11 and Artemis (Huertas, 2010). MRE11 exhibits a 3' to 5' exonuclease activity and plays a critical role in homologous recombination, but its function in non-homologous end-joining is still to be determined. On the other hand, Artemis shows a 5' to 3' exonuclease activity, and it is suggested to be involved in a subset of DNA double-strand breaks. In fact, cells defective in both nucleases do not show significant radiation sensitivity. Processing of broken ends might create DNA single-strand breaks, which are amended by the DNA polymerase X family, such as polymerase mu and polymerase lambda, and terminal deoxyribonucleotidyltransferase. DNA double-strand breaks are finally rejoined by a complex composed of DNA ligase IV, XRCC4, and XLF.
Until now, several mutants defective in DNA double-strand break repair have been cloned (Jeggo, 1998). They are highly sensitive to radiation and show chromosome instability in response to DNA damaging agents. As shown in Table 1, at least four independent groups were identified. XR-1 mutant belong to X-ray repair complementing defective repair in Chinese hamster cells 4 (XRCC4) group holds mutations in the XRCC4 gene. Both xrs-5 and xrs-6 cells are the members of the XRCC5 group, and they show profound defect in the Ku80 function (Singleton et al., 1997). In xrs-5 cells, the expression of the Ku80 gene is significantly compromised. In xrs-6 cells, a 13-base pair insertion causes a truncation of KU80 protein, which accelerates degradation of KU80 protein. The responsible gene for the XRCC7 group is the DNA-PKcs (Zdzienicka, 1999). Both scid and V-3 mutants harbor premature termination of the protein in the C-terminus. In irs-20 a mutation that causes substitution of the amino acid located in the C-terminal region.

Mutants	Complementation group	Gene
XR-1	XRCC4	*XRCC4*
xrs-5, xrs-6	XRCC5	*Ku80*
-	XRCC6	*Ku70*
scid, V3	XRCC7	*DNA-PKcs*

Table 1. Rodent cell mutants with defective non-homologous end-joining repair.

Radiation sensitivity of these mutants was determined by colony formation assay. A single cell is able to form a cluster of progenitor cells, namely, a colony, when it is incubated for 10 days or more. After X-irradiation, numbers of colonies are decreased in a dose dependent manner. Consequently, cell survival can be calculated by dividing the number of colonies after X-irradiation by the number of colonies formed by the control cells. As shown in Figure 2, both xrs-5 (closed diamond), xrs-6 (closed triangle), and scid (closed square) cells show significant reduction of cell survival as compared to CHO cells (open circle). These cells lose the shoulder of the survival curve observed in CHO cells, indicating that they lose DNA repair capacity. To compliment the defect in xrs5 cells, the human Ku86 gene was introduced by electroporation, and as a result, radiation sensitivity was significantly recovered (open diamond), confirming that a single gene mutation causes profound DNA repair defect.

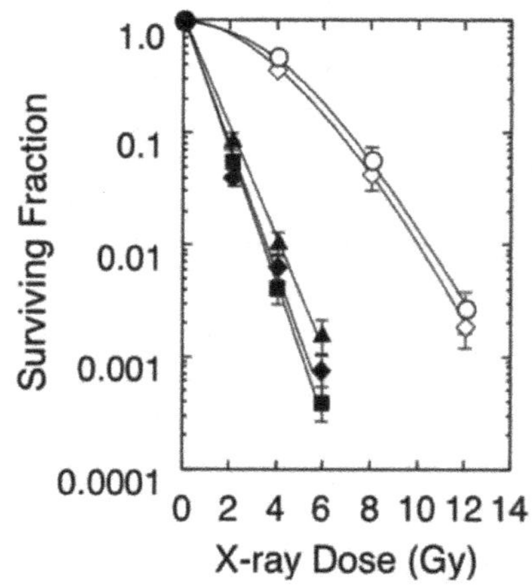

Fig. 2. Survival curves of CHO cells and Ku80-deficient cells.

These cells were irradiated with X-rays from an X-ray generator at 150 kVp and 5 mA with a 0.1-mm copper. The dose rate was 0.44 Gy/min. Dose rates were determined with an ionization chamber.

4. Induction of delayed phenotypes in DNA repair-deficient cells

4.1 Methods for detection of delayed phenotypes

Since radiation-induced genomic instability is manifested as the expression of delayed effects in the progeny of surviving cells, most of the study isolated colonies formed by the cells surviving X-irradiation. The primary colonies were cloned 10 days after irradiation. The cells obtained from each colony have already passed 15 to 20 population doublings. Then, the primary clones were subjected to the secondary colony formation. After 10 day, the secondary clones were isolated, and the cells were at 30 to 35 population doubling levels after irradiation. Delayed reproductive death was examined by colony-forming ability. Colonies derived from the surviving cells often contain giant cells, which occupied an area in the colony several times greater than the rest of the cells. Colonies containing at least one giant cell were judged as giant cell-positive colony. Delayed chromosomal bridges were detected between two dividing daughter nuclei in the anaphase cells in the surviving colonies. Delayed chromosomal aberrations were examined in metaphase cells derived from the primary and the secondary clones. Both chromatid- and chromosome-type aberrations were analyzed, and total 200 metaphases were counted per each sample.

Delayed induction of DNA double strand breaks was determined by 53BP1 foci by immunofluorescence. 53BP1 is a protein, which was originally discovered as a p53-binding protein. Lately, it turns to be clear that 53BP1 is a critical component of DNA damage signalling pathway (Polo and Jackson, 2011). ATM-dependent DNA damage checkpoint plays a central role in protecting integrity of the genome (Kastan and Bartek, 2004, Lavin, 2008, Shiloh and Kastan, 2001, Shiloh, 2003). ATM, which forms dimer or oligomer in the control cells, dissociates into monomer through autophosphorylation at serine 1981 in response to ionizing radiation (Bakkenist and Kastan, 2003). Activated ATM transduces DNA damage signal through phosphorylation of down-stream factors, including histone H2AX, MDC1 and 53BP1 (Ciccia and Elledge, 2010, Kastan and Lim, 2000)(Figure 3), and DNA damage signal is amplified through the formation of ionizing radiation-induced foci

(Bonner et al., 2008). Activated ATM also phosphorylates p53 and CHK2/Cds1, which result in an induction of apoptosis as well as cell cycle arrest. Furthermore, ATM phosphorylates MRE11, NBS1, and Artemis, by which DNA repair ability may be regulated. Previously, it was demonstrated that the number of DNA double-strand breaks and the number of foci are well correlated, and since then, ionizing radiation-induced foci have been treated as a trustable marker for DNA double-strand breaks (Bonner et al., 2008). Foci of phosphorylated histone H2AX at serine 139 were the first ones to be used as DNA damage marker (Paull et al., 2000). Subsequently, foci of phosphorylated ATM at serine 1981 were demonstrated to illustrate low level of DNA double-strand breaks (Suzuki et al., 2006). Compared to these foci, 53BP1 foci create larger discrete foci, which can be detected even in tissue specimens (Nakashima et al., 2008). Thus, 53BP1 foci have been treated as DNA damage marker.

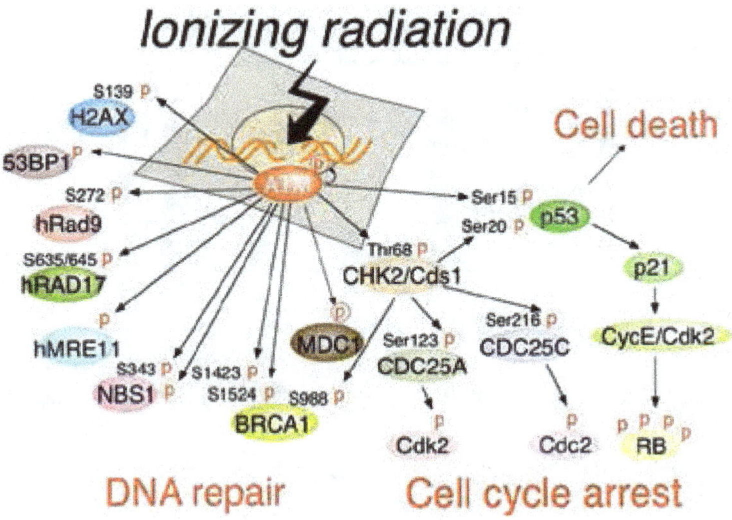

Fig. 3. ATM-dependent DNA damage checkpoint signalling.

53BP1 foci were detected by a specific antibody against the human 53BP1 protein. The primary antibody was visualized by Alexa594-labelled anti-rabbit IgG antibody. The nuclei were counterstained with DAPI. The samples were examined with an Olympus fluorescence microscope. Digital images were captured by a cooled CCD camera, and the images were analyzed by image analysis software.

4.2 Manifestation of delayed phenotypes

Radiation-induced genomic instability needs to be examined at the same survival levels, so that 8 Gy and 10 Gy of X-rays were irradiated to CHO, while 2 and 4 Gy of X-rays were exposed to xrs-5 and xrs-6 cells, respectively. The primary clones were isolated, and they were subjected to the secondary colony formation. As shown in Figure 4, colony-forming ability is significantly reduced in CHO cells derived from surviving clones compared with those derived from the control clones. In contrast, no such difference is observed in both xrs-5 and xrs-6 cells, indicating that delayed reproductive death was completely absent in both xrs-5 and xrs-6 cells. In CHO cells, the frequency of giant cells and chromosomal bridges is also increased only in surviving clones, whereas, delayed induction of these phenotypes was completely abrogated in xrs-5 and xrs-6 cells (Figures 5 and 6).

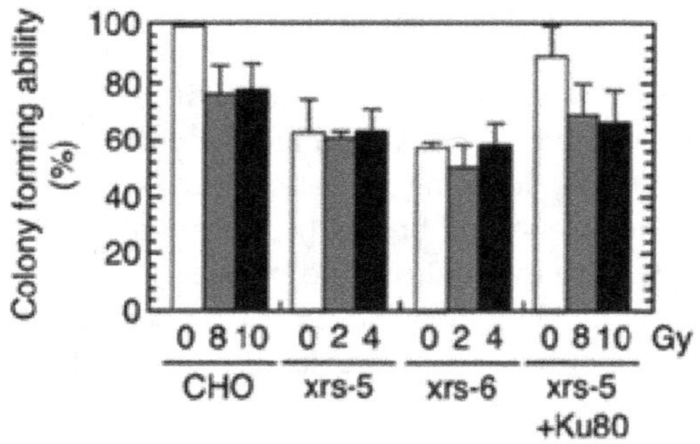

Fig. 4. Delayed reproductive death at 30-35 population doublings post-irradiation.

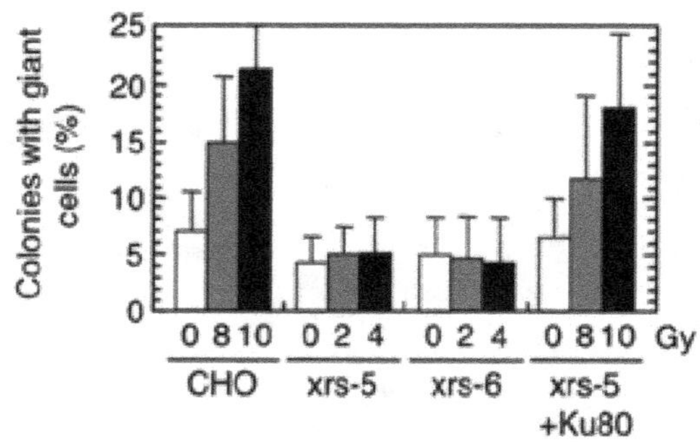

Fig. 5. Delayed giant cell formation at 30-35 population doublings post-irradiation.

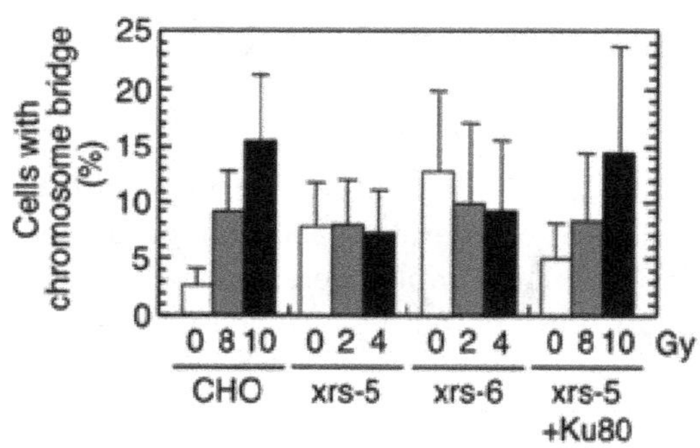

Fig. 6. Delayed chromosome bridge (right) at 30-35 population doublings post-irradiation.

In order to confirm that defective induction of these delayed phenotypes are caused by the simple Ku80-deficiency, the human Ku86 gene was introduced into xrs-5 cells. Expression of human KU80 protein was confirmed by western blotting, and sufficient amount of KU80 protein was detected in the complimented cells. Accordingly, it was confirmed that complementation of the defective Ku80 function in xrs-5 cells simultaneously restored delayed reproductive death, giant cell formation and delayed chromosomal bridge formation to the levels observed in CHO cells. Thus, the results clearly indicated that Ku80-dependent rejoining is involved in the manifestation of delayed phenotypes in the progenies of X-ray-surviving cells.

4.3 Delayed induction of DNA double-strand breaks

It is possible that delayed phenotypes are caused by delayed DNA double strand breaks and Ku80-dependent mis-rejoining. Delayed induction of DNA double strand breaks were examined by 53BP1 foci in cells at 30-35 PDL post-irradiation (Figure 7). Since the primary antibody against 53BP1 is visualized by the secondary antibody labeled with Alexa594, 53BP1 foci are detected as discrete large red dots within the blue nuclei. Upon X-irradiation, the foci of DNA damage checkpoint factors become detectable within a few minutes after exposure. At 1 to 2 hours after X-irradiation, the initial foci are detectable in all exposed cells. Many small foci, most of which diameter distributed between 0.4 and 1.0 micrometer, were observed. The number of foci is decreased thereafter, indicating DNA repair. While the number of the initial foci reduced significantly during the first 6 to 10 hours, some fraction of the initial foci is remained as residual foci. Diameter of these residual foci increased time-dependently, and they are quite large in size after 24 hours (Yamauchi et al., 2008). The number of foci shows no significant change thereafter, however, the cells with large residual foci are diluted out, when the foci-negative cells dominate the population. Thus, the background foci is rarely detectable even in the cells surviving 10 Gy of X-rays. While the frequency of 53BP1 foci per cell in the control CHO cells was approximately 0.14 ± 0.07, it was increased to 0.41 ± 0.19 in 10 Gy-surviving cells. The frequency of 53BP1 foci in the unirradiated xrs5 cells were relatively higher (0.18 ± 0.08) compared to the CHO cells, and it was about 0.51 ± 0.27 in 4 Gy-surviving cells.

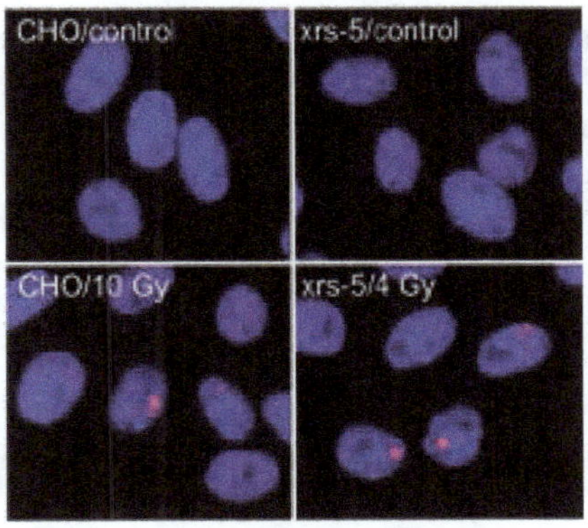

Fig. 7. Delayed induction of 53BP1 foci in CHO and xrs-5 cells at 30-35 population doublings post-irradiation.

Previously, a few studies including ours have suggested that delayed DNA double strand breaks are induced several generations after the initial insult (Barber et al., 2006, Huang et al., 2007, Suzuki et al., 2003), which has been proven by examining the delayed induction of foci of DNA damage checkpoint factors, such as phosphorylated histone H2AX. While phosphorylated histone H2AX foci are frequently used as biochemical markers for DNA double strand breaks, the foci of other DNA damage checkpoint factors, such as phosphorylated ATM foci and 53BP1 foci, are colocalized with phosphorylated histone H2AX foci, and they could also be used as alternative markers for DNA damage. In the present study, we demonstrated that the frequency of 53BP1 foci was higher in the progenies of surviving cells compared to unirradiated cells. Thus, it is confirmed that delayed induction of DNA double strand breaks in the progeny of surviving cells associated with pleiotropic manifestation of radiation-induced genomic instability.

4.4 Mis-rejoining of delayed DNA double-strand breaks

Although the number of spontaneous foci per cell in the foci-positive cells is 1, we found multiple numbers of foci in not a small numbers of surviving cells. Therefore, it is possible that mis-rejoining of delayed DNA double-strand breaks results in delayed chromosomal instability. We tested this possibility by examining delayed induction of dicentric chromosomes at 30-35 PDL post irradiation (Figure 8).

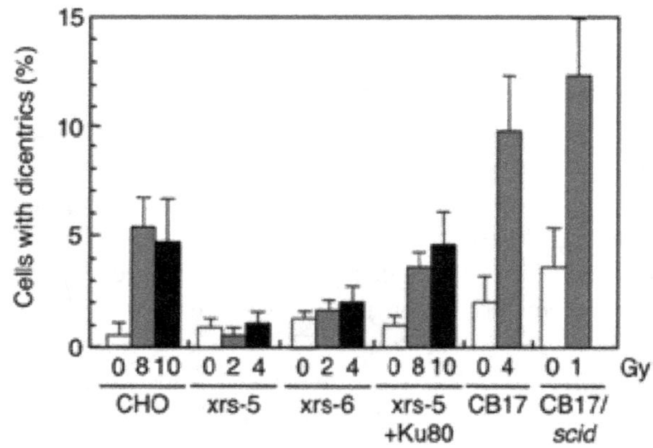

Fig. 8. Delayed chromosomal instability at 30-35 population doublings post-irradiation.

We found that delayed formation of dicentric chromosomes was significantly increased in CHO cells. Whereas, it is absent in xrs5 and xrs6 cells, while the control levels of dicentric chromosome were comparable among those cells. To confirm whether defective induction of dicentric chromosomes is related to Ku80-deficiency, delayed chromosomal instability was examined in the complimented xrs5 cells. We observed that delayed induction of dicentric chromosomes was increased to the level observed in CHO cells. Delayed chromosomal instability was also examined in cells derived from DNA-PKcs-defective *scid* mouse (Figure 8). Cells were irradiated with equivalent 10% survival doses and delayed induction of dicentric chromosomes was analyzed 30-35 PDL post-irradiation. The frequency of dicentric chromosomes in the unirradiated *scid* was higher than that in the wild-type cells, and increased dicentric frequencies in surviving cells were observed.

5. Role of non-homologous end-joining on radiation-induced genomic instability

Radiation-induced genomic instability has been reported commonly in various cell systems including human and rodent cells (Little, 2003, Lorimore et al., 2003, Morgan et al., 1996, Suzuki et al., 2003). However, Chang and Little demonstrated that delayed reproductive death, one characteristic manifestation of radiation-induced genomic instability, was not observed in Ku80-deficient xrs5 cells (Chang and Little, 1992a). The authors suggested that the cellular processing of DNA double strand breaks during repair must play a role in delayed reproductive death. In fact, our current study confirmed their results and found that not only delayed cell death but also delayed induction of giant cells and chromosome bridge were absent in xrs-5 cells (Figures 5 and 6). Furthermore, other Ku80-deficient cell line, xrs6, also revealed deficiency in the induction of those delayed phenotypes. Thus, it becomes clear that Ku80-dependent non-homologous end-joining is involved in the manifestation of radiation-induced genomic instability. Then the question should be about the mechanism. One possible explanation of the defective induction of some delayed phenotypes is that error-free DNA repair, such as homologous recombination, reduced the incidence of transmissible damage in the absence of error-prone non-homologous end-joining repair. If so, delayed induction of DNA double strand breaks should be lower in Ku80-defective cells than the control CHO cells. Therefore, we checked whether delayed DNA damage was less frequent in xrs5 cells. The results clearly indicated that it was not the case. Thus, even without Ku80-dependent repair, genomic instability by itself could be induced in the progenies of surviving cells. The second possibility is that defective DNA repair in xrs5 cells decreased the chance of mis-rejoining of the broken ends that occurred many generations after the initial insult. In fact, delayed induction of chromosome bridges between two daughter cells was significantly reduce in xrs-5 and xrs-6 cells (Figure 6). Furthermore, delayed induction of dicentric chromosomes was completely absent in both xrs-5 and xrs-6 cells (Figure 8). Although several studies have reported that chromosome breakages are more frequent in Ku80-deficient cells (Darroudi and Natarajan, 1987, Kemp and Jeggo, 1986), the frequency of dicentric chromosome was relatively low considering the frequency of chromosome breaks. These results support our conclusion that the formation of dicentric chromosome caused by delayed DNA damage was compromised in Ku80-deficient cells. Although a back-up non-homologous end-joining may undertake mis-rejoining of broken ends in the absence of Ku80-dependent DNA repair (Iliakis et al., 2004), it is highly likely that a major pathway of illegitimate rejoining the DNA breaks is Ku80-dependent process (Liang et al., 1996). We also confirmed that radiation-induced genomic instability was manifested in cells derived from DNA-PKcs-defective *Scid* mouse. Moreover, delayed dicentric formation was normally detected in *Scid* cells. Therefore, DNA-PK-independent rejoining, which was suggested previously (Gao et al., 1998), is involved in delayed dicentric formation. Recently, it has been postulated that XRCC4/DNA Ligase IV-dependent but DNA-PKcs-independent rejoining needs Ku80/70 complex. Thus, it is highly possible that Ku80-dependent mis-rejoining is involved in delayed generation of dicentric chromosomes, by which chromosome bridges is generated. Such mis-rejoining inhibits segregation of two daughter cells, which results in delayed induction of giant cells as well as delayed reproductive death.

It has been well described that genomic instability, which is known as gross chromosomal rearrangement, is commonly observed in yeast. Gross chromosomal rearrangements manifest as translocations, chromosomal deletions, and inversions, indicating that they could be means to accelerate multiple genetic alterations associated with carcinogenesis (Kolodner et al., 2002). Although multiple pathways cooperate to suppress gross chromosomal rearrangement, homologous recombination plays a pivotal role in avoiding gross chromosomal rearrangement (Myung et al., 2001). Moreover, the restrained recruitment of homologous recombination proteins has been reported to promote gross chromosomal rearrangement. Thus, non-homologous end-joining has little effect on gross chromosomal rearrangement in yeast.

It should be very interesting to know the consequence of cells harboring mis-rejoined chromosomes. Previously, it was reported that ionizing radiation induced genomic instability in the progeny of surviving CHO cells, which resulted in a heritable mutator phenotypes. For example, mutation frequency at the hypoxanthine-guanine phosphoribosyltransferase locus in surviving clones was persistently higher than the unirradiated progenies (Lim et al., 2000). It was expected that such mis-rejoining caused large deletions at the gene locus, however, multiplex polymerase chain reaction analysis revealed that point mutations are the predominant type of genetic alterations in the mutants (Chang and Little, 1992b). Because cells with micronuclei were frequently observed among the surviving cells, persistent break induction, which may not be involved in delayed cell death under the p53-dysfunctional condition (Tzang et al., 1999), may be resulted from mis-rejoined chromosomes. In fact, previous study demonstrated that delayed chromosomal instability was mediated by bridge-breakage-fusion cycle, which could also be involved in the perpetuation of radiation-induced genomic instability. It has been proved that ionizing radiation induces delayed genomic instability, which accumulates genetic alterations including gene mutations, loss of heterozygosity, and chromosome rearrangements, concurrently with delayed reproductive death. As Ku80-deficiency compromised delayed cell death through the formation of dicentric chromosomes, it is likely that such cells with defective DNA repair capacity are more susceptible to carcinogenesis induced by DNA damaging agents.

6. Molecular nature of radiation signature involved in radiation-induced genomic instability

Radiation-induced genomic instability is transmitted through many generations after the initial X-irradiation, indicating that there should be some mechanism(s), by which the initial radiation insults are memorized (Suzuki, 1997). As delayed DNA double-strand breaks are identified in surviving cells, persistent DNA damage is one candidate for radiation signature. In fact, a recent study has proved that DNA double-strand breaks induced by very low dose of X-rays remain unrepaired for many days in confluent cells (Rothkamm and Lobrich, 2003). Furthermore, if persistent DNA is radiation signature, radiation-induced genomic instability is more prevailing in xrs-5 and xrs-6 cells compared with CHO cells. But, we observed radiation-induced genomic instability at similar level between these cells (Suzuki et al., 2009). Thus, these results exclude the possibility that radiation signature is DNA double-strand breaks *per se*. Previously, we compared delayed aberrations of X chromosome with or without large deletion at the hypoxanthine-quanine-phosphorybosyltransferase gene, which is located at Xq26.1 (Toyokuni et al., 2009, Suzuki et al., 2003). Because cells defective in the gene were able to grow in the presence of 6-thioguanine, we cloned 6-thioguanine resistant clones after 3 Gy of X-rays, and examine gene deletion. We found some of the resistant clones had large deletions expanding over several megabases. Interestingly, these clones with large deletions showed higher probability to induce delayed chromosomal instability. Thus, altered higher-order chromatin structure could be a candidate for radiation signature. It is possible that such altered higher-order chromatin structure results in replication stress, which causes DNA double-strand breaks.

7. Conclusion

Ionizing radiation induces delayed destabilization of the genome in the progenies of surviving cells. This phenomenon, which is called radiation-induced genomic instability, is manifested by delayed induction of radiation effects, such as cell death, chromosome aberration, and mutation in the progeny of cells surviving radiation exposure. Previously, it was reported that delayed cell death was absent in Ku80-deficient cells. We have proved that this is because delayed induction of dicentric chromosomes is significantly compromised in those cells. In fact, reintroduction of the human Ku86 gene complimented the defective DNA repair and recovered delayed induction of dicentric chromosomes and delayed cell death. Thus, our current study demonstrated that DNA repair pathway is an important determinant of cellular response to ionizing radiation not only in the immediate response but also in cells surviving radiation exposure. Survived cells induced DNA double strand breaks many generations after the initial insult. Although the mechanism of delayed DNA damage induction has to be determined, delayed dicentric formation indicated that delayed DNA damage was induced in G1 phase. Such delayed DNA damage could be repaired by NHEJ repair, but it also provided a chance to engender mis-rejoining. These results should bring a new insight into how DNA repair protects the integrity of the genome from the insults of DNA damaging agents.

8. Acknowledgements

This work was supported in part by grants for scientific research and by Nagasaki University Global COE program from the Ministry of Education, Culture, Sports, Science, and Technology, Japan. The authors greatly appreciated Dr. Penny A. Jeggo for providing the plasmid containing the human Ku86 gene.

9. References

Azzam, E.I.; de Toledo, S.M. & Little, J.B. (2003). Oxidative metabolism, gap junctions and the ionizing radiation-induced bystander effect. *Oncogene*, Vol.22, No.45, (October 2003), pp. 7050-7057, ISSN 0950-9232

Bakkenist, C.J. & Kastan M.B. (2003). DNA damage activates ATM through intermolecular autophosphorylation and dimer dissociation. *Nature*, Vol.421, No.6922, (January 2003), pp. 499-506, ISSN 0028-0836

Barber, R.C.; Hickenbotham, P., Hatch, T., Kelly, D., Topchiy, N., Almeida, G.M., Jones, G.D., Johnson, G.E., Parry, J.M., Rothkamm, K. & Dubrova, Y.E. (2006). Radiation-induced transgenerational alterations in genome stability and DNA damage. *Oncogene*, Vol.25, No. 56, (November 2006), pp. 7336-7342, ISSN 0950-9232

Bonner, W.M.; Redon, C.E., Dickey, J.S., Nakamura, A.J., Sedelnikova, O.A., Solier, S. & Pommier, Y. (2008). GammaH2AX and cancer. *Nature Review of Cancer*, Vol. 8, No.12, (December 2008), pp. 957-967, ISSN 1474-175X

Burma, S.; Chen, B.P. & Chen, D.J. (2006). Role of non-homologous end joining (NHEJ) in maintaining genomic integrity. *DNA Repair*, Vol.5, No.9-10, (September 2006), pp. 1042-1048, ISSN 1568-7864

Chang, W.P. & Little, J.B. (1992a). Evidence that DNA double-strand breaks initiate the phenotype of delayed reproductive death in Chinese hamster ovary cells. *Radiation Research*, Vol.131, No.1, (July 1992), pp. 53-59, ISSN 0033-7587

Chang, W.P. & Little, J.B. (1992b). Persistent elevated frequency of spontaneous mutations in progeny of CHO clones surviving X-irradiation: association with delayed reproductive death phenotypes. *Mutation Research*, Vol.270, No.2, (November 1992), pp. 191-199, ISSN 0027-5107

Ciccia, A. & Elledge, S.J. (2010). The DNA damage response: making it safe to play with knives. *Molecular Cell*, Vol.28, No.2, (October 2007), pp. 739-745, ISSN 1097-2765

Coates, P.J.; Rundle, J.K., Lorimore, S.A. & Wright, E.G. (2008). Indirect macrophage responses to ionizing radiation: implications for genotype-dependent bystander signaling. *Cancer Research*, Vol.68, No.2 ,(January 2008), pp. 450-456, ISSN 0008-5472

Darroudi, F. & Natarajan, A.T. (1987). Cytogenetical characterization of Chinese hamster ovary X-ray-sensitive mutant cells xrs 5 and xrs 6. I. Induction of chromosomal aberrations by X-irradiation and its modulation with 3-aminobenzamide and caffeine. *Mutation Research*, Vol.177, No.1, (March 1987), pp. 133-148, ISSN 0027-5107

Downs, J.A.; Nussenzweig, M.C. & Nussenzweig, A. (2007). Chromatin dynamics and the preservation of genetic information. *Nature*, Vol.447, No.7147, (June 2007), pp. 951-958, ISSN 0028-0836

Gao, Y.; Chaudhuri, J., Zhu, C., Davidson, L., Weaver, D.T. & Alt, F.W. (1998). A targeted DNA-PKcs-null mutation reveals DNA-PK-independent functions for KU in V(D)J recombination. *Immunity*, Vol.9, No.3, (September 1998), pp. 367-376, ISSN 1074-7613

Hartlerode, A.J. & Scully, R. (2009). Mechanisms of double-strand break repair in somatic mammalian cells. *The Biochemical Journal*, Vol.423, (September 2009), pp. 157-168, ISSN 0264-6021

Huang, L.; Snyder, A.R. & Morgan, W.F. (2003). Radiation-induced genomic instability and its implications for radiation carcinogenesis. *Oncogene*, Vol.22, No.45, (October 2003), pp. 5848-5854, ISSN 0950-9232

Huang, L.; Kim, P.M., Nickoloff, J.A. & Morgan, W.F. (2007). Targeted and nontargeted effects of low-dose ionizing radiation on delayed genomic instability in human cells. *Cancer Research*, Vol.67, No.3, (February 2007), pp. 1099-1104, ISSN 0008-5472

Huertas, P. (2010). DNA resection in eukaryotes: deciding how to fix the break. *Nature Structual and Molecular Biology*, Vol.17, No. 1, (January 2010), pp. 11-16, ISSN 1545-9993

Iliakis, G.; Wang, H., Perrault, A.R., Boecker, W., Rosidi, B., Windhofer, F., Wu, W., Guan, J., Terzoudi, G. & Pantelias, G. (2004). Mechanisms of DNA double strand break repair and chromosome aberration formation. *Cytogenetic Genome Research*, Vol.104, No.1-4, (November 2004), pp. 14-20, ISSN 1424-8581

Jackson S.P. & Bartek, J. (2009). The DNA-damage response in human biology and diseases. *Nature*, Vo.461, No.7267, (October 2009), pp. 1071-1078, ISSN 0028-0836

Jeggo, P.A. (1998). Identification of genes involved in repair of DNA double-strand breaks in mammalian cells. *Radiation Research*, Vol.150, No.5, (November 1998), pp. 80-91, ISSN 0033-7587

Kadhim, M.A.; MacDonald, D.A., Goodhead, D.T., Lorimore, S.A., Marsden, S.J. & Wright, E.G. (1992). Transmission of chromosomal instability after plutonium alpha-particle irradiation. *Nature*, Vol.355, No.6362, (February 1992), pp. 738-740, ISSN 0028-0836

Kastan, M.B. & Lim, D.S. (2000). The many substrates and functions of ATM. *Nature Reviews. Molecular and Cellular Biology*, Vol.1, No.3, (December 2000), pp. 179-186, ISSN 1471-0072

Kastan, M.B. & Bartek, J. (2004). Cell-cycle checkpoints and cancer. *Nature*, Vol.432, No.7015, (November 2004), pp. 316-323, ISSN 0028-0836

Kemp, L.M. & Jeggo, P.A. (1986). Radiation-induced chromosome damage in X-ray-sensitive mutants (xrs) of the Chinese hamster ovary cell line. *Mutation Research*, Vol.166, No.3, (November 1986), pp. 255-263, ISSN 0027-5107

Kim, G.J.; Chandrasekaran, K. & Morgan, W.F. (2006a). Mitochondrial dysfunction, persistently elevated levels of reactive oxygen species and radiation-induced genomic instability: a review. *Mutagenesis*, Vol.21, No.6, (October 2006), pp. 361-368, ISSN 0267-8357

Kim, G.J.; Fiskum, G.M. & Morgan, W.F. (2006b). A role for mitochondrial dysfunction in perpetuating radiation-induced genomic instability. *Cancer Research*, Vol.66, No.21, (November 2006), pp. 10377-10383, ISSN 0008-5472

Kolodner, R.D.; Putnam, C.D., Myung, K. (2002) Maintenance of genome stability in *Saccharomyces cerevisiae*. *Science*, Vol.297, (July 2002), pp. 552-557, ISSN 0193-4511

Lavin, M.F. (2008). Ataxia-telangiectasia: from a rare disorder to a paradigm for cell signalling and cancer. *Nature Reviews. Molecular and Cellular Biology*, Vol.9, No.10, (October 2008), pp. 759-769, ISSN 1471-0072

Leonhardt, E.A.; Trinh, M., Chu, K. & Dewey, W.C. (1999). Evidence that most radiation-induced HPRT mutants are generated directly by the initial radiation exposure. *Mutation Research*, Vol.426, No.1, (May 1999), pp. 23-30, ISSN 0027-5107

Liang, F.; Romanienko, P.J., Weaver, D.T., Jeggo, P.A. & Jasin, M. (1996). Chromosomal double-strand break repair in ku80-deficient cells. *Proceedings of the National Academy of Science USA*, Vol.93, No.17, (August 1996), pp. 8929-8933, ISSN 0027-8424

Lieber, M.R. (2010). The mehanism of Double-strand DNA break repair by the nonhomologous DNA end-joining pathway. *Annual review of Biochemistry*, Vol.79, No.1, (July 2010), pp. 181-211, ISSN 0066-4154

Lim, D.S.; Vogel, H., Willefrod, D.M., Sands, A.T., Platt, K.A. & Hasty, P. (2000). Analysis of ku80-mutant mice and cells with deficient levels of p53. *Molecular and Cellular Biology*, Vol.20, No.11, (June 2000), pp. 3772-3780, ISSN 0270-7306

Limoli, C.L.; Giedzinski, E., Morgan, W.F., Swarts, S.G., Jones, G.D. & Hyun, W. (2003). Persistent oxidative stress in chromosomally unstable clones. *Cancer Research*, Vol.63, No.12, (June 2003), pp. 3107-3111, ISSN 0008-5472

Little, J.B. (2003). Genomic instability and bystander effects: a historical perspective. *Oncogene*, No.22, Vol.45, (October 2003), pp. 6978-6987, ISSN 0950-9232

Lorimore, S.A.; Coates, P.J. & Wright, E.G. (2003). Radiation-induced genomic instability and bystander effects: inter-related nontargeted effects of exposure to ionizing radiation. *Oncogene*, Vol.22, No.45 (October 2003), pp. 7058-7069, ISSN 0950-9232

Rothkamm, K. & Löbrich, M. (2003). Evidence for a lack of DNA double-strand break repair in human cells exposed to very low x-ray doses. *Proceedings of the National Academy of Science U S A*, Vol.100, No. 9, (April 2003), pp. 5057-5062, ISSN 0027-8424

Mahaney, B.L.; Meek, K. & Lees-Miller, S.P. (2009). Repair of ionizing radiation-induced DNA double-strand breaks by non-homologous end-joining. *The Biochemical Journal*, Vol.417, No.3, (February 2009), pp. 639-650, ISSN 0264-6021

Miller, J.H.; Jin, S., Morgan, W.F., Yang, A., Wan, Y., Aypar, U., Peters, J.S. & Springer, D.L. (2008). Profiling mitochondrial proteins in radiation-induced genome-unstable cell lines with persistent oxidative stress by mass spectrometry, *Radiation Research*, Vol.169, No.6, (June 2008), pp. 700-706, ISSN 0033-7587

Morgan, W.F.; Day, J.P., Kaplan, M.I., McGhee, E.M. & Limoli, C.L. (1996). Genomic instability induced by ionizing radiation. *Radiation Research*, Vol.146, No.3, (September 1996), pp. 247-258, ISSN 0033-7587

Morgan W.F. (2003). Non-targeted and delayed effects of exposure to ionizing radiation: I. Radiation-induced genomic instability and bystander effects in vitro. *Radiation Research*, Vol.159, No.5, (May 2003), pp. 567-580, ISSN 0033-7587

Mothersill, C. & Seymour, C. (2004). Radiation-induced bystander effects--implications for cancer. *Nature Review of Cancer*, Vol.4, No.2, (February 2004), pp. 158-164, ISSN 1474-175X

Myung, K.; Chen, C., Kolodner, R.D. (2001) Multiple pathways cooperate in the suppression of genomic instability in *Saccharomyces cerevisiae*. *Nature*, Vol.411, No.6841, (June 2001), pp. 1073-1076, ISSN 0028-0836

Nakashima, M.; Suzuki, K., Meirmanov, S., Naruke, Y., Matsuu-Matsuyama, M., Shichijo, K., Saenko, V., Kondo, H., Hayashi, T., Ito, M., Yamashita, S. & Sekine, I. (2008). Foci formation of p53-binding protein 1 in thyroid tumors: activation of genomic instability during thyroid carcinogenesis. *International Journal of Cancer*, Vol.122, No.5, (March 2008), pp. 1082-1088, ISSN 0828-6924

Niwa, O. (2003). Induced genomic instability in irradiated germ cells and in the offspring; reconciling discrepancies among the human and animal studies. *Oncogene*, Vol.22, No.45, (October 2003), pp. 7078-7086, ISSN 0950-9232

Niwa, O. (2006). Radiation induced dynamic mutations and transgenerational effects. *Journal of Radiation Research*, Vol.47, No.1, (January 2006), pp. 25-30, ISSN 0449-3060

O'Driscoll, M. & Jeggo, P.A. (2006). The role of double-strand break repair - insights from human genetics. *Nature Review of Genetics*, Vol.7, No.1, (January 2006), pp. 45-54, ISSN 1471-0056

Pastink, A.; Eeken, J.C. & Lohman, P.H. (2001). Genomic integrity and the repair of double-strand breaks. *Mutation Research*, Vol.480-481, (September 2001), pp. 37-50, ISSN 0027-5107

Paull, T.T.; Rogakou. E.P., Yamazaki, V., Kirchgessner, C.U., Gellert, M. & Bonner WM. (2000). A critical role for histone H2AX in recruitment of repair factors to nuclear foci after DNA damage. *Current Biology*, Vol.10, No. 15, (July 2000), pp. 886-895, ISSN 0960-9822

Polo, S.E. & Jackson, S.P. (2011). Dynamics of DNA damage response proteins at DNA breaks: a focus on protein modifications. *Genes and Development*, Vol.25, No. 5, (March 2011), pp. 409-433, ISSN 0890-9369

Prise, K. & O'Sullivan, J.M. (2009). Radiation-induced bystander signalling in cancer therapy. *Nature Review of Cancer*, Vol.9, No.5, (May 2009), pp. 351-360, ISSN 1474-175X

Roy, K.; Kodama, S., Suzuki, K., Fukase, K. & Watanabe, M. (2000). Hypoxia relieves X-ray-induced delayed effects in normal human embryo cells. *Radiation Research*, Vol.154, No.6, (December 2000), pp. 659-666, ISSN 0033-7587

Shiloh, Y. & Kastan, M.B. (2001). ATM: genome stability, neuronal development, an cancer cross paths. *Advances in Cancer Research*, Vol.83, (January 2001), pp. 209-254, ISSN 0065-230X

Shiloh, Y. (2003). ATM and related protein kinases: safeguarding genome integrity. *Nature Review of Cancer*, Vol.3, No.3, (March 2003), pp. 155-168, ISSN 1474-175X

Singleton, B.K.; Priestley, A., Steingrimsdottir, H., Gell, D., Blunt, T., Jackson, S.P., Lehmann, A.R. & Jeggo, P.A. (1997). Molecular and biochemical characterization of xrs mutants defective in Ku80. *Molecular and Cellular Biology*, Vol.17, No.3, (March 1997), pp. 1264-1273, ISSN 0270-7360

Sonoda, E.; Hochegger, H., Saberi, A., Taniguchi, Y. & Takeda, S. (2006). Differential usage of non-homologous end-joining and homologous recombination in double strand break repair. *DNA Repair*, Vol.5, No.9-10, (September 2006), pp. 1021-2129, ISSN 1568-7864

Sowa Resat, M.B. & Morgan, W.F. (2004). Radiation-induced genomic instability: a role for secreted soluble factors in communicating the radiation response to non-irradiated cells. *Journal of Cell Biochemistry*, Vol.92, No.5, (August 2004), pp. 1013-1019, ISSN 0730-2312

Suzuki, K. (1997). Multistep nature of X-ray-induced neoplastic transformation in mammalian cells: genetic alteration and instability. Journal of Radiation Research, Vol.38, No.1, (March 1997), pp. 55-63, ISSN0449-3060

Suzuki, K.; Ojima, M., Kodama, S. & Watanabe, M. (2003). Radiation-induced DNA damage and delayed induced genomic instability. *Oncogene*, Vol.22, No.45, (October 2003), pp. 6988-6993 ISSN 0950-9232

Suzuki, K.; Yokoyama, S., Waseda, S., Kodama, S. & Watanabe, M. (2003). Delayed reactivation of p53 in the progeny of cells surviving ionizing radiation. *Cancer Research*, Vol.63, No.5, (March 2003), pp. 936-941, ISSN 0008-5472

Suzuki, K.; Okada, H., Yamauchi, M., Oka, Y., Kodama, S. & Watanabe, M. (2006). Qualitative and quantitative analysis of phosphorylated ATM foci induced by low-dose ionizing radiation. *Radiation Research*, Vol.165, No. 5, (May 2006), pp. 499-504, ISSN 0033-7587

Suzuki, K.; Kodama, S. & Watanabe, M. (2009). Role of Ku80-dependent end-joining in delayed genomic instability in mammalian cells surviving ionizing radiation. *Mutation Research*, Vol.683, No.1-2, (January 2009), pp. 29-34, ISSN 0027-5107

Toyokuni, H.; Maruo, A., Suzuki, K. & Watanabe, M. (2009). The contribution of radiation-induced large deletion of the genome to chromosomal instability. *Radiation Research*, Vol.171, No.2, (February 2009), pp. 198-203, ISSN 0033-7587

Tzang, B.S.; Lai, Y.C., Hsu, M., Chang, H.W., Chang, C.C., Huang, P.C. & Liu, Y.C. (1999). Function and sequence analysis of tumor suppressor gene p53 of CHO.K1 cells.*DNA and Cell Biology*, Vol.18, No.4, (April 1999), pp. 315-321, ISSN 1044-5498

van Gent, D.C.; Hoeijmakers, J.H. & Kanaar, R. (2001). Chromosomal stability and the DNA double-stranded break connection. *Nature Review of Genetics*, Vol.2, No.3, (March 2001), pp. 196-206, ISSN 1471-0056

Weterings, E. & Chen, D.J. (2007). DNA-dependent protein kinase in nonhomologous end joining: a lock with multiple keys? The *Journal of Cell Biology*, Vol.179, No. 2, (October 2007), pp. 183-186, ISSN 0021-9525

Wright, E.G. (2007). Microenvironment and genetic factors in haemopoietic radiation responses. *International Journal of Radiation Biology*, Vol.83, No.11-12, (November-December 2007), pp. 813-818, ISSN 0955-3002

Wright, E.G. (2010). Manifestations and mechanisms of non-targeted effects of ionizing radiation. *Mutation Research*, Vol.687, No.1-2, (May 2010), pp. 28-33, ISSN 0027-5107

Wynman, C. & Kannar, R. (2006). DNA double strand break repair: all's well that ends well. *Annual Review of Genetics*, Vol.40, No.1, (December 2006), pp. 363-383, ISSN 0066-4197

Yamauchi, M.; Oka, Y., Yamamoto, M., Niimura, K., Uchida, M., Kodama, S., Watanabe, M., Sekine, I., Yamashita, S. & Suzuki, K. (2008). Growth of persistent foci of DNA damage checkpoint factors is essential for amplification of G1 checkpoint signaling. *DNA Repair*, Vol.7, No.3, (March 2008), pp. 405-17, ISSN 1568-7864

Zdzienicka, M.Z. (1999). Mammalian X-ray-sensitive mutants which are defective in non-homologous (illegitimate) DNA double-strand break repair. *Biochimie*, Vol.81, No.1-2, (January-February 1999), pp. 107-116, ISSN 0300-9084

5

UV Damaged DNA Repair & Tolerance in Plants

Ashwin L. Ganpudi and Dana F. Schroeder
University of Manitoba,
Canada

1. Introduction

In both natural and agricultural conditions, plants are frequently subjected to unfavourable environments, resulting in varying degrees of stress. UV irradiation, drought, heat shock, chilling/freezing, salinity and oxygen deficiency are a few of the major abiotic factors restricting plant growth and development. An important consequence of stratospheric ozone depletion is increased transmission of solar Ultra Violet (UV) radiation through the earth's atmosphere. This increased incidence of UV irradiation causes detrimental effects to all life forms on earth.

1.1 UV irradiation

The spectrum of solar electromagnetic radiation striking the earth's atmosphere ranges from 100 nm to 1 mm. This includes the UV spectrum (100-400 nm), visible spectrum (380-780 nm) and infrared spectrum (700 nm-1 mm). The UV spectrum is further subdivided into three catogories: UV-C (100-280 nm), UV-B (280-315 nm), and UV-A (315-400 nm) (Ballaré, 2003). The shortest of these wavelengths, UV-C, is blocked completely by the ozone layer and atmospheric oxygen. In contrast, UV-A is weakly absorbed and directly transmitted to the earth's surface. Wavelengths in the UV-B range are absorbed efficiently though not completely by ozone, as a very small percentage may pass through holes in the ozone. UV-C is extremely harmful, followed by UV-B, while UV-A has milder effects (Batschauer et al., 1999).

1.2 Plants and UV radiation

Plants, due to their non-motile nature, generally have a higher rate of UV tolerance than animals. Plant secondary metabolites aid in defence against both abiotic and biotic stress factors. Plants are capable of reflecting or absorbing harmful UV rays via thick layers of waxy cutin or submerin on the cell walls and intracellular accumulation of chemical substances such as flavanols or phenolics. The biological effects of UV radiation on plants include altered growth responses, reproductive deformities, epigenetic variations, plant susceptibly to biotic factors, premature senescence, damage to the photosynthetic apparatus, and altered conformation of membrane structures. A wide array of genes were found to be induced upon prolonged exposure to low doses of UV-B in the model plant *Arabidopsis thaliana* (Frohnmeyer & Staiger, 2003; Mackerness, 2000; Ries et al., 2000). Upregulated transcripts include: antioxidant/free radical scavenging enzymes, proteins involved in: DNA repair, translation, E3 ligase system, cell cycle, signal transduction, and secondary metabolites, as well as several other genes with unknown function (Brosché et al., 2002; Jansen et al., 2008). UV-B also results in numerous changes in plant morphology. This signalling cascade is well reviewed elsewhere (Jenkins, 2009). Here we focus on plant responses to UV-induced DNA damage.

1.3 UV induced DNA damage

UV-C/B radiation is directly absorbed by DNA, inducing lesions which inhibit vital cellular functions such as transcription and DNA replication. UV-A is comparatively less efficient in lesion induction but triggers the production of reactive oxygen species (ROS) (Kunz et al., 2006). The primary UV induced DNA lesions include cyclobutane pyrimidine dimers (adjacent pyrimidines covalently linked between C-5 and C-6 carbon atoms) and secondary lesions 6-4 pyrimidine-pyrimidone photoproducts (6-4 PP) (covalent linkage between the C-4 position of a pyrimidine to the C-6 position of an adjacent pyrimidine) (Fig. 1). In order to respond to this damage, plants employ specific mechanisms (Britt, 1999). In light conditions, photoreactivation catalyses dimer monomerizations while during dark conditions, Nucleotide Excision Repair (NER) excises these helix-distorting lesions. Finally, residual lesions are bypassed via translesion synthesis (TLS).

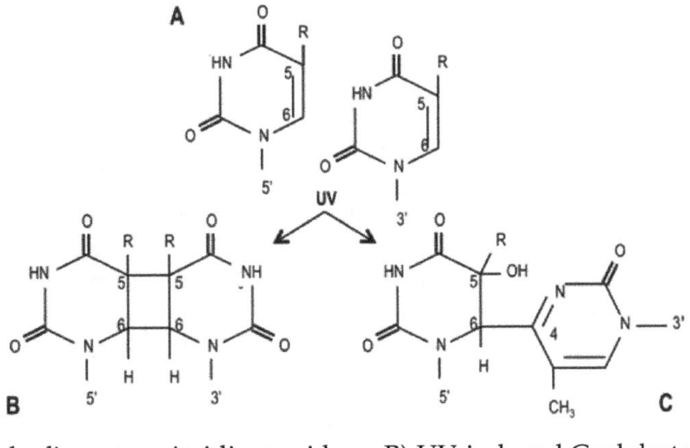

Fig. 1. A) Normal adjacent pyrimidine residues. B) UV-induced Cyclobutane Pyrimidine Dimer (CPD) and C) 6-4 Pyrimidine-Pyrimidone photoproduct (6-4 PP).

2. Photoreactivation

Photoreactivation is a blue light dependant DNA repair mechanism catalysed by the photolyase (E.C 4.1.99.3) class of enzymes. Pyrimidine dimers are split by the action of two photoactive damage specific DNA repair enzymes - CPD photolyase and 6-4 PP photolyase. Both classes of photolyase require two co-factors, one being the two electron reduced form of Flavin Adenine Dinucleotide (FAD) and the second chromophore, a blue light harvesting photoantenna, being either 5,10- methenyltretrahydrofolate (MTHF) or 8-hydroxy-7,8-didemethyl-5-deazariboflavin (8-HDF). FAD is an essential co-factor for regulating DNA binding and repair. In contrast, the second chromophore has a higher extinction co-efficient and an absorption maximum at longer wavelengths, hence regulates the rate of repair depending on the external light intensity. MTHF or 8-HDF absorbs the photoreactivating blue light photons and transfers this excitation energy to the reduced FAD. The $FADH^-$ in turn transfers electrons to the lesions, catalyzing the cleavage of the cyclobutane rings and dimer monomerization (Deisenhofer, 2000; Sancar, 2003, 2008). Multiple sequence alignment reveals that conserved homology between prokaryotic and eukaryotic CPD photolyases is limited to the C-terminal FAD binding site. It has been suggested that a common ancestor gave rise to both type I and type II photolyases but diverged at an early evolutionary stage (Yasui et al., 1994). CPD photolyases have been classified into Class I (microbial) and Class II (higher eukaryotes excluding placental mammals) groups, respectively. The 6–4 photolyases from *Drosophila* and *Arabidopsis* have strong sequence similarity to class I CPD photolyases (Nakajima et al., 1998; Todo et al., 1996). Similarly cryptochromes, the plant blue light photoreceptors, are 30% similar to the class I microbial photolyases, but demonstrate no photolyase activity (Ahmad & Cashmore, 1993). Thus, microbial Class I CPD photolyases, eukaryotic 6–4 photolyases, and blue light photoreceptors constitute the class I photolyase/photoreceptor family.

Genes encoding CPD photolyases and 6-4 PP photolyases have been identified and characterized in a range of prokaryotic and eukaryotic systems (Sancar, 2003). In plants genes encoding CPD photolyases have been identified in *Arabidopsis thaliana (*Ahmed et al., 1997*)*, cucumber (Takahashi et al., 2002), rice (Hirouchi et al., 2003), spinach (Yoshihara et al., 2005), and soybean (Yamamoto et al., 2008). Genes encoding 6-4 PP photolyases have been identified in *Arabidopsis* and rice (Chen et al., 1994; Singh et al., 2010). In *Arabidopsis,* the highest levels of both photolyases are associated with floral tissues, which may presumably serve to minimize lesions in germline cells. While expression of the CPD photolyase is light/UV-B regulated, 6-4 PP photolyase is constitutively expressed (Takahashi et al., 2002; Waterworth et al., 2002). The *Arabidopsis* CPD photolyase gene (*AtPHR1*) encodes a class II CPD photolyase. An *Arabidopsis* mutant (*uvr2*) lacking this gene is hypersensitive to UV. AtPHR1 is efficient in CPD photoreactivation but deficient in 6-4 photoproduct repair (Ahmed et al., 1997; Landry et al., 1997). *AtPHR1* is upregulated several fold in a UV insensitive mutant of *Arabidopsis* (*uvi1*) irrespective of light conditions, conferring constitutive protection (Tanaka et al., 2002). Overexpression of CPD photolyase in *Arabidopsis* and rice resulted in enhanced CPD removal (Hidema et al., 2007; Kaiser et al., 2009; Ueda et al., 2005). Genetic complementation of photolyase deficient *E.coli* strains with soybean, rice, spinach and *Arabidopsis* CPD photolyase genes restored photoreactivation activity (Yamamoto et al., 2007, 2008; Yoshihara et al., 2005). CPD photolyase activity in *Arabidopsis* (Pang & Hays, 1991; Waterworth et al., 2002), soybean (Yamamoto et al., 2008) and rice (Hidema et al., 2000) has been reported to be temperature sensitive. Rice CPD photolyase, encoded by a single copy gene in the nuclear genome, translocates to chloroplasts, mitochondria and nuclei to repair UV-induced CPDs in all three genomes (Takahashi et al., 2011), a phenomenon not observed in spinach chloroplasts (Hada et al., 2000) or young *Arabidopsis* seedlings (Chen et al., 1996). However, upon exposure to photoreactivating blue light, *Arabidopsis* seedlings did exhibit efficient repair of CPDs in the extracellular organelles (Draper & Hays, 2000). The *Arabidopsis* 6-4 PP photolyase, encoded by the *UVR3* gene, encodes a 62 kDa protein with 45% identity to *Drosophila* 6-4 PP photolyase and 17% identity to the Class II CPD photolyases. AtUVR3 is proficient in 6-4 photoproduct removal but deficient in CPD repair. Both *uvr2* and *uvr3* are nonsense mutations, and the double mutants are extremely sensitive to UV relative to the single mutants (Nakajima et al., 1998). Photolyases appear to be the sole repair mechanism active in non-proliferating plant tissues (Kimura et al., 2004). Hence, photolyases play an important role in plant repair of UV damaged DNA.

3. Nucleotide excision repair

Nucleotide excision repair (NER) is a light independent repair process involving a series of reactions: initial damaged DNA recognition, DNA unwinding, dual incision bracketing the lesion, repair synthesis and final ligation to seal the repaired site. NER initiates with specific sub-pathways for transcriptionally active (Transcription Coupled Repair (TC-NER)) or silent (Global Genomic Repair (GG-NER)) DNA. TC-NER and GG-NER exhibit different damage recognition strategies followed by a common repair pathway (Gillet & Scharer, 2006) (Fig. 2). Defects in human NER genes result in the photosensitive syndromes Xeroderma pigmentosum (XP) or Cockayne syndrome (CS). Eight genetic complementation groups for XP have been identified (XPA-G, V) as well as two for CS (CSA and CSB). While XP-V mutation uniquely results in defects in translesion synthesis, XP -A, -B, -D, -F, and -G mutation results in both TC-NER and GG-NER defects, while XP –C and -E mutation results in GG-NER defects only. CSA and CSB mutation results exclusively in TC-NER defects (Hoeijmakers, 2001; Svejstrup, 2002). Bioinformatic analysis of the plant NER protein machinery suggests the molecular mechanisms are largely but not entirely conserved with that of the extensively studied yeast *S. cerevisiae* and mammalian cells (Kimura & Sakaguchi, 2006; Kunz et al., 2005, 2006). NER in plants has been studied primarily in rice and *Arabidopsis* (Singh et al., 2010). Many *Arabidopsis* NER related genes were initially isolated by analysis of UV hypersensitive (*uvh*) and UV repair defective (*uvr*) mutants which were subsequently mapped to homologues of the human XP genes (Table 1).

3.1 Global genomic repair
3.1.1 Damage recognition
3.1.1.1 DDB1 & DDB2

In mammalian systems, damage detection in the GG-NER pathway involves UV-Damaged DNA Binding protein 1 and 2 (DDB1 and DDB2) followed by the XPC-HR23B-CEN2 complex. In humans DDB2 complements the *XPE* mutation and plays a role in recognition of the UV-induced lesion, while DDB1 is required for high affinity interaction of the DDB1-DDB2 complex (Groisman et al., 2003; Luijsterburg et al., 2007; Rapic-Otrin et al., 2002). *S. pombe* Ddb1 knockouts result in chromosomal segregation defects, UV sensitivity and slow S phase progression leading to defects in meiosis (Holmberg et al., 2005). DDB1 and DDB2 homologues have been identified in rice, where they are UV-induced in proliferating tissues (Ishibashi et al., 2003). *Arabidopsis thaliana* encodes two homologs of DDB1 - DDB1A and DDB1B. These proteins are 91% identical with redundant function. Although *ddb1b* null alleles appear lethal, a viable partial loss of function allele exhibits no developmental or UV sensitive phenotypes (Bernhardt et al., 2010; Schroeder et al., 2002). Overexpression of DDB1A in *Arabidopsis* confers enhanced UV resistance and *ddb1a* knockouts exhibit mild UV sensitivity (Al Khateeb & Schroeder, 2009; Molinier et al., 2008). *AtDDB2* encodes a 48 kDa nuclear localized protein with upregulated expression upon UV-induction. *AtDDB2* loss of function results in UV sensitivity while overexpression increases UV tolerance (Biedermann & Hellmann, 2010; Koga et al., 2006; Molinier et al., 2008).

3.1.1.2 Cullin based E3 ligases

The 127 kDa DDB1 homologs function as substrate adaptors for CULLIN4 based E3 ubiquitin (Ub) ligases (Groisman et al., 2003). E3 Ub ligases are multimeric complexes that add ubiquitin moieties to target proteins and contain CULLIN proteins as scaffolding

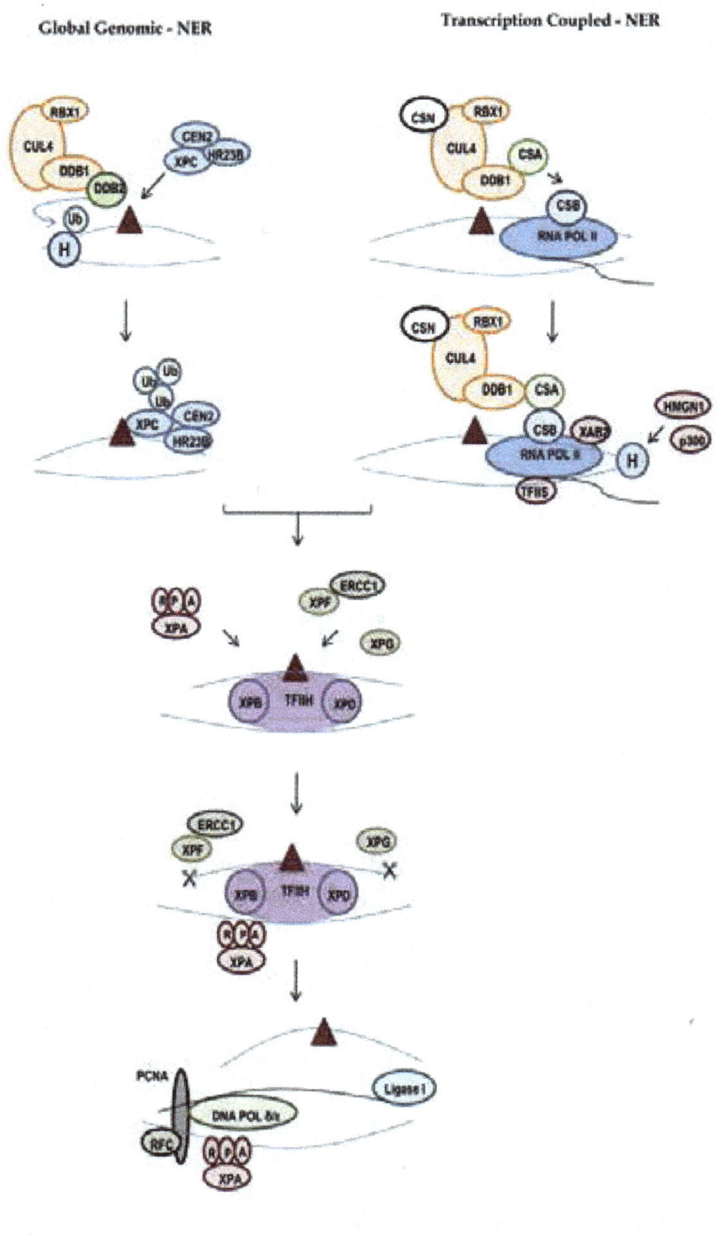

Fig. 2. Overview of mammalian nucleotide excision repair. In GG-NER, DDB2-CUL4 mediated histone (H) and XPC ubiquitination facilitates lesion binding. In TC-NER, stalled RNA POL II recruits CSB and the CSA-CUL4-CSN complex, followed by recruitment of other TC-NER specific factors. In both cases, NER core players follow suit: XPB and XPD helicases of the TFIIH complex, XPF-ERCC1 and XPG endonucleases, and the ssDNA binding XPA-RPA complex. The fragment encompassing the lesion is excised, followed by repair synthesis and ligation. Repair synthesis requires DNA POL δ/ε in concert with accessory proteins PCNA, RFC and RPA. See text for details.

subunits (Hua & Vierstra, 2011). CUL4 based E3 ubiquitin ligases consist of three core subunits: CULLIN4 (CUL4), RING finger protein REGULATOR OF CULLINS1 (ROC1)/RING-BOX1 (RBX1), and DDB1. The CUL4 - RBX1 - DDB1 complex interacts with a large number of proteins containing WD40 motifs referred to as DCAF proteins (DDB1-CUL4 Associated Factor) or DWD proteins (DDB1 binding WD40 proteins) (Lee & Zhou, 2007). DDB2 is an example of a WD40 domain containing DCAF protein. WD40 motifs are characterized by 40 amino acid repeats initiated by a glycine-histidine dipeptide and terminated by a tryptophan-aspartate (WD) dipeptide facilitating protein-protein interactions. DDB1 is composed of three β propeller domains (BPA, BPB and BPC) and DDB2, in addition to the WD40 domain, contains a helix loop helix (HLX) segment in the N terminal. While the clam shaped BPA-BPC of DDB1 mediates interaction with the HLX motif of DDB2 and other DCAF substrates, BPB exhibits exclusive interactions with CUL4 (Scrima et al., 2008).

AtCUL4 is a 91 kDa protein with a conserved CH motif and an extended N terminal region of 65 amino acids that shares close sequence similarity to its human/mouse orthologs. *AtCUL4* loss of function results in abnormal plant development (Bernhardt et al., 2006; Chen et al., 2006) and UV sensitivity (Molinier et al., 2008). Examples of DCAF proteins interacting with the *Arabidopsis* CUL4–DDB1A/B complex include AtDDB2 (Bernhardt et al., 2006), AtCSA-1&2 (Biedermann & Hellmann, 2010; Zhang et al., 2010), as well as the negative regulator of photomorphogenesis DET1 (De-etiolated1) (Schroeder et al., 2002), and many other DWD proteins (Lee et al., 2008). Recent results have shed light on the cross talk between photomorphogenesis regulation and repair of UV damaged DNA. HY5, a positive regulator of photomorphogenesis, has been shown to regulate gene sets connected to UV tolerance, such as the *UVR3* and *PHR1* photolyases, as well as secondary metabolite transcriptional regulators (Oravecz et al., 2006; Ulm et al., 2004). DET1, initially identified as a nuclear localized negative regulator of photomorphogenesis, exhibits a constitutively light grown phenotype in addition to increased levels of flavanoids (Pepper et al., 1994). Recent papers show that *det1* mutants exhibit enhanced UV tolerance through increased levels of secondary metabolites reflecting/absorbing UV irradiation as well as by upregulation of photolyase genes. Further it appears that DET1 protein dosage influences UV sensitivity of plants as DET1 overexpressing lines exhibit increased UV sensitivity (Castells et al., 2010, 2011).

3.1.1.3 Histone ubiquitination facilitates NER machinery entry

In mammals, in the absence of UV irradiation, DDB2-DDB1-CUL4-RBX1 (DDB2 complex) was found to be associated with the COP9 Signalosome complex (CSN). CSN shares significant structural homology with the 19S lid of 26S proteosome. The CSN deconjugates neddylation (Nedd8) from CULLINs, thereby regulating the activation, stability or the disassembly of CULLIN based E3 ligase activity (Parry & Estelle, 2004; Schwechheimer & Deng, 2001). The DDB2 - CSN complex show no ubiquitin ligase activity, but upon UV irradiation, these complexes disassociate in parallel with increased neddylation and activation of CUL4 (Groisman et al., 2003). Core histone proteins have been identified as potential targets for DDB2-DDB1-CUL4-RBX1 mediated proteosomal degradation. Kapetanaki et al. (2006) and Wang et al. (2006) describe the ubiquitination of H2A, H3 and H4 histone proteins. Reduction of histone H3 and H4 ubiquitination by knockdown of *cul4* impairs recruitment of the repair protein XPC to the damaged foci and inhibits the repair process. Thus biochemical studies indicate that DDB-CUL4-RBX1-mediated histone

Human	Yeast	Function	ATG no.	Arabidopsis
Photoreactivation:				
ND	*ND*	6-4 PP Photolyase	At3g15620	*UVR3*
ND	*PHR1*	Class II CPD Photolyase	At1g12370	*PHR1/UVR2*
Nucleotide Excision Repair:				
DDB1	*ND*	Substrate adaptor for CUL4. Interacts with DCAF proteins	At4g05420 At4g21100	*AtDDB1a* *AtDDB1b*
DDB2/XPE	*ND*	Damaged DNA binding (DCAF)	At5g58760	*AtDDB2*
CUL4	*CUL4*	Scaffolding subunit of E3 Ub ligase	At5g46210	*AtCUL4*
XPC	*RAD4*	GG-NER damage recognition	At5g16630	*AtXPC*
HR23B	*RAD23*	Binds to XPC	At1g79650 At1g16190 At3g02540 At5g38470	*AtRAD23A* *AtRAD23B* *AtRAD23C* *AtRAD23D*
CEN2	*CEN2*	Stabilizes XPC-HR23B complex	At3g50360	*AtCEN2*
XPB	*RAD25*	Subunit of TFIIH. 3′->5′ helicase	At5g41370 At5g41360	*AtXPB1* *AtXPB2*
XPD	*RAD3*	Subunit of TFIIH. 5′->3′ helicase	At1g03190	*AtXPD/UVH6*
GTF2H1 *GTF2H2* *GTF2H3* *GTF2H4* *GTF2H5*	*TFB1* *SSL1* *TFB4* *TFB2* *TFB5*	Core TFIIH subunits	At1g55750 At3g61420 At1g05055 At1g18340 At4g17020 At1g12400 At1g62886	*AtTFB1-1* *AtTFB1-2* *Atp44* *AtTFB4* *AtTFB2* *AtTFB5-1* *AtTFB5-2*
XPA	*RAD14*	ssDNA binding	ND	*ND*
XPG	*RAD2*	3′ endonuclease	At3g28030	*AtXPG/UVH3*
ERCC1	*RAD10*	5′ endonuclease with XPF	At3g05210	*AtERCC1/UVR7*
XPF	*RAD1*	5′ endonuclease with ERCC1	At5g41150	*AtXPF/UVH1*
PCNA	*PCNA*	RFC dependant sliding clamp	At1g07370 At2g29570	*AtPCNA1* *AtPCNA2*
RFC1 *RFC2* *RFC3* *RFC4* *RFC5*	*RFC1* *RFC2* *RFC3* *RFC4* *RFC5*	DNA-dependent ATPase required for DNA replication and repair	At5g22010 At1g21690 At1g77470 At1g63160 At5g27740	*AtRFC1* *AtRFC2* *AtRFC3* *AtRFC4* *AtRFC5*
RPA70 *RPA32* *RPA14*	*RFA1* *RFA2* *RFA3*	ssDNA binding protein required for architectural role in dual lesion incision and repair synthesis	At2g06510 At4g19130 At5g08020 At5g45400 At5g61000 At2g24490 At3g02920 At3g52630 At4g18590	*AtRPA70A* *AtRPA70B* *AtRPA70C* *AtRPA70D* *AtRPA70E* *AtRPA32A* *AtRPA32B* *AtRPA14A* *AtRPA14B*
CSA	*RAD28*	TC-NER specific DCAF protein	At1g27840 At1g19750	*AtCSA1A* *AtCSA1B*

Human	Yeast	Function	ATG no.	Arabidopsis
CSB	*RAD26*	SWI/SNF2 like ATPase	At2g18760	*AtCSB*
XAB2	*SYF1*	Complex stabilization	At5g28740	*AtXAB2*
TFIIS	*TFIIS*	TC-NER elongation factor	At2g38560	*AtTFIIS*
HMGN1	*ND*	Nucleosome binding	ND	*ND*
EP300/CBP	*ND*	Histone acetyl transferase	At1g79000 At1g67220 At1g55970 At3g12980 At1g16710	*HAC1* *HAC2* *HAC4* *HAC5* *HAC12*
Translesion Synthesis				
POLH/XPV	*RAD30*	Y-family DNA polymerase	At5g44740	*AtPOLH*
REV1	*REV1*	Y-family DNA polymerase	At5g44750	*AtREV1*
POLZ	*REV3*	B-family DNA polymerase	At1g67500	*AtREV3*
REV7	*REV7*	REV3 accessory subunit	At1g16590	*AtREV7*
POLK	*ND*	Y-family DNA polymerase	At1g49980	*AtPOLK*

Table 1. Genes involved in UV damaged DNA repair and tolerance. ND=not detected.

ubiquitination weakens the interaction between histones and DNA to further facilitate the recruitment of repair proteins to damaged DNA (Guerrero-Santoro et al., 2008; Higa et al., 2006). The activated DDB2 complex recruits XPC via protein-protein interactions, followed by ubiquitination of XPC and DDB2. Polyubiquitinated DDB2 exhibits reduced affinity for damaged DNA and is subsequently displaced from the damaged foci, whereas polyubiquitinated XPC enhances its binding to DNA (Sugasawa et al., 2005). In *Arabidopsis,* DDB2 turnover is abrogated in *cul4, ddb1a, atr* and *det1* mutants suggesting that ATR and DET1 may co-operate with the CUL4-DDB1 E3 ligase complex in regulating NER (Castells et al., 2011; Molinier et al., 2008).

3.1.1.4 XPC-HR23B-CEN2

The next step in GG-NER involves the homologous heterodimers hXPC-hHR23B (in Humans) and RAD4-RAD23 (in yeast). In addition to hXPC-hHR23B, Araki et al. (2001) identified hCEN2, a Ca^{2+} binding protein contributing to the stability of the hXPC-hHR23B complex. Hence in mammalian systems the identified protein recognition complex is hXPC-hHR23B-hCEN2, however neither hHR23B nor hCEN2 bind to damaged DNA but enhance both the affinity and specificity of hXPC binding to damaged DNA (Fitch et al., 2003; Nishi et al., 2005). AtCEN2 shares 49% identity with hCEN2, *Atcen2* mutants are UV sensitive, and AtCEN2 overexpression resulted in enhanced repair. Upon UV irradiation, AtCEN2 level increases and it rapidly translocates to the nucleus. AtCEN2-AtXPC interaction in *Arabidopsis thaliana* has also been demonstrated (Liang et al., 2006; Molinier et al., 2004). Potential homologs of HR23B/RAD23 have been identified in *Arabidopsis thaliana, Oryza sativa* and *Daucus carota* (Schultz & Quatrano, 1997; Sturm & Leinhard, 1998). The *Arabidopsis* genome has 4 loci encoding RAD23 homologs (RAD23a, RAD23b, RAD23c, RAD23d), and although mutants exhibit multiple pleotrophic developmental defects (Farmer et al., 2010), UV sensitivity or complex interactions with the *Arabidopsis* NER machinery have not yet been reported.

3.1.2 DNA unwinding complex assembly

Following recognition, the damaged region is unwound by the TFIIH transcription factor which joins the XPC-CEN2-HR23B complex. TFIIH is a complex of 10 proteins, seven of which are players in the NER pathway (helicases XPB and XPD, p62, p44, p34, p52, and p8). The last five proteins are encoded by GTF2H1, GTF2H2, GTF2H3, GTF2H4, GTF2H5 (Frit et al., 1999). TFIIH not only participates in NER of transcriptionally active and inactive DNA, but also in RNA POL II dependant transcription, cell cycle control and regulation of nuclear receptor activity (Chen & Suter, 2003). ATP dependant 5′->3′ and 3′->5′ helicase activities associated with XPD/RAD3 and XPB/RAD25 respectively unwind the DNA encompassing the lesion with the concomitant release of the recognition complex. Human XPB and the corresponding yeast RAD25 knockouts are lethal. *Arabidopsis thaliana,* unlike the sugarcane, rice or mammalian genomes, encodes two homologs of XPB - AtXPB1 and AtXPB2. These proteins are 95% identical with redundant functions and are expressed constitutively throughout plant development (Morgante et al., 2005; Ribeiro et al., 1998). Despite this redundancy, *xpb1* mutants exhibit delayed germination and flowering phenotypes but are not UV sensitive (Costa et al., 2001). Phenotypes of *Arabidopsis xpb2* or double mutants have not yet been reported. *Arabidopsis* XPD is 56% and 50% identical to human and yeast sequences. *Arabidopsis XPD/RAD3* null mutations are lethal, however viable point mutation alleles are UV sensitive and were identified as *uvh6* (*uv hypersensitive 6*) mutants. (Jenkins et al., 1997; Liu et al., 2003). Another component of the of TFIIH complex, p44, was identified in *Arabidopsis* as ATGTF2H2 and was found to interact in vivo with AtXPD (Vonarx et al., 2006).

3.1.3 Endonuclease recruitment following unwinding

TFIIH further recruits additional factors such as XPA and heterotrimeric Replication Protein A (RPA), composed of 70, 32 and 14 kDa subunits, to promote and stabilize the formation of an open intermediate essential for the dual incision by XPG and XPF-ERCC1 (Excision Repair Complementing defective repair in Chinese hamster 1) (RAD1/RAD10) endonucleases at the 3′ and 5′ sites respectively (Tapais et al., 2004). The RPA-XPA complex exhibits interactions with both endonucleases (He et al., 1995; Wold, 1997), however the specific function of XPA is still not evident. Initially it was thought to function as a lesion recognition complex in concert with XPC, but was later determined to be recruited after TFIIH entry and facilitate XPC complex departure (Hey et al., 2002; Volker et al., 2001). In addition, XPA homologues do not exist in plants (Kunz et al., 2005). The dual incisions catalyzed by the endonucleases excise oligonucleotides of about 20-30 bases containing the lesion (Reidl et al., 2003).

Potential homologs of ERCC1, XPF, XPG and RPA have been identified in plants. Although ERCC1 was first cloned from male germ line cells of *Lilium longiforum,* southern blots confirmed the presence of ERCC1 across diverse plant species such as *A. thaliana, B. napus, Z. mays, L. esculentum, N. tobacum,* and *O. sativa* (Xu et al., 1998). Hefner et al. (2003) mapped the *Arabidopsis uvr7* mutant to *AtERCC1. Atercc1* knockouts are phenotypically normal in contrast to the lethal mammalian counterparts (Weeda et al., 1997). *Atercc1* mutants are extremely sensitive to DNA damaging chemicals such as mitomycin and ionizing agents such as UV and γ - radiation (Hefner et al., 2003). More recent studies in *Arabidopsis* indicate significant roles of *AtERCC1* in concert with *AtXPF* in homologous recombination and chromosomal stability (Dubest et al., 2002, 2004; Vannier et al., 2009). Gallego et al. (2000) and Liu et al. (2000) characterized the single copy AtXPF which is 37% and 29% identical to human XPF and *S. cerevisiae* RAD1 respectively. *AtXPF* is homogenously expressed, was mapped to the *uvh1* mutant in *Arabidopsis,* and partially complements the yeast *rad1* mutant (Gallego et al., 2000). *AtXPF* point mutations result in sensitivity to ionizing radiation and mitomycin C, and impaired removal of photoproducts (Fidanstef et al., 2000; Vonarx et al., 2002). *AtXPG* was mapped to the *UVH3* locus and knockouts result in UV sensitivity as well as premature senescence and reduced seed production (Liu et al., 2001). The *XPG* rice homolog, *OsSEND-1,* exhibits upregulated mRNA levels in response to UV and DNA damaging agents (Furukawa et al., 2003a).

ssDNA binding RPA proteins in plants were first identified in rice (Ishibashi et al., 2001). Unlike most eukaryotic organisms, *Arabidopsis* and rice possess multiple copies of the RPA homologs. In addition to participating in DNA repair, RPA proteins play a role in homologous recombination and DNA replication in humans and yeast (Sakaguchi et al., 2009). The rice genome encodes three OsRPA70 (OsRPA70A, OsRPA70B, OsRPA70C), three OsRPA32 (OsRPA32-1, OsRPA32-2, OsRPA32-3) and one OsRPA14. *In vivo* interactions in rice confirms three different complex formations: OsRPA70A-OsRPA32-2-OsRPA14 (Type1); OsRPA70B-OsRPA32-1-OsRPA14 (Type2); and OsRPA70C-OsRPa32-3-OsRPA14 (Type3). Subcellular localization of all three OsRPA32 was detected in both the nucleus and chloroplasts. OsRPA70A was only in the chloroplast whereas OsRPA70B and OsRPA70C were exclusively to the nucleus. This data suggest that while the Type1 complex may participate in chloroplast DNA repair, Type2 and Type3 complexes concentrate on nuclear DNA repair (Ishibashi et al., 2006). OsRPA70A and OsRPa70B share only 33% sequence homology and exhibit differences in expression pattern (Ishibashi et al., 2001). A T-DNA insertion in *OsRPA70A* resulted in partial male sterility, complete female sterility and hypersensitivity to DNA mutagens (Chang et al., 2009). OsRPA32 protein abundance is regulated by both UV irradiation and cell cycle phase (Marwedal et al., 2002). *Arabidopsis,* on the other hand, encodes five putative RPA70 genes and two copies each of RPA32 and RPA14 (Shultz et al., 2007). *Arabidopsis* RPA70A interacts preferentially with AtRPA32A rather than AtRPA32B. Knockouts of both AtRPA70A and AtRPA70B exhibited UV sensitivity when irradiated, but exhibited wildtype characteristics under normal conditions (Ishibashi et al., 2005; Takashi et al., 2009).

3.1.4 Repair synthesis and ligation

In mammals, the gap formed by the excision is filled via PCNA (Proliferating Cell Nuclear Antigen) and RFC dependant DNA synthesis by DNA POL δ/ε. These components are likely recruited by XPG and RPA as RFC exhibits interaction with RPA (Yuzhakov et al., 1999). RFC catalyzes the ATP dependant loading of PCNA to DNA at the 3′ OH. PCNA is a homotrimeric protein which forms a sliding clamp-like complex (Gulbis et al., 1996) and interacts with the DNA POL to ensure replication occurs processively (Mocquet et al., 2008). The final phase of NER is completed by phosphodiester backbone rejoining of the repaired DNA strand by DNA Ligase I.

Although PCNA and RFC homologues have been identified in plants, their specific role in nucleotide excision repair has not yet been elucidated (Furukawa et al., 2003b; Strzalka & Ziemienowicz, 2011). Recently, Roy et al. (2011) cloned and characterized a homolog of mammalian DNA POLλ in *Arabidopsis.* AtPOLλ was upregulated upon UV induction under dark conditions, and *Atpolλ* mutants exhibited UV sensitivity and decreased DNA repair. Thus, this report suggests a role for DNA POLλ in plant NER.

3.2 Transcription coupled repair

The emerging picture of mammalian TC-NER is of a complex mechanism requiring two essential assembly factors (CSA and CSB), certain TC-NER specific proteins (P300, HMGN1, XAB2 and TFIIS), as well as core NER proteins. UV induced DNA damage is initially recognised by RNA POL II, which stalls when it encounters helix-distorting lesions on the template strand during transcription. Stalled RNA POL II backtracks a few nucleotides and is recognised by the CSB protein which in turn co-ordinates the recruitment of the repair factors required to accomplish Transcription Coupled NER (Mellon, 2005).

Cloning and characterization of the mammalian CSB gene revealed a nuclear protein of 168 kDa with a region of homology to the SWI2/SNF2 family of helicases. CSB has been shown to interact with RNA POL II and this interaction is enhanced and prolonged by UV exposure (van den Boom et al., 2004). Studies propose that functional CSB in the absence of UV could also serve as a component of the transcriptional machinery promoting elongation (Fousteri & Mullenders, 2008; Hanawalt & Spivak, 2008). Further, CSB facilitates the entry of the core NER factors XPA, XPG and TFIIH through complex interactions (Laine & Egly, 2006; Saxowsky & Doetsch, 2006; Svejstrup, 2002). Mammalian CSA on the other hand is a 46 kDa DWD protein containing seven WD40 repeats that associates with DDB1-CUL4 type E3 ligases and is recruited to the damaged site after CSB. CSA physically interacts with the CSB-RNA POL II complex in a UV dependant manner (Groisman et al., 2003; Fousteri et al., 2006). Interestingly, unlike the DDB2 complex, the CSA-CUL4 Ub ligase complex is active under normal conditions but is rapidly inactivated upon UV irradiation by CSN. Hence CSN plays a differential and dynamic role in regulating both pathways of Nucleotide Excision Repair. The stable CSN-CSA-CSB complex is required for the recruitment of the other NER factors. Following repair, CSN dissociates, reactivating CSA Ub ligase activity and resulting in CSB degradation. Clearance of CSB is required for the reinitiation of transcription by RNA POL II (Groisman et al., 2003, 2006).

Several papers over the years propose the fate of RNA POL II during the coupling process: either ubiquitinated and degraded, translocated or bypassed from the lesion site, or simply stalled during the entire repair process, is still a matter of debate (Reviewed in Tornaletti, 2009). XAB2 (XPA binding protein 2) is a RNA-binding protein with 15 tetratricopeptide repeats. In addition to interacting with XPA, XAB2 is capable of interacting with CSA, CSB and RNA POL II (Nakatsu et al., 2000). XAB2 is thought to stabilize protein assemblies by functioning as a scaffolding subunit. XAB2 knockouts in mammalian cells exhibit hypersensitivity and decreased recovery of mRNA synthesis post UV irradiation (Kuraoka et al., 2008). Increased amounts of histone acetyl transferase p300 and High Mobility Group Nucleosome binding domain containing protein 1 (HMGN1) interact with RNA POL II in a CSB-dependant manner upon UV irradiation but exhibit weak interactions under normal conditions (Fousteri et al., 2006). Both HMGN1 and p300 are nucleosome interacting proteins which remodel the chromatin structure behind the arrested polymerase and facilitating the backward translocation of RNA POL II (Hanawalt & Spivak, 2008). TFIIS, functioning as a transcription elongation factor, stimulates the arrested RNA POL II to restart elongation. This TFIIS-RNA POL II interaction is significantly increased upon UV irradiation (Fousteri et al., 2006). Hence it is proposed that TFIIS facilitates resumption of transcription post DNA lesion removal in a CSA/B-dependent manner.

Elucidation of the TC-NER mechanism in plants is still at its infancy. While there is no plant homologue for HMGN1, the *Arabidopsis* genome encodes homologues of XAB2,

TFIIS, and five p300/CBP homologues, however the role of these genes in DNA repair has not been assessed (Grasser et al., 2009; Kunz et al., 2005; Pandey et al., 2002). Only recently was the homolog of human CSA cloned and characterized in *Arabidopsis*. In contrast to mammalian systems, the *Arabidopsis* genome encodes two homologs of CSA - AtCSA1A and AtCSA1B, 92% identical DWD proteins with overlapping subcellular localization and expression patterns. These proteins exist as heterotetramers in planta and are capable of interacting with the DDB1-CUL4 E3 complex. Knockouts of either gene result in UV sensitivity and decreased photoproduct removal (Zhang et al., 2010). Concurrently, another group overexpressed AtCSA1A, which surprisingly also resulted in increased UV sensitivity. This result is hypothesised to be due to competition between CSA and with other DWD proteins to interact with the DDB1-CUL4 complex. Interestingly AtCSA1A levels remained constant upon UV induction (Biedermann & Hellmann, 2010). RNAi of a putative *Arabidopsis* CSB homolog resulted in a UV sensitive phenotype (Shaked et al., 2006). Hence, taken as a whole, these results confirm the role of the CUL4-DDB1-CSA and CSB pathway in plants.

4. Translesion synthesis

Despite the available repair mechanisms, there are times when UV damage persists and DNA replication proceeds past UV lesions via translesion synthesis (TLS). This synthesis proceeds via one of several DNA polymerases: Polη, Rev1, Polζ, Polκ or Polι. Polη (eta) is encoded by the *POLH* locus in humans and is homologous to yeast RAD30. Polη performs error-free bypass of CPDs, and loss of function results in increased mutation and xeroderma pigmentosa (XP-V) in humans. REV1 exhibits dCMP transferase activity but is required for 6-4 PP bypass independent of this activity, suggesting its role may be in recruitment of other polymerases. Polζ is composed of REV3 and REV7 and exhibits error prone repair. REV3 is a B-family polymerase (unlike the other TLS polymerases which are all Y-family polymerases) and REV7 an accessory subunit that enhances REV3 activity (Waters et al., 2009). Polκ activity is specific to N2-dG lesions in both animals and plants, while plants do not have a Polι homologue (Garcia-Diaz & Bebenek, 2007; Garcia-Ortiz et al., 2007).

Homologues of REV1, REV3 and REV7 as well as Polη have been identified in *Arabidopsis* (Sakamoto et al., 2003; Santiago et al., 2006; Takahashi et al., 2005). Mutant alleles of *REV3, REV1* and *REV7* all result in UV sensitivity, although *rev1* only weakly and *rev7* only to long-term UV exposure (Sakamoto et al., 2003; Takahashi et al., 2005). Interestingly, AtREV1 cannot insert nucleotides across from UV-induced DNA lesions, suggesting that its role is primarily in the recruitment of other TLS polymerases (Takahashi et al., 2007). The UV sensitivity of the *rev1 rev3* double mutant is similar to that of *rev3*, additional evidence that the role of REV1 may be in REV3 recruitment (Takahashi et al., 2005). Analysis of mutation frequency in *rev1* and *rev3* mutants shows a reduction relative to wildtype rate, evidence that these genes contribute to error-prone repair (Nakagawa et al., 2011).

Polη is encoded by the *Arabidopsis POLH* gene. The *POLH* transcript is ubiquitously expressed and alternatively spliced, and AtPolη exhibits similar levels of activity *in vitro* as the human protein (Hoffman et al., 2008; Santiago et al., 2008a, 2009). *AtPOLH* overexpression results in increased UV tolerance, while *AtPOLH* loss of function results in weak UV sensitivity, but enhances the sensitivity of the *rev3* mutant, evidence that Polη is acting independently of Polζ (Curtis & Hays, 2007; Santiago et al., 2008b). *POLH* mutants exhibit an increased mutation frequency, indicating a role in error-free repair. Interestingly, this increased mutation rate is suppressed in the *rev3 polh* double mutant, indicating that REV3 is required for the increased mutations in *polh* (Nakagawa et al., 2011). AtPolη interacts with the *Arabidopsis* PCNA homologues PCNA1 and PCNA2. In yeast the interaction with PCNA2 was found to be functionally important and require the PCNA-interacting protein (PIP) box and Ubiquitin-binding motif (UBM) of AtPolη (Anderson et al., 2008).

In other systems, PCNA monoubiquitination by RAD6/RAD18 is implicated in polymerase switching during translesion synthesis (Waters et al., 2009). While the *Arabidopsis* genome contains *RAD6* homologues (*AtUBC1-3*), no obvious *RAD18* homologue exists (Kraft et al., 2005). Interestingly, in mammalian cells, the CUL4-DDB1-CDT2 E3 ubiquitin ligase was recently shown to also monoubiquitinate PCNA and promote translesion synthesis (Terai et al., 2010). The CUL4-DDB1-CDT2 complex also ubiquitinates Polη (Kim & Micheal, 2008; Soria & Gottifredi, 2010), suggesting that this complex may be a key regulator of translesion synthesis (Abbas & Dutta, 2011). All components of the CUL4-DDB1-CDT2 complex exist in plants (Lee et al., 2008), so it will be interesting to examine the role of this complex in translesion synthesis.

5. Other responses

In addition to DNA repair and TLS, UV-damaged DNA also triggers other cellular responses such as cell cycle arrest and cell death (Batista et al., 2009). In general, relatively little is known about the molecular basis of these responses in plants. As in mammalian systems, in plants the initial damage sensors include ATM (double strand breaks), ATR (ssDNA) and ATR-interacting protein ATRIP (Culligan et al., 2004; Furukawa et al., 2010; Sakamoto et al., 2009). Plants do not have a p53 homologue, in contrast damage signalling pathways converge on the SOG1 transcription factor, resulting in cell cycle arrest and cell death (Furukawa et al., 2010; Preuss & Britt, 2003; Yoshiyama et al., 2009). UV-induced cell death in plants also involves topoismerase I (Balestrazzi et al., 2010), metacaspase-8 and caspase-3-like activities (Danon et al., 2004; He et al., 2008; Zhang et al., 2009), as well as changes in reactive oxygen species and mitochrondria (Gao et al., 2008).

6. Conclusions

Thus, despite the barrage of damage resulting from solar UV exposure plants face every day, they have a variety of mechanisms which allow them to survive. UV induced DNA damage is repaired by direct photoreactivation via photolyases, or by dark repair (NER) in both transcribed (TC-NER) or non-transcribed regions (GG-NER). Finally, rather than repair UV damage, plants can tolerate its presence and proceed with DNA replication via translesion synthesis, although there can be mutagenic consequences of this activity. The continued study of these pathways and the interplay between them in plants is sure to bring additional insight.

7. Acknowledgements

Research in our laboratory is supported by a grant from the Natural Sciences & Engingeering Research Council of Canada (NSERC).

8. References

Abbas, T. & Dutta, A. (2011). CRL4Cdt2: master coordinator of cell cycle progression and genome stability. *Cell Cycle,* 10(2):241-9

Ahmad, M. & Cashmore, A.R. (1993). *HY4* gene of *A. thaliana* encodes a protein with characteristics of a blue-light photoreceptor. *Nature,* 366 (6451):162-6

Ahmad, M., Jarillo, J.A., Klimczak, L.J., Landry, L.G., Peng, T., Last, R.L. & Cashmore, A.R. (1997). An enzyme similar to animal type II photolyases mediates photoreactivation in *Arabidopsis. Plant Cell,* 9(2):199-207

Al Khateeb, W.M. & Schroeder, D.F. (2009). Overexpression of *Arabidopsis* damaged DNA binding protein 1A (DDB1A) enhances UV tolerance. *Plant Mol Biol.,* 70(4):371-83

Anderson, H.J., Vonarx, E.J., Pastushok, L., Nakagawa, M., Katafuchi, A., Gruz, P., Di Rubbo, A., Grice, D.M., Osmond, M.J., Sakamoto, A.N., Nohmi, T., Xiao, W. & Kunz, B.A. (2008). *Arabidopsis thaliana* Y-family DNA polymerase eta catalyses translesion synthesis and interacts functionally with PCNA2. *Plant J.,* 55(6):895-908

Araki, M., Masutani, C., Takemura, M., Uchida, A., Sugasawa, K., Kondoh, J., Ohkuma, Y. & Hanaoka, F. (2001). Centrosome protein centrin 2/caltractin 1 is part of the xeroderma pigmentosum group C complex that initiates global genome nucleotide excision repair. *J Biol Chem.,* 276(22):18665-72

Balestrazzi, A., Locato, V., Bottone, M.G., De Gara, L., Biggiogera, M., Pellicciari, C., Botti, S., Di Gesù, D., Donà, M. & Carbonera, D. (2010). Response to UV-C radiation in topo I-deficient carrot cells with low ascorbate levels. *J Exp Bot.,* 61(2):575-85

Ballaré, C.L. (2003). Stress under the sun: spotlight on ultraviolet-B responses. *Plant Physiol.,* 132:1725-1727

Batista, L.F., Kaina, B., Meneghini, R. & Menck, C.F. (2009). How DNA lesions are turned into powerful killing structures: insights from UV-induced apoptosis. *Mutat Res.,* 681(2-3):197-208

Batschauer, A. (1999). Light perception in higher plants. *Cell Mol Life Sci.,* 55:153-165

Bernhardt, A., Lechner, E., Hano, P., Schade, V., Dieterle, M., Anders, M., Dubin, M.J., Benvenuto, G., Bowler, C., Genschik, P. & Hellmann, H. (2006). CUL4 associates with DDB1 and DET1 and its downregulation affects diverse aspects of development in *Arabidopsis thaliana. Plant J.,* 47(4):591-603

Bernhardt, A., Mooney, S. & Hellmann, H. (2010). *Arabidopsis* DDB1a and DDB1b are critical for embryo development. *Planta,* 232(3):555-566

Biedermann, S. & Hellmann, H. (2010). The DDB1a interacting proteins ATCSA-1 and DDB2 are critical factors for UV-B tolerance and genomic integrity in *Arabidopsis thaliana. Plant J.,* 62(3):404-15

Biedermann, S. & Hellmann, H. (2011). WD40 and CUL4-based E3 ligases: lubricating all aspects of life. *Trends Plant Sci.,* 16(1):38-46

Britt, A.B. (1999). Molecular genetics of DNA repair in higher plants. *Trends Plant Sci.,* 4(1):20-25

Brosché, M., Schuler, M.A., Kalbina, I., Connor, L. & Strid, A. (2002). Gene regulation by low level UV-B radiation: identification by DNA array analysis. *Photochem Photobiol Sci.,* 1(9):656-64

Castells, E., Molinier, J., Drevensek, S., Genschik, P., Barneche, F. & Bowler, C. (2010). *det1-1*-induced UV-C hyposensitivity through *UVR3* and *PHR1* photolyase gene over-expression. *Plant J.,* 63:392–404

Castells, E., Molinier, J., Benvenuto, G., Bourbousse, C., Zabulon, G., Zalc, A., Cazzaniga, S., Genschik, P., Barneche, F. & Bowler, C. (2011). The conserved factor DE-ETIOLATED 1 cooperates with CUL4-DDB1(DDB2) to maintain genome integrity upon UV stress. *EMBO J.*, 30(6):1162-72

Chang, Y., Gong, L., Yuan, W., Li, X., Chen, G., Li, X., Zhang, Q. & Wu, C. (2009). Replication protein A (RPA1a) is required for meiotic and somatic DNA repair but is dispensable for DNA replication and homologous recombination in rice. *Plant Physiol.*, 151(4):2162-73

Chen, H., Shen, Y., Tang, X., Yu, L., Wang, J., Guo, L., Zhang, Y., Zhang, H., Feng, S., Strickland, E., Zheng, N. & Deng, X. W. (2006). *Arabidopsis* CULLIN4 Forms an E3 Ubiquitin Ligase with RBX1 and the CDD Complex in Mediating Light Control of Development. *Plant Cell,* 18(8):1991-2004

Chen, J.J., Mitchell, D.L. & Britt, A.B. (1994). A Light-Dependent Pathway for the Elimination of UV-Induced Pyrimidine (6-4) Pyrimidinone Photoproducts in *Arabidopsis. Plant Cell,* 6(9):1311-1317

Chen, J.J., Jiang, C.Z. & Britt, A.B. (1996). Little or no repair of cyclobutyl pyrimidine dimers is observed in the organellar genomes of the young *Arabidopsis* seedlings. *Plant Physiol.*, 111(1):19–25

Chen, J. & Suter, B. (2003). Xpd, a structural bridge and a functional link. *Cell Cycle,* 2(6):503-6

Costa, R.M., Morgante, P.G., Berra, C.M., Nakabashi, M., Bruneau, D., Bouchez, D., Sweder, K.S., Van Sluys, M.A. & Menck, C.F. (2001). The participation of AtXPB1, the XPB/RAD25 homologue gene from *Arabidopsis thaliana,* in DNA repair and plant development. *Plant J.*, 28(4):385-95

Culligan, K., Tissier, A. & Britt, A. (2004). ATR regulates a G2-phase cell-cycle checkpoint in *Arabidopsis thaliana. Plant Cell,* 16(5):1091-104

Curtis, M.J. & Hays, J.B. (2007). Tolerance of dividing cells to replication stress in UVB-irradiated *Arabidopsis* roots: requirements for DNA translesion polymerases eta and zeta. *DNA Repair (Amst).*, 6(9):1341-58

Danon, A., Rotari, V.I., Gordon, A., Mailhac, N. & Gallois, P. (2004). Ultraviolet-C overexposure induces programmed cell death in *Arabidopsis,* which is mediated by caspase-like activities and which can be suppressed by caspase inhibitors, p35 and Defender against Apoptotic Death. *J Biol Chem.*, 279(1):779-87

Deisenhofer, J. (2000). DNA photolyases and cryptochromes. *Mutat Res.*, 460(3-4):143-9

Draper, C.K. & Hays, J.B. (2000). Replication of chloroplast, mitochondrial and nuclear DNA during growth of unirradiated and UVB-irradiated *Arabidopsis* leaves. *Plant J.*, 23(2):255-65

Dubest, S., Gallego, M.E. & White, C.I. (2002). Role of the AtRad1p endonuclease in homologous recombination in plants. *EMBO Rep.*, 3(11):1049-54

Dubest, S., Gallego, M.E. & White, C.I. (2004). Roles of the AtErcc1 protein in recombination. *Plant J.*, 39(3):334-42

Farmer, L.M., Book, A.J., Lee, K.H., Lin, Y.L., Fu, H. & Vierstra, R.D. (2010). The RAD23 family provides an essential connection between the 26S proteasome and ubiquitylated proteins in *Arabidopsis. Plant Cell,* 22(1):124-42

Fidantsef, A.L., Mitchell, D.L. & Britt, A.B. (2000). The *Arabidopsis UVH1* gene is a homolog of the yeast repair endonuclease RAD1. *Plant Physiol.*, 124(2):579-86

Fitch, M.E., Nakajima, S., Yasui, A. & Ford, J.M. (2003). In vivo recruitment of XPC to UV-induced cyclobutane pyrimidine dimers by the DDB2 gene product. *J Biol Chem.,* 278(47):46906-10

Fousteri, M., Vermeulen, W., van Zeeland, A.A. & Mullenders, L.H. (2006). Cockayne syndrome A and B proteins differentially regulate recruitment of chromatin remodeling and repair factors to stalled RNA polymerase II in vivo. *Mol Cell,* 23(4):471-82

Fousteri, M. & Mullenders, L.H. (2008). Transcription-coupled nucleotide excision repair in mammalian cells: molecular mechanisms and biological effects. *Cell Res.,* 18(1):73-84

Frit, P., Bergmann, E. & Egly, J.M. (1999). Transcription factor IIH: a key player in the cellular response to DNA damage. *Biochimie,* 81(1-2):27-38

Frohnmeyer, H. & Staiger, D. (2003). Ultraviolet-B Radiation-Mediated Responses in Plants. Balancing Damage and Protection. *Plant Physiol.,* 133(4):1420–1428

Furukawa, T., Kimura, S., Ishibashi, T., Mori, Y., Hashimoto, J. & Sakaguchi, K. (2003a). OsSEND-1: a new RAD2 nuclease family member in higher plants. *Plant Mol Biol.,* 51(1):59-70

Furukawa, T., Ishibashi, T., Kimura, S., Tanaka, H., Hashimoto, J. & Sakaguchi, K. (2003b). Characterization of all the subunits of replication factor C from a higher plant, rice (Oryza sativa L.), and their relation to development. *Plant Mol Biol.,* 53(1-2):15-25

Furukawa, T., Curtis, M.J., Tominey, C.M., Duong, Y.H., Wilcox, B.W., Aggoune, D., Hays, J.B. & Britt, A.B. (2010). A shared DNA-damage-response pathway for induction of stem-cell death by UVB and by gamma irradiation. *DNA Repair (Amst).,* 9(9):940-8

Gallego, F., Fleck, O., Li, A., Wyrzykowska, J. & Tinland, B. (2000). AtRAD1, a plant homologue of human and yeast nucleotide excision repair endonucleases, is involved in dark repair of UV damages and recombination. *Plant J.,* 21(6):507-18

Gao, C., Xing, D., Li, L. & Zhang, L. (2008). Implication of reactive oxygen species and mitochondrial dysfunction in the early stages of plant programmed cell death induced by ultraviolet-C overexposure. *Planta,* 227(4):755-67

Garcia-Diaz, M. & Bebenek, K. (2007). Multiple functions of DNA polymerases. *CRC Crit Rev Plant Sci.,* 26(2):105-122

García-Ortiz, M.V., Roldán-Arjona, T. & Ariza, R.R. (2007). The noncatalytic C-terminus of AtPOLK Y-family DNA polymerase affects synthesis fidelity, mismatch extension and translesion replication. *FEBS J.,* 274(13):3340-50

Gillet, L.C.J. & Scharer, O.D. (2006). Molecular mechanisms of mammalian global genome nucleotide excision repair. *Chem. Rev.,* 106(2):253-276

Grasser, M., Kane, C.M., Merkle, T., Melzer, M., Emmersen, J. & Grasser, K.D. (2009). Transcript elongation factor TFIIS is involved in *Arabidopsis* seed dormancy. *J Mol Biol.,* 386(3):598-611

Groisman, R., Polanowska, J., Kuraoka, I., Sawada, J., Saijo, M., Drapkin, R., Kissilev, A.F., Tanaka, K. & Nakatani, Y. (2003). The ubiquitin ligase activity in the DDB2 and CSA complexes is differentially regulated by the COP9 signalosome in response to DNA damage. *Cell,* 113(3): 357-367

Groisman, R., Kuraoka, I., Chevallier, O., Gaye, N., Magnaldo, T., Tanaka, K., Kisselev, A.F., Harel-Bellan, A. & Nakatani, Y. (2006). CSA-dependent degradation of CSB by the ubiquitin-proteasome pathway establishes a link between complementation factors of the Cockayne syndrome. *Genes Dev.,* 20(11):1429-34

Guerrero-Santoro, J., Kapetanaki, M.G., Hsieh, C.L., Gorbachinsky, I., Levine, A.S. & Rapić-Otrin, V. (2008). The cullin 4B-based UV-damaged DNA-binding protein ligase binds to UV-damaged chromatin and ubiquitinates histone H2A. *Cancer Res.*, 68(13):5014-22

Gulbis, J.M., Kelman, Z., Hurwitz, J., O'Donnell, M. & Kuriyan, J. (1996). Structure of the C-terminal region of p21(WAF1/CIP1) complexed with human PCNA. *Cell*, 87(2):297-306

Hada, M., Hino, K., Buchholz, G., Goss, J., Wellmann, E. & Shin, M. (2000). Assay of DNA photolyase activity in spinach leaves in relation to cell compartmentation-evidence for lack of DNA photolyase in chloroplasts. *Biosci Biotechnol Biochem.*, 64:1288–1291

Hanawalt, P.C. & Spivak, G. (2008). Transcription-coupled DNA repair: two decades of progress and surprises. *Nat Rev Mol Cell Biol.*, 9(12):958-70

He, R., Drury, G.E., Rotari, V.I., Gordon, A., Willer, M., Farzaneh, T., Woltering, E.J. & Gallois, P. (2008). Metacaspase-8 modulates programmed cell death induced by ultraviolet light and H2O2 in *Arabidopsis. J Biol Chem.*, 283(2):774-83

He, Z., Henricksen, L.A., Wold, M.S. & Ingles, C.J. (1995). RPA involvement in the damage-recognition and incision steps of nucleotide excision repair. *Nature*, 374: 566–569

Hefner, E., Preuss, S.B. & Britt, A.B. (2003). *Arabidopsis* mutants sensitive to gamma radiation include the homologue of the human repair gene ERCC1. *J Exp Bot.*, 54(383):669-80

Hey, T., Lipps, G., Sugasawa, K., Iwai, S., Hanaoka, F. & Krauss, G. (2002). The XPC-HR23B complex displays high affinity and specificity for damaged DNA in a true-equilibrium fluorescence assay. *Biochemistry*, 41(21): 6583–6587

Hidema, J., Kumagai, T. & Sutherland, B.M. (2000). UV radiation-sensitive norin 1 rice contains defective cyclobutane pyrimidine dimer photolyase. *Plant Cell*, 12(9):1569-78

Hidema, J., Taguchi, T., Ono, T., Teranishi, M., Yamamoto, K. & Kumagai, T. (2007). Increase in CPD photolyase activity functions effectively to prevent growth inhibition caused by UVB radiation. *Plant J.*, 50(1):70-9

Higa, L.A., Wu, M., Ye, T., Kobayashi, R., Sun, H. & Zhang, H. (2006). CUL4-DDB1 ubiquitin ligase interacts with multiple WD40-repeat proteins and regulates histone methylation. *Nat Cell Biol.*, 8(11):1277-83

Hirouchi, T., Nakajima, S., Najrana, T., Tanaka, M., Matsunaga, T., Hidema, J., Teranishi, M., Fujino, T., Kumagai, T. & Yamamoto, K. (2003). A gene for a Class II DNA photolyase from *Oryza sativa*: cloning of the cDNA by dilution-amplification. *Mol Genet Genomics*, 269(4):508-16

Hoeijmakers, J.H. (2001). Genome maintenance mechanisms for preventing cancer. *Nature*, 411: 135-141

Hoffman, P.D., Curtis, M.J., Iwai, S. & Hays, J.B. (2008). Biochemical evolution of DNA polymerase eta: properties of plant, human, and yeast proteins. *Biochemistry*, 47(16):4583-96

Holmberg, C., Fleck, O., Hansen, H.A., Liu, C., Slaaby, R., Carr, A.M. & Nielsen, O. (2005). Ddb1 controls genome stability and meiosis in fission yeast. *Genes Dev.*,19:853–862

Hua, Z. & Vierstra, R.D. (2011). The Cullin-RING Ubiquitin-Protein Ligases. *Annu Rev Plant Biol.*, 62:299-334

Ishibashi, T., Kimura, S., Furukawa, T., Hatanaka, M., Hashimoto, J. & Sakaguchi, K. (2001). Two types of replication protein A 70 kDa subunit in rice, *Oryza sativa*: molecular cloning, characterization, and cellular & tissue distribution. *Gene*, 272(1-2):335-43

Ishibashi, T., Kimura, S., Yamamoto, T., Furukawa, T., Takata, K., Uchiyama, Y., Hashimoto, J. & Sakaguchi, K. (2003). Rice UV-damaged DNA binding protein homologues are most abundant in proliferating tissues. *Gene*, 308:79-87

Ishibashi, T., Koga, A., Yamamoto, T., Uchiyama, Y., Mori, Y., Hashimoto, J., Kimura, S. & Sakaguchi, K. (2005). Two types of replication protein A in seed plants. *FEBS J.*, 272(13):3270-81

Ishibashi, T., Kimura, S. & Sakaguchi, K. (2006). A higher plant has three different types of RPA heterotrimeric complex. *J Biochem.*, 139(1):99-104

Jansan, M.A.K., Hectors, K., O'Brien, N.M., Guisez, Y. & Potters, G. (2008). Plant stress and human health: Do human consumers benefit from UV-B acclimated crops? *Plant Science*, 175:449–458

Jenkins, G.I. (2009). Signal transduction in responses to UV-B radiation. *Annu Rev Plant Biol.*, 60:407-31

Jenkins, M.E., Suzuki, T.C. & Mount, D.W. (1997). Evidence that heat and ultraviolet radiation activate a common stress-response program in plants that is altered in the *uvh6* mutant of *Arabidopsis thaliana*. *Plant Physiol.*, 115(4):1351-8

Kaiser, G., Kleiner, O., Beisswenger, C. & Batschauer, A. (2009). Increased DNA repair in *Arabidopsis* plants overexpressing CPD photolyase. *Planta*, 230(3):505-15

Kapetanaki, M.G., Guerrero-Santoro, J., Bisi, D.C., Hsieh, C.L., Rapić-Otrin, V. & Levine, A.S. (2006). The DDB1-CUL4ADDB2 ubiquitin ligase is deficient in xeroderma pigmentosum group E and targets histone H2A at UV-damaged DNA sites. *Proc Natl Acad Sci U S A.*, 103(8):2588-93

Kim, S.H. & Michael, W.M. (2008). Regulated proteolysis of DNA polymerase eta during the DNA-damage response in *C. elegans*. *Mol Cell*, 32(6):757-66

Kimura, S., Tahira, Y., Ishibashi, T., Mori, Y., Mori, T., Hashimoto, J. & Sakaguchi, K. (2004). DNA repair in higher plants; photoreactivation is the major DNA repair pathway in non-proliferating cells while excision repair (nucleotide excision repair and base excision repair) is active in proliferating cells. *Nucleic Acids Res.*, 32(9):2760-7

Kimura, S. & Sakaguchi, K. (2006). DNA repair in plants. *Chem Rev.*, 106(2):753-66

Koga, A., Ishibashi, T., Kimura, S., Uchiyama, Y. & Sakaguchi, K. (2006). Characterization of T-DNA insertion mutants and RNAi silenced plants of *Arabidopsis thaliana* UV-damaged DNA binding protein 2 (AtUV-DDB2). *Plant Mol Biol.*, 61(1-2):227-40

Kraft, E., Stone, S.L., Ma, L., Su, N., Gao, Y., Lau, O.S., Deng, X.W. & Callis, J. (2005). Genome analysis and functional characterization of the E2 and RING-type E3 ligase ubiquitination enzymes of *Arabidopsis*. *Plant Physiol.*, 139(4):1597-611

Kunz, B.A., Anderson, H.J., Osmond, M.J. & Vonarx, E.J. (2005). Components of nucleotide excision repair and DNA damage tolerance in *Arabidopsis thaliana*. *Environ Mol Mutagen.*, 45(2-3):115-27

Kunz, B.A., Cahill, D.M., Mohr, P.G., Osmond, M.J. & Vonarx, E.J. (2006). Plant responses to UV radiation and links to pathogen resistance. *Int Rev Cytol.*, 255:1-40

Kuraoka, I., Ito, S., Wada, T., Hayashida, M., Lee, L., Saijo, M., Nakatsu, Y., Matsumoto, M., Matsunaga, T., Handa, H., Qin, J., Nakatani, Y. & Tanaka, K. (2008). Isolation of

XAB2 complex involved in pre-mRNA splicing, transcription, and transcription-coupled repair. *J Biol Chem.*, 283(2):940-50

Lainé, J.P. & Egly, J.M. (2006). Initiation of DNA repair mediated by a stalled RNA polymerase IIO. *EMBO J.*, 25(2):387-97

Landry, L.G., Stapleton, A.E., Lim, J., Hoffman, P., Hays, J.B., Walbot, V. & Last, R.L. (1997). An *Arabidopsis* photolyase mutant is hypersensitive to ultraviolet-B radiation. *Proc Natl Acad Sci U S A.*, 94(1):328-32

Lee, J. & Zhou, P. (2007). DCAFs, the missing link of the CUL4-DDB1 ubiquitin ligase. *Mol Cell*, 26(6):775-80

Lee, J.H., Terzaghi, W., Gusmaroli, G., Charron, J.B., Yoon, H.J., Chen, H., He, Y.J., Xiong, Y. & Deng, X.W. (2008). Characterization of *Arabidopsis* and rice DWD proteins and their roles as substrate receptors for CUL4-RING E3 ubiquitin ligases. *Plant Cell*, 20(1):152-67

Liang, L., Flury, S., Kalck, V., Hohn, B. & Molinier, J. (2006). CENTRIN2 interacts with the *Arabidopsis* homolog of the human XPC protein (AtRAD4) and contributes to efficient synthesis-dependent repair of bulky DNA lesions. *Plant Mol Biol.*, 61(1-2):345-56

Liu, Z., Hossain, G.S., Islas-Osuna, M.A., Mitchell, D.L. & Mount, D.W. (2000). Repair of UV damage in plants by nucleotide excision repair: *Arabidopsis* UVH1 DNA repair gene is a homolog of *Saccharomyces cerevisiae* Rad1. *Plant J.*, 21(6):519-28

Liu, Z., Hall, J.D. & Mount, D.W. (2001). *Arabidopsis UVH3* gene is a homolog of the *Saccharomyces cerevisiae* RAD2 and human XPG DNA repair genes. *Plant J.*, 26(3):329-38

Liu, Z., Hong, S.W., Escobar, M., Vierling, E., Mitchell, D.L., Mount, D.W. & Hall, J.D. (2003). *Arabidopsis* UVH6, a homolog of human XPD and yeast RAD3 DNA repair genes, functions in DNA repair and is essential for plant growth. *Plant Physiol.*, 132(3):1405-14

Luijsterburg, M.S., Goedhart, J., Moser, J., Kool, H., Geverts, B., Houtsmuller, A.B., Mullenders, L.H., Vermeulen, W. & van Driel, R. (2007). Dynamic in vivo interaction of DDB2 E3 ubiquitin ligase with UV-damaged DNA is independent of damage-recognition protein XPC. *J Cell Sci.*, 120(15):2706-16

Mackerness, S. (2000). Plant responses to ultraviolet-B (UV-B:280–320 nm) stress: What are the key regulators? *Plant Growth Regul.*, 37:27-39

Marwedel, T., Ishibashi, T., Lorbiecke, R., Jacob, S., Sakaguchi, K. & Sauter, M. (2003). Plant-specific regulation of replication protein A2 (OsRPA2) from rice during the cell cycle and in response to ultraviolet light exposure. *Planta.*, 217(3):457-65

Mellon, I. (2005). Transcription-coupled repair: a complex affair. *Mutat Res.*, 577(1-2):155-61

Mocquet, V., Lainé, J.P., Riedl, T., Yajin, Z., Lee, M.Y. & Egly, J.M. (2008). Sequential recruitment of the repair factors during NER: the role of XPG in initiating the resynthesis step. *EMBO J.*, 27(1):155-67

Molinier, J., Ramos, C., Fritsch, O. & Hohn, B. (2004). CENTRIN2 modulates homologous recombination and nucleotide excision repair in *Arabidopsis*. *Plant Cell*, 16(6):1633-43

Molinier, J., Lechner, E., Dumbliauskas, E. & Genschik, P. (2008). Regulation and role of *Arabidopsis* CUL4-DDB1A-DDB2 in maintaining genome integrity upon UV stress. *PloS Genetics*, 4(6):e10000

Morgante, P.G., Berra, C.M., Nakabashi, M., Costa, R.M., Menck, C.F. & Van Sluys, M.A. (2005). Functional XPB/RAD25 redundancy in *Arabidopsis* genome: characterization of AtXPB2 and expression analysis. *Gene*, 344:93-103

Nakagawa, M., Takahashi, S., Tanaka, A., Narumi, I. & Sakamoto, A.N. (2011). Role of AtPol{zeta}, AtRev1, and AtPol{eta} in UV light-induced mutagenesis in *Arabidopsis*. *Plant Physiol.*, 155(1):414-20

Nakajima, S., Sugiyama, M., Iwai, S., Hitomi, K., Otoshi, E., Kim, S.T., Jiang, C.Z., Todo, T., Britt, A.B. & Yamamoto, K. (1998). Cloning and characterization of a gene (*UVR3*) required for photorepair of 6-4 photoproducts in *Arabidopsis thaliana*. *Nucleic Acids Res.*, 26(2):638-44

Nakatsu, Y., Asahina, H., Citterio, E., Rademakers, S., Vermeulen, W., Kamiuchi, S., Yeo, J.P., Khaw, M.C., Saijo, M., Kodo, N., Matsuda, T., Hoeijmakers, J.H. & Tanaka, K. (2000). XAB2, a novel tetratricopeptide repeat protein involved in transcription-coupled DNA repair and transcription. *J Biol Chem.*, 275(45):34931-7

Nishi, R., Okuda, Y., Watanabe, E., Mori, T., Iwai, S., Masutani, C., Sugasawa, K. & Hanaoka, F. (2005). Centrin2 stimulates nucleotide excision repair by interacting with xeroderma pigmentosum group C protein. *Mol Cell Biol.*, 25(13):5664-74

Oravecz, A., Baumann, A., Máté, Z., Brzezinska, A., Molinier, J., Oakeley, E.J., Adám, E., Schäfer, E., Nagy, F. & Ulm, R. (2006). CONSTITUTIVELY PHOTOMORPHOGENIC1 is required for the UV-B response in *Arabidopsis*. *Plant Cell*, 18(8):1975-90

Pandey, R., Müller, A., Napoli, C.A., Selinger, D.A., Pikaard, C.S., Richards, E.J., Bender, J., Mount, D.W. & Jorgensen, R.A. (2002). Analysis of histone acetyltransferase and histone deacetylase families of *Arabidopsis thaliana* suggests functional diversification of chromatin modification among multicellular eukaryotes. *Nucleic Acids Res.*, 30(23):5036-55

Pang, Q. & Hays, J.B. (1991). UV-B-Inducible and Temperature-Sensitive Photoreactivation of Cyclobutane Pyrimidine Dimers in *Arabidopsis thaliana*. *Plant Physiol.*, 95(2):536-43

Parry, G. & Estelle, M. (2004). Regulation of Cullin based ubiquitin ligases by the Nedd8/RUB ubiquitin like proteins. *Semin Cell Dev. Biol.*, 15: 221-229

Pepper, A., Delaney, T., Washburn, T., Poole, D. & Chory, J. (1994). DET1, a negative regulator of light-mediated development and gene expression in *Arabidopsis*, encodes a novel nuclear-localized protein. *Cell*, 78(1):109-16

Preuss, S.B. & Britt, A.B. (2003). A DNA-damage-induced cell cycle checkpoint in *Arabidopsis*. *Genetics*, 164(1):323-34

Rapić-Otrin, V., McLenigan, M.P., Bisi, D.C., Gonzalez, M. & Levine, A.S. (2002). Sequential binding of UV DNA damage binding factor and degradation of the p48 subunit as early events after UV irradiation. *Nucleic Acids Res.*, 30(11):2588-98

Ribeiro, D.T., Machado, C.R., Costa, R.M., Praekelt, U.M., Van Sluys, M.A. & Menck, C.F. (1998). Cloning of a cDNA from *Arabidopsis thaliana* homologous to the human XPB gene. *Gene*, 208(2):207-13

Riedl, T., Hanaoka, F. & Egly, J.M. (2003). The comings and goings of nucleotide excision repair factors on damaged DNA. *EMBO J.*, 22(19):5293-303

Ries, G., Heller, W., Puchta, H., Sandermann, H., Seidlitz, H.K. & Hohn, B. (2000). Elevated UV-B radiation reduces genome stability in plants. *Nature*, 406(6791):98-101

Roy, S., Choudhury, S.R., Singh, S.K. & Das, K.P. (2011). AtPolλ, A Homolog of Mammalian DNA Polymerase λ in *Arabidopsis thaliana*, is Involved in the Repair of UV-B Induced DNA Damage through the Dark Repair Pathway. *Plant Cell Physiol.*, 52(2): 448-467

Sakaguchi, K., Ishibashi, T., Uchiyama, Y. & Iwabata, K. (2009). The multi-replication protein A (RPA) system--a new perspective. *FEBS J.*, 276(4):943-63

Sakamoto, A., Lan, V.T., Hase, Y., Shikazono, N., Matsunaga, T. & Tanaka, A. (2003). Disruption of the *AtREV3* gene causes hypersensitivity to ultraviolet B light and gamma-rays in *Arabidopsis*: implication of the presence of a translesion synthesis mechanism in plants. *Plant Cell,* 15(9):2042-57

Sakamoto, A.N., Lan, V.T., Puripunyavanich, V., Hase, Y., Yokota, Y., Shikazono, N., Nakagawa, M., Narumi, I. & Tanaka, A. (2009). A UVB-hypersensitive mutant in *Arabidopsis thaliana* is defective in the DNA damage response. *Plant J.*, 60(3):509-17

Sancar, A. (2003). Structure and function of DNA photolyase and cryptochrome blue-light photoreceptors. *Chem Rev.*, 103(6):2203-37

Sancar, A. (2008). Structure and function of photolyase and in vivo enzymology: 50th anniversary. *J Biol Chem.*, 283(47):32153-7

Santiago, M.J., Alejandre-Durán, E. & Ruiz-Rubio, M. (2006). Analysis of UV-induced mutation spectra in *Escherichia coli* by DNA polymerase eta from *Arabidopsis thaliana. Mutat Res.*, 601(1-2):51-60

Santiago, M.J., Ruiz-Rubio, M., Dio, L.D., González-Reyes, J.A. & Alejandre-Durán, E. (2008a). Ubiquitous expression of two translesion synthesis DNA polymerase genes in *Arabidopsis. Planta,* 227(6):1269-77

Santiago, M.J., Alejandre-Durán, E., Muñoz-Serrano, A. & Ruiz-Rubio, M. (2008b). Two translesion synthesis DNA polymerase genes, *AtPOLH* and *AtREV1*, are involved in development and UV light resistance in *Arabidopsis. J Plant Physiol.*, 165(15):1582-91

Santiago, M.J., Alejandre-Durán, E. & Ruiz-Rubio, M. (2009). Alternative splicing of two translesion synthesis DNA polymerases from *Arabidopsis thaliana. Plant Science,* 176(4):591-596

Saxowsky, T.T. & Doetsch, P.W. (2006). RNA polymerase encounters with DNA damage: transcription-coupled repair or transcriptional mutagenesis? *Chem Rev.*, 106(2):474-88

Schroeder, D.F., Gahrtz, M., Maxwell, B.B., Cook, R.K., Kan, J.M., Alonso, J.M., Ecker, J.R. & Chory, J. (2002). De-etiolated1 and Damaged DNA Binding Protein 1 interact to regulate *Arabidopsis* photomorphogenesis. *Curr Biol.*, 12(17):1462-72

Schultz, T.F. & Quatrano R.S. (1997). Characterization and expression of a rice *RAD23* gene. *Plant Mol Biol.*, 34: 557-562

Schwechheimer, C. & Deng, X.W. (2001). COP9 signalosome revisited: a novel mediator of protein degradation. *Trends Cell Biol.*, 11(10):420-426

Scrima, A., Konícková, R., Czyzewski, B.K., Kawasaki, Y., Jeffrey, P.D., Groisman, R., Nakatani, Y., Iwai, S., Pavletich, N.P. & Thomä, N.H. (2008). Structural basis of UV DNA-damage recognition by the DDB1-DDB2 complex. *Cell,* 135(7):1213-23

Shaked, H., Avivi-Ragolsky, N. & Levy, A.A. (2006). Involvement of the *Arabidopsis* SWI2/SNF2 chromatin remodeling gene family in DNA damage response and recombination. *Genetics,* 173(2):985-94

Shultz, R.W., Tatineni, V.M., Hanley-Bowdoin, L. & Thompson, W.F. (2007). Genome-wide analysis of the core DNA replication machinery in the higher plants *Arabidopsis* and rice. *Plant Physiol.*, 144(4):1697-714

Singh, S.K., Roy, S., Choudhury, S.R. & Sengupta, D.N. (2010). DNA repair and recombination in higher plants: insights from comparative genomics of *Arabidopsis* and rice. *BMC Genomics*, 11:443

Soria, G. & Gottifredi, V. (2010). PCNA-coupled p21 degradation after DNA damage: The exception that confirms the rule? *DNA Repair (Amst)*, 9(4):358-64

Strzalka, W. & Ziemienowicz, A. (2011). Proliferating cell nuclear antigen (PCNA): a key factor in DNA replication and cell cycle regulation. *Ann Bot.* 107(7):1127-40

Sturm, A. & Leinhard, S. (1998). Two isoforms of plant RAD 23 complement a UV sensitive rad23 mutant in yeast. *Plant J.*, 13(6): 815-821

Sugasawa, K., Okuda, Y., Saijo, M., Nishi, R., Matsuda, N., Chu, G., Mori, T., Iwai, S., Tanaka, K., Tanaka, K. & Hanaoka, F. (2005). UV-induced ubiquitylation of XPC protein mediated by UV-DDB-ubiquitin ligase complex. *Cell*, 121(3):387-400

Svejstrup, J.Q. (2002). Mechanisms of Transcription coupled repair. *Nat Rev Mol Cell Biol.*, 3(1):21-29

Takahashi, M., Teranishi, M., Ishida, H., Kawasaki, J., Takeuchi, A., Yamaya, T., Watanabe, M., Makino, A. & Hidema, J. (2011). Cyclobutane pyrimidine dimer (CPD) photolyase repairs ultraviolet-B-induced CPDs in rice chloroplast and mitochondrial DNA. *Plant J.*, 66(3):433-42

Takahashi, S., Nakajima, N., Saji, H. & Kondo, N. (2002). Diurnal change of cucumber CPD photolyase gene (*CsPHR*) expression and its physiological role in growth under UV-B irradiation. *Plant Cell Physiol.*, 43(3):342-9

Takahashi, S., Sakamoto, A., Sato, S., Kato, T., Tabata, S. & Tanaka, A. (2005). Roles of *Arabidopsis* AtREV1 and AtREV7 in translesion synthesis. *Plant Physiol.*, 138(2):870-81

Takahashi, S., Sakamoto, A.N., Tanaka, A. & Shimizu, K. (2007). AtREV1, a Y-family DNA polymerase in *Arabidopsis*, has deoxynucleotidyl transferase activity in vitro. *Plant Physiol.*, 145(3):1052-60

Takashi, Y., Kobayashi, Y., Tanaka, K. & Tamura, K. (2009). *Arabidopsis* replication protein A 70a is required for DNA damage response and telomere length homeostasis. *Plant Cell Physiol.*, 50(11):1965-76

Tanaka, A., Sakamoto, A., Ishigaki, Y., Nikaido, O., Sun, G., Hase, Y., Shikazono, N., Tano, S. & Watanabe, H. (2002). An ultraviolet-B resistant mutant with enhanced DNA repair in *Arabidopsis*. *Plant Physiol*, 129(1):64–71

Tapias, A., Auriol, J., Forget, D., Enzlin, J.H., Schärer, O.D., Coin, F., Coulombe, B. & Egly, J.M. (2004). Ordered conformational changes in damaged DNA induced by nucleotide excision repair factors. *J Biol Chem.*, 279(18):19074-83

Terai, K., Abbas, T., Jazaeri, A.A. & Dutta, A. (2010). CRL4(Cdt2) E3 ubiquitin ligase monoubiquitinates PCNA to promote translesion DNA synthesis. *Mol Cell*, 37(1):143-9

Todo, T., Ryo, H., Yamamoto, K., Toh, H., Inui, T., Ayaki, H., Nomura, T. & Ikenaga, M. (1996). Similarity among the Drosophila (6-4)photolyase, a human photolyase homolog, and the DNA photolyase-blue-light photoreceptor family. *Science*, 272(5258):109-12

Tornaletti, S. (2009). DNA repair in mammalian cells: Transcription-coupled DNA repair: directing your effort where it's most needed. *Cell Mol Life Sci.*, 66(6):1010-20

Ueda, T., Sato, T., Hidema, J., Hirouchi, T., Yamamoto, K., Kumagai, T. & Yano, M. (2005). qUVR-10, a major quantitative trait locus for ultraviolet-B resistance in rice, encodes cyclobutane pyrimidine dimer photolyase. *Genetics*, 171(4):1941-50

Ulm, R., Baumann, A., Oravecz, A., Máté, Z., Adám, E., Oakeley, E.J., Schäfer, E. & Nagy, F. (2004). Genome-wide analysis of gene expression reveals function of the bZIP transcription factor HY5 in the UV-B response of *Arabidopsis*. *Proc Natl Acad Sci U S A.*, 101(5):1397-402

Vannier, J.B., Depeiges, A., White, C. & Gallego, M.E. (2009). ERCC1/XPF protects short telomeres from homologous recombination in *Arabidopsis thaliana*. *PLoS Genet.*, 5(2):e1000380

van den Boom, V., Citterio, E., Hoogstraten, D., Zotter, A., Egly, J.M., van Cappellen, W.A., Hoeijmakers, J.H., Houtsmuller, A.B. & Vermeulen, W. (2004). DNA damage stabilizes interaction of CSB with the transcription elongation machinery. *J Cell Biol.*, 166(1):27-36

Volker, M., Mone, M.J., Karmakar, P., van Hoffen, A., Schul, W., Vermeulen, W., Hoeijmakers, J.H., van Driel, R., van Zeeland, A.A. & Mullenders, L.H. (2001). Sequential assembly of the nucleotide excision repair factors in vivo. *Mol Cell*, 8(1):213–224

Vonarx, E.J., Howlett, N.G., Schiestl, R.H. & Kunz, B.A. (2002). Detection of *Arabidopsis thaliana* AtRAD1 cDNA variants and assessment of function by expression in a yeast rad1 mutant. *Gene*, 296(1-2):1-9

Vonarx, E.J., Tabone, E.K., Osmond, M.J., Anderson, H.J. & Kunz, B.A. (2006). *Arabidopsis* homologue of human transcription factor IIH/nucleotide excision repair factor p44 can function in transcription and DNA repair and interacts with AtXPD. *Plant J.*, 46(3):512-21

Wang, H., Zhai, L., Xu, J., Joo, H.Y., Jackson, S., Erdjument-Bromage, H., Tempst, P., Xiong, Y. & Zhang, Y. (2006). Histone H3 and H4 ubiquitylation by the CUL4-DDB-ROC1 ubiquitin ligase facilitates cellular response to DNA damage. *Mol Cell*, 22(3):383-94

Waters, L.S., Minesinger, B.K., Wiltrout, M.E., D'Souza, S., Woodruff, R.V. & Walker, G.C. (2009). Eukaryotic translesion polymerases and their roles and regulation in DNA damage tolerance. *Microbiol Mol Biol Rev.*, 73(1):134-54

Waterworth, W.M., Jiang, Q., West, C.E., Nikaido, M. & Bray, C.M. (2002). Characterization of *Arabidopsis* photolyase enzymes and analysis of their role in protection from ultraviolet-B radiation. *J Exp Bot.*, 53(371):1005-15

Weeda, G., Donker, I., De Wit, J., Morreau, H. Janssens, R., Vissers, C.J., Nigg, A., van Steeg, H., Bootsma, D. & Hoeijmakers, J.H. (1997). Disruption of mouse ERCC1 results in a novel repair syndrome with growth failure, nuclear abnormalities and senescence. *Curr Biol.*, 7(6): 427-39

Wold, M.S. (1997). Replication protein A: a heterotrimeric, single-stranded DNA-binding protein required for eukaryotic DNA metabolism. *Annu Rev Biochem.*, 66:61-92

Xu, H., Swoboda, I., Bhalla, P.L., Sijbers, A.M., Zhao, C., Ong, E.K., Hoeijmakers, J.H. & Singh, M.B. (1998). Plant homologue of human excision repair gene ERCC1 points to conservation of DNA repair mechanisms. *Plant J.*, 13(6):823-9

Yamamoto, A., Hirouchi, T., Mori, T., Teranishi, M., Hidema. J., Morioka, H., Kumagai, T. & Yamamoto, K. (2007). Biochemical and biological properties of DNA photolyases derived from utraviolet-sensitive rice cultivars. *Genes Genet Syst.*, 82(4):311-9

Yamamoto, A., Tanbir, N., Hirouchi, T., Teranishi, M., Hidema, J., Morioka, H. & Yamamoto, K. (2008). Temperature-sensitive photoreactivation of cyclobutane thymine dimer in soybean. *J Radiat Res (Tokyo)*, 49(2):189-96

Yasui, A., Eker, A.P., Yasuhira, S., Yajima, H., Kobayashi, T., Takao, M. & Oikawa, A. (1994). A new class of DNA photolyases present in various organisms including aplacental mammals. *EMBO J.*, 13(24):6143-51

Yoshihara, R., Imaki, T., Hori, M., Watanabe, C., Yamamoto, K. & Takimoto, K. (2005). CPD photolyase gene from *Spinacia oleracea*: repair of UV-damaged DNA and expression in plant organs. *J Radiat Res (Tokyo)*, 46(2):157-64

Yoshiyama, K., Conklin, P.A., Huefner, N.D. & Britt, A.B. (2009). Suppressor of gamma response 1 (SOG1) encodes a putative transcription factor governing multiple responses to DNA damage. *Proc Natl Acad Sci USA*, 106(31):12843-8

Yuzhakov, A., Kelman, Z., Hurwitz, J. & O'Donnell, M. (1999). Multiple competition reactions for RPA order the assembly of the DNA polymerase delta holoenzyme. *EMBO J.*, 18(21):6189-99

Zhang, C., Guo, H., Zhang, J., Guo, G., Schumaker, K.S. & Guo, Y. (2010). *Arabidopsis* cockayne syndrome A-like proteins 1A and 1B form a complex with CULLIN4 and damage DNA binding protein 1A and regulate the response to UV irradiation. *Plant Cell*, 22(7):2353-69

Zhang, L., Xu, Q., Xing, D., Gao, C. & Xiong, H. (2009). Real-time detection of caspase-3-like protease activation in vivo using fluorescence resonance energy transfer during plant programmed cell death induced by ultraviolet C overexposure. *Plant Physiol.*, 150(4):1773-83

6

DNA Damage Caused by Polycyclic Aromatic Hydrocarbons: Mechanisms and Markers

Balam Muñoz and Arnulfo Albores
Departamento de Toxicología,
Centro de Investigación y de Estudios Avanzados del I.P.N.
México

1. Introduction

Polycyclic Aromatic Hydrocarbons (PAHs) are a group of chemicals that occur naturally in coal, crude oil and gasoline. Incomplete combustion of organic material results in emission of PAHs (ATSDR, 1996). These molecules consist of two or more aromatic rings fused in linear, angular or cluster arrangements (Fig. 1) and by definition are composed of hydrogen and carbon. PAHs containing up to six fused aromatic rings are often known as "small" PAHs while those containing more than six aromatic rings are called "large" PAHs. As pure chemicals, these compounds are colorless, white or pale yellow solids. Their physicochemical properties, vapor pressure and solubility vary according to their molecular weight. PAHs possess a highly characteristic UV absorbance spectra although some may be fluorescent (Fetzer & Biggs, 1994). PAHs are ubiquitous and persistent as a consequence of natural (forest fires and volcanic eruptions) and human activities (Jongeneelen, 2001). PAHs may distribute in water, soil and the atmosphere according to different weather and geographical factors. Although industrial activity such as coke manufacturing or asphalt production are major contributors to PAH emissions, incineration, power generation and several mobile sources also emit a considerable amount of PAHs. Significant sources of PAHs in surface waters include deposition of airborne PAHs, municipal wastewater discharge, urban storm-water runoff, and industrial waste. Food groups that tend to have the highest levels of PAHs include charcoal broiled or smoked meats, leafy vegetables, grains, and vegetable fats and oils (Yu, 2005). Therefore, workers of these industries and the general population are continually exposed to different concentrations of PAH mixtures. The Agency for Toxic Substances and Disease Registry (ATSDR) has grouped 17 PAHs according to their health effects (ATSDR, 1996). The United States Environmental Protection Agency (EPA) has designated 28 PAH compounds as priority pollutants (EPA, 2009) (Table 1). The International Agency for Research on Cancer (IARC) has classified some these compounds as carcinogenic (group 1) or likely carcinogenic (group 2A) to humans, for example benzo[*a*]pyrene and dibenz[*a,h*]anthracene, respectively (IARC, 2010). Finally, the National Institute of Standards and Technology has created a classification of PAHs according to their symbols, molecular formulas, class and notation among other properties (NIST, 2010).

The most common mechanism of carcinogenesis induced by PAHs is DNA damage through the formation of adducts. Alternatively, in the presence of reactive oxidative species, DNA damage can also result. In this chapter, we review the mechanisms of damage caused by exposure to PAHs, factors involved in repairing the damage, and the important role of biomarkers.

2. Metabolism of PAHs

Once PAHs enter the body they are metabolized in a number of organs (including liver, kidney, lungs), excreted in bile, urine or breast milk and stored to a limited degree in adipose tissue. The principal routes of exposure are: inhalation, ingestion, and dermal contact. The lipophilicity of PAHs enables them to readily penetrate cellular membranes (Yu, 2005). Subsequent metabolism renders them more water-soluble making them easier for the body to remove. However, PAHs can also be converted to more toxic or carcinogenic metabolites.

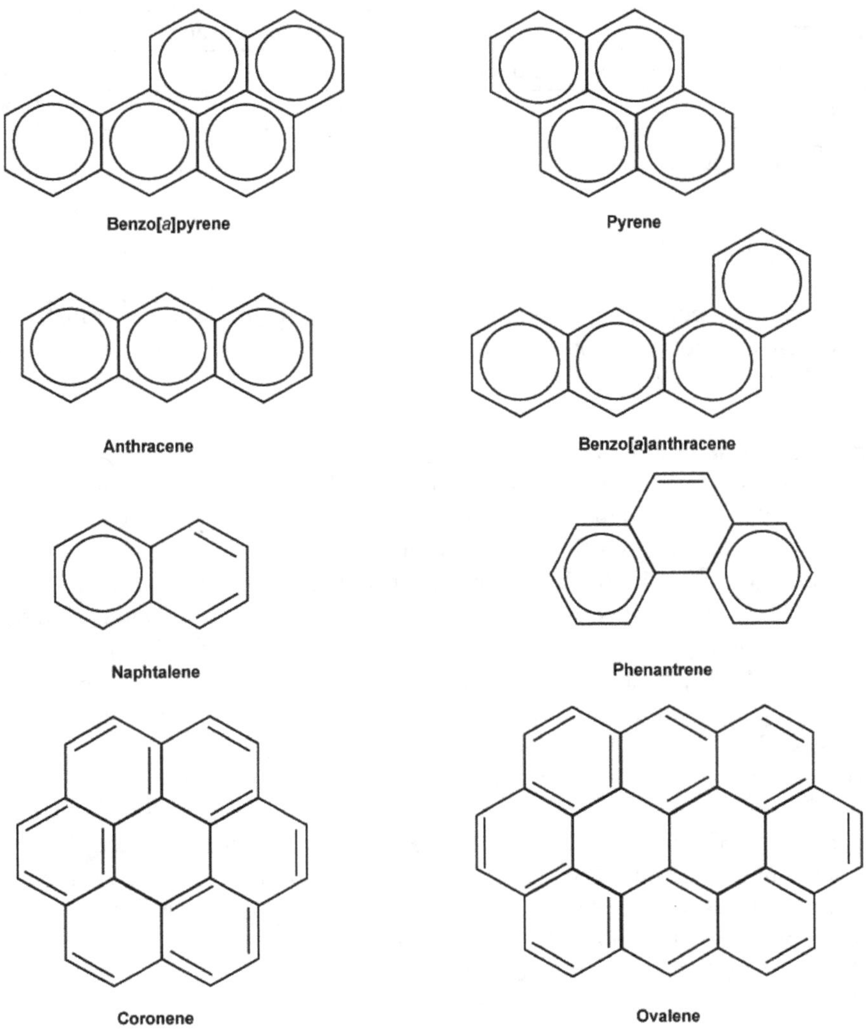

Fig. 1. Structures of some polycyclic aromatic hydrocarbons.

Name	CAS[1]	Name	CAS
Acenaphthene	83-32-9	Dibenz(a,j)acridine,	224-42-0
Acenaphtylene	208-96-8	Dibenzo(a,h)anthracene	53-70-3
Benzo(a)anthracene	56-55-3	Dibenzo(a,e)fluoranthene	5385-75-1
Benzo(a)phenanthrene (chrysene)	218-01-9	Dibenzo(a,e)pyrene	192-65-4
Benzo(a)pyrene	50-32-8	Dibenzo(a,h)pyrene	189-64-0
Benzo(b)fluoranthene	205-99-2	Dibenzo(a,l)pyrene	191-30-0
Benzo(j)fluoranthene	205-82-3	7H-Dibenzo(c,g)carbazole	194-59-2
Benzo(k)fluoranthene	207-08-9	7,12-Dimethylbenz(a)anthracene	57-97-6
Benzo(g,h,i)perylene	191-24-2	Fluorene	86-73-7
Benzo(j,k)fluorene (fluoranthene)	206-44-0	Indeno(1,2,3-cd)pyrene	193-39-5
Benzo(r,s,t)pentaphene	189-55-9	3-Methylcholanthrene	56-49-5
Dibenz(a,h)acridine	226-36-8	5-Methylchrysene	3697-24-3
Phenanthrene	85-01-8	Pyrene	129-00-0
1-Nitropyrene	5222-43-0	Anthracene	120-12-7

Table 1. US EPA priority polycyclic aromatic hydrocarbons.

After exposure, these molecules induce expression of phase I and II metabolizing enzymes (Shimada, 2006) including aldo-ketone reductases, cytochrome P-450s, catechol-O-methyltransferase, epoxide hydrolase, peroxidases, glutathione S-transferases, N-acetyltransferases, sulfotransferases, and other enzymes catalyzing conjugation reactions (Williams & Phillips, 2000).

2.1 Phase I metabolism of PAHs

There are three main pathways for activation of PAHs: the formation of a PAH radical cation in a metabolic oxidation process involving cytochrome P450 peroxidase, the formation of PAH-o-quinones by dihydrodiol dehydrogenase-catalyzed oxidation and finally the creation of dihydrodiol epoxides, catalyzed by cytochrome P450 enzymes (Guengerich, 2000). The most common mechanism of metabolic activation of PAHs, such as benzo[a]pyrene (B[a]P), is via the formation of bay-region dihydrodiol epoxides e.g. benzo[a]pyrene-7,8-dihydrodiol-9,10-epoxide (BPDE), via CYP450 and epoxide hydrolase (EH) (Fig. 2). The most important enzymes in the metabolism of PAHs are CYPs 1A1, 1A2, 1B1 and 3A4. CYP1A1 is highly inducible by PAHs such as B[a]P and some polyhalogenated hydrocarbons. Recombinant human CYP1A1 metabolizes compounds such as B[a]P, 2-acetylaminofluorene and 7,8-diol,7-12-dimethylbenz[a]anthracene (Kim, et al., 1998). CYP1A2 and CYP1B2 are also inducible by the exposure to PAHs. In fact, these enzymes share the same mechanism with which PAH molecules interact with, the aryl hydrocarbon receptor (AhR). The AhR is present in the cytoplasm as a complex with other proteins such as heat shock protein 90 (Hsp90), p23 and AhR-interacting protein. After forming a complex with PAHs, the Hsp90 is released and the AhR-PAH complex translocates to the nucleus (Fig 3). Here, it creates a heterodimer with a ARNT (Ah Receptor Nuclear Translocator) and

[1] CAS (Chemical Abstracts Service) registry number

afterwards binds to DNA via the xenobiotic response element (XRE) situated in the promoter region of CYP1A and CYP1B genes (Shimada, et al., 2002)). CYP3A4 and CYP3A5 are known to activate PAHs present in cigarette smoke, such that increased protein levels and activity of these enzymes in cells exposed to smoke have been detected (Piipari, et al., 2000)). Furthermore, genetic variants of CYPs are associated with risk of carcinogenesis. Some polymorphisms of CYP1A1 are associated with adduct formation and mutagenesis in several populations and species (Ichiba, et al., 1994, Rojas, et al., 2000, Shields, et al., 1992). This fact is related to the metabolizing rate and the subsequent repair mechanism associated with DNA damage. Polycyclic aromatic hydrocarbons are activated by a pathway that involves both CYP enzymes and epoxide hydrolase.

Other phase I enzymes related to PAHs metabolism are the aldo-keto reductases. These enzymes oxidize polycyclic aromatic (PAH) trans-dihydrodiols to reactive and redox-active o-quinones *in vitro* (Quinn & Penning, 2006). Specifically, AKR1A1, and members of the AKR1C dihydrodiol/hydroxysteroid dehydrogenase subfamily, AKR1C1-AKR1C4 are involved in metabolic activation of PAH trans-dihydrodiol. Production of o-quinone metabolites by these enzymes has been shown *in vitro* and in cell lines to amplify ROS and oxidative damage to DNA bases to form the highly mutagenic lesion 8-oxo-dGuo and render damaged and carcinogenic DNA (Quinn, et al., 2008).

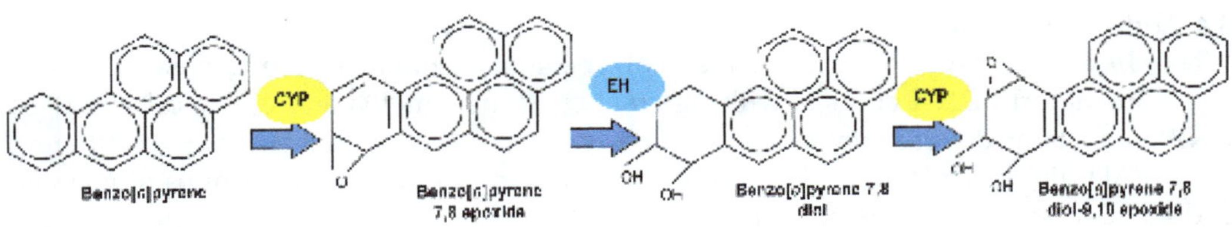

Fig. 2. Mechanism of activation of BaP by cytochrome P450 (CYP) and epoxide hydrolase (EH).

2.2 Phase II metabolism of PAHs

Phase II metabolism includes conjugation of metabolites from phase I with small molecules catalyzed by specific enzymes such as sulfotransferases (SULTs), UDP-glucuronyl transferases (UGTs) or glutathione S-transferases (GSTs). SULTs have been shown to activate some metabolites of PAHs such as 7,12-dimethylbenz[a]anthracene and its methyl-hydroxylated derivatives, in different tissues (Chou, et al., 1998). Polymorphisms of SULT1A1 have been associated with PAH-DNA adduct levels (Tang, et al., 2003). Glucuronidation is also a main pathway for PAH detoxification metabolism. Like sulfation, glucuronidation produces polar conjugates that are readily excreted. Oxygenated benzo[*a*]pyrene derivatives are common substrates of UDP-glucuronyltransferase (Bansal, et al., 1981), the resulting metabolite, 1-hydroxypyrene glucuronide, and the parental 1-hydroxypyrene are used as biomarkers of PAH exposure (Strickland, et al., 1994). Finally, GSTs are also involved in conjugation of PAH derivatives. The importance of this activity has been demonstrated *in vitro* using the corresponding diol epoxides of dibenzo[*a,l*]pyrene and benzo[*a*]pyrene as substrates for these enzymes (Sundberg, et al., 2002). Activity of GSTs is related to their glutathione redox status and genotoxic damage, at least in placenta tissue, therefore this status can be used as biomarker of PAH exposure (Obolenskaya, et al., 2010). On the other hand, polymorphisms of phase II metabolism are associated with carcinogenesis and with DNA damage. For instance, there is an important association between GSTM1 gene polymorphism and the DNA adduct levels (Binkova, et al., 2007). GSTs are also important for quenching and detoxifying ROS and their derivatives (Bonner, et al., 2005).

3. Mechanisms of damage

PAHs undergo metabolic activation to diol-epoxides as we discussed before, which bind covalently to DNA. Afterwards, they form adducts or induce oxidative stress that provokes mutations. If DNA repair mechanisms are afflicted by the adduct formation rate the result is an accumulation of mutations in DNA that may induce carcinogenesis. Several studies indicate that the number of adducts formed is related to the degree of PAH exposure. However, is also important to consider the effect of life stage of the organism at exposure to PAHs (Bolognesi, et al., 1991), as well as concentration and genetic profiles of PAHs, among other factors. PAH exposure induces several molecular and cellular responses that modify the endogenous environment. Exposure to PAHs induces genes involved in apoptosis, cell cycle control and DNA repair (Castorena-Torres, et al., 2008).

3.1 Adduct formation

When PAHs are metabolized reactive diol epoxide enantiomers are generated. These enantiomers form DNA adducts with different structures, motifs and biological activities. DNA adducts of diverse conformations are excised by DNA repair enzymes at different rates. PAH diol epoxides (PAHDEs) bind covalently to exocyclic amino groups of guanine and adenine, forming stable adducts within DNA (Lin, et al., 2001). Futhermore, there are correlations between DNA adduct levels and mutagenesis. The structure of some PAHDEs forms a region called "Fjord", which some studies indicate is a region that is highly involved with high tumorigenicity. These molecules are mostly non-planar, reactive, and bind preferentially to adenine nucleotides. On the other hand, PAHDES with a "bay" region are planar, less reactive and bind to guanine nucleotides (Fig. 4). Geacintov and colleagues (1997) have described several structural motifs by nuclear magnetic resonance analysis. These structural types are divided into: (a) minor groove, when the PAH is partially accessible to the solvent; (b) classical intercalation, when the PAH is protected from the environment and forms a "sandwich structure" and (c) base-displaced intercalation, when PAHs substitute the healthy base (Buterin, et al., 2000, Geacintov, et al., 1997).

Molecular studies have revealed that adducts in DNA block polymerase replication activity, contributing to increased DNA damage by reducing repair activity (Hsu, et al., 2005). An example of adduct formation between adenine or guanine and benzopyrene diol epoxide (BPDE) is shown in Figure 5. Interestingly, some compounds present in food are capable of preventing adducts such as ellagic acid (EA) by the formation of adducts previous to DNA binding (Lagerqvist, et al., 2011). The presence of adducts have been evaluated in marine and aquatic species as an indicator of environmental occurrence of PAHs. Some studies have revealed, by X-ray crystallography, structures of PAH-adducted oligonucleotides bound to bacterial DNA polymerases (Hsu, et al., 2005, Ling, et al., 2004).

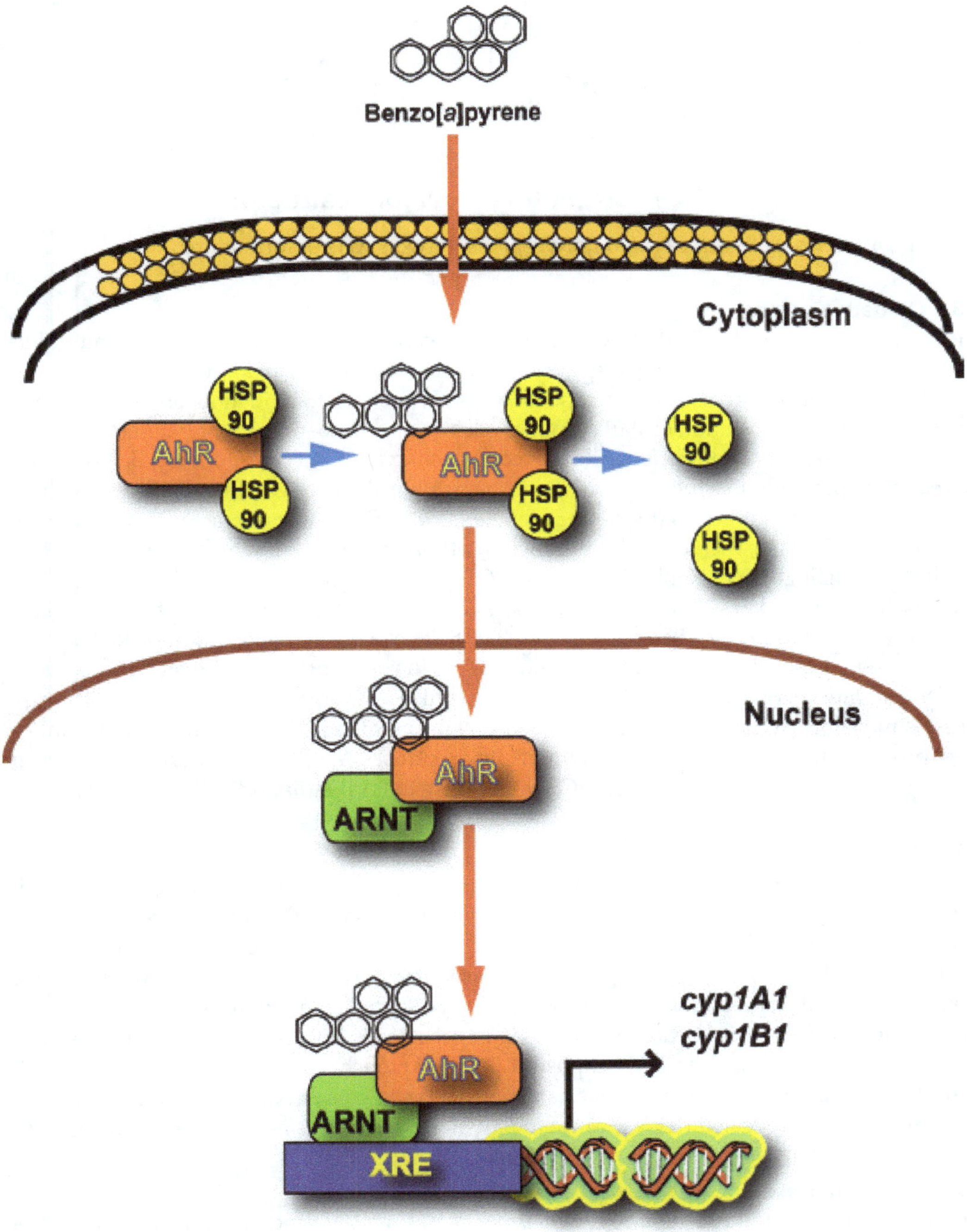

Fig. 3. Aryl hydrocarbon receptor (AhR) pathway activated by BaP induces expression of *cyp1A1* and *cyp1B1*.

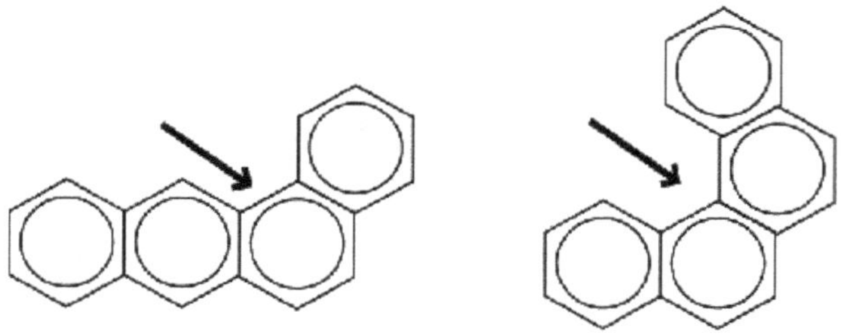

Fig. 4. Difference between bay and fjord regions in two PAH conformations.

3.2 Oxidative stress

It has been reported that BaP derivatives have the capacity to enter redox cycles and induce the production of reactive oxygen species (ROS), thereby causing oxidative stress (An, et al., 2011). BaP radical-cations are precursors for 6-OH-BaP. Auto-oxidation of this derivative may result in the formation of BaP quinones such as 6, 12-, 1,6- and 3,6-BaP dione (Briede, et al., 2004). These metabolites can undergo redox-cycling to their corresponding BaP diols and produce superoxide reactive oxygen species which are then converted to hydroxyl radicals by the Haber-Weiss reaction (Lesko & Lorentzen, 1985). Free radicals react with guanine and cause DNA damage, including the production of 7-hydro-8-oxo-20-deoxyguanosine (8-oxo-dG) (Chatgilialoglu & O'Neill, 2001). The OGG1 gene codes for a DNA glycosylase involved in base excision repair of 8-oxo-dG that arises from ROS. When this system fails there is an increase in mutation rate (Bonner, et al., 2005). Balance between generation of ROS species and scavenging of these molecules is fundamental in repairing DNA damage. If the rate of ROS generation is greater than their removal it is likely that more DNA damage will result. PAHs may absorb light energy in UVR (280–400 nm) region and may induce DNA damage by production of ROS. For example, chrysene, induces apoptosis and DNA damage in human keratinocytes by generating ROS in response to UVB radiation (Ali, et al., 2011).

3.3 Mutations

The failure of repair mechanisms and constant exposure to PAHs induce mutagenesis in cells. These mutations are present in multiple genes including those that participate in cell survival. In particular, p53 mutations are associated with risk of carcinogenesis in PAH-exposed individuals. Since the p53 protein is a transcription factor that regulates cell proliferation, differentiation, apoptosis, and DNA repair, mutations induced in this important protein could lead to severe damage in cells and genes. Some studies have associated p53 mutations to PAH exposure (Mordukhovich, et al., 2010, Yoon, et al., 2003). Another common target of mutagenesis is the ras gene (Ross & Nesnow, 1999). A study by Gray et al. (2001) revealed that exposure to BaP in mice increases mutation of the K-ras gene.

3.4 Carcinogenesis

Forming adducts in DNA repair-related genes is not the only mechanism by which PAHs induce carcinogenesis. An additional danger amounts from their resemblance to steroid hormones allowing PAHs the ability to activate estrogen receptors and metabolism. The ability of several PAHs to displace natural estrogens and occupy ER binding sites, at least to some extent, implies a potential mechanism of action in endocrine tissues that is ER-mediated (Santodonato, 1997). Nevertheless, the most important mechanism of carcinogenesis is a deficient DNA repair system in key genes involved in cell cycle control. Since chronic exposure to PAHs is related to a high rate of mutagenesis it is probable that damage to DNA is cumulative. Several studies have associated chronic occupational PAH exposure to multiple types of cancer including cancer of the bladder, lung, kidney, liver, and breast (Boffetta, et al., 1997, Dickey, et al., 1997, Karami, et al., 2011, Shen, et al., 2003).

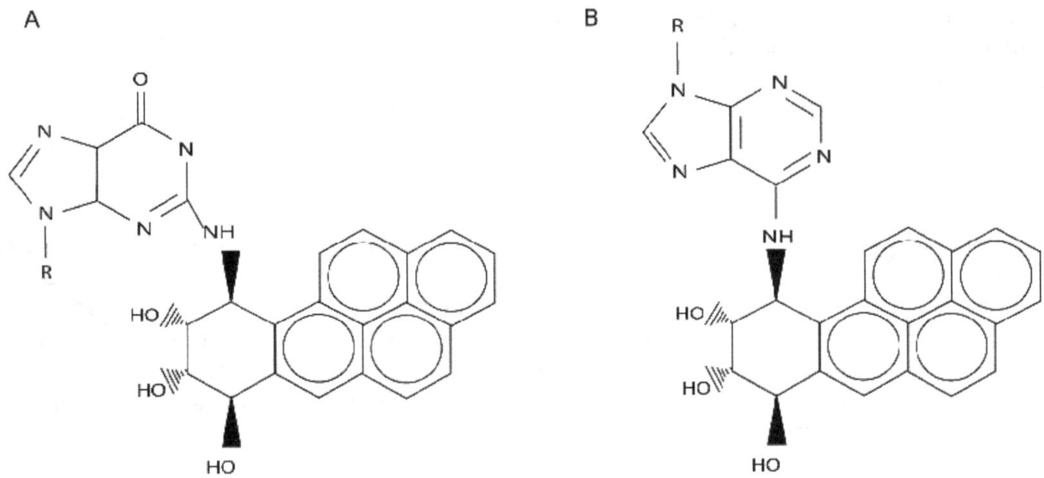

Fig. 5. Structures and interaction of two common adducts: (A) BPDE-dG adduct and (B) BPDE-dA adduct.

4. Mechanisms of repair

Several molecular processes exist in cells that repair damage caused from PAH exposure, adduct formation, and ROS production. If the damage is repaired by these mechanisms no further consequences should result. However, if the lesions escape repair and survive to the next round of DNA replication faulty translesion bypass can occur causing mutagenesis and carcinogenesis. The most common mechanisms of repair used by cells exposed to PAHs are: nucleotide excision repair (NER), base excision repair (BER), non-homologous end joining (NHEJ) of DNA double-strand breaks (DSBs), homologous recombinational repair (HRR) and transcription coupled repair (TCR). On the other hand, some studies indicate that DNA damage induced by PAHs is preferentially repaired by NER or BER (Braithwaite, et al., 1998), and to a lesser extent by HRR (Meschini, et al., 2010).

4.1 Nucleotide excision repair (NER)

In this process, cells recognize damaged DNA regions based on their abnormal structure or chemistry, then excise and replace them. This pathway is complex, requiring more than 20 different proteins. NER is considered the main pathway for removal of bulky DNA adducts (Braithwaite, et al., 1998). There are two distinct forms of NER: GG-NER (Global Genomic-NER) and TC-NER (Transcription Coupled-NER). The first corrects damage in transcriptionally silent areas of the genome, while the second repairs lesions on the actively transcribed strand of the DNA. In GG-NER, the XPC (Xeroderma Pigmentosum Complementation Group-C)/hHR23B (Rad23 homolog B) protein complex is responsible for the initial detection of damaged DNA. On the other hand, TC-NER does not require XPC, however the stalled RNA Polymerase complex is displaced in order to allow the NER proteins to access the damaged DNA. After this process, TC-NER and GG- NER proceed in identical ways. XPA and RPA (Replication Protein-A) then bind at the location of injury and further aid in damage detection. Subsequently, the XPB and XPD helicases unwind the DNA duplex in the surrounding area of the lesion. The endonucleases XPG and ERCC1 (Excision Repair Cross-Complementing group-1)/XPF then cleave one strand of the DNA at positions 3' and 5' to the damage, respectively, generating a 30 base oligonucleotide containing the lesion. This oligonucleotide is displaced, permitting gap repair synthesis (performed by DNA Pol Delta/Epsilon, and other accessory proteins). Finally, DNA ligase seals the nick in the repaired strand (Fig. 6). Several studies demonstrate that certain polymorphisms in NER genes alter the efficiency of DNA repair (Shen, et al., 2006, Vodicka, et al., 2004). Four polymorphisms, XPA - 4G/A (rs1800975), ERCC1 C8092A (rs3212986), XPD Lys751Gln (rs1052559), and XPF Ser835Ser (rs1799801), are associated with a reduced capacity for DNA repair and an increased susceptibility to various cancers (Hu, et al., 2004, Monzo, et al., 2007). However, a recent study reports that significant opportunities exist for an interaction between the XPA-4 G/A polymorphism and PAH exposure on sperm DNA damage (Gu, et al., 2010). Although some PAHs lack "bay" and/or "fjord" regions, such as anthracene for example, this molecule also induces DNA damage, activating repair mechanisms, and has in fact has been shown to induce NER and MMR pathways (Desler, et al., 2009).These findings provide support for the importance of NER pathway in DNA damage induced by PAHs.

4.2 Base excision repair (BER)

BER involves the combined activity of some specific proteins that recognize and excise DNA damage, replacing the damaged moiety with normal nucleotides. PAH adducts are repaired by this mechanism. BER consists of three important steps: first, removal of the incorrect base by an appropriate DNA N-glycosylase to create an AP site (apurinic/apyrimidinic site); second, cutting off the damaged DNA strand by AP endonuclease upstream of the AP site, therefore creating a 3'-OH terminus adjacent to the AP site and finally, extension of the 3'-OH terminus by DNA polymerase, accompanied by excision of the AP site. Several enzymes are required to complete these three steps. In humans, there are at least six different glycosylases that bind specifically to a target base and hydrolyze the N-glycosylic bond generating the AP or abasic site. Next, the AP site is processed by the APE1 system (AP Endonuclease-1, or HAP1/REF1/APEX), which cuts the phosphodiester backbone adjacent to the 5' end of the AP site, resulting in a 3' hydroxyl group and a transient 5′ dRP (abasic deoxyribose phosphate). The removal of the dRP is accomplished by DNA Pol Beta (polymerase beta) activity, which adds one nucleotide to the 3′ end of the nick and removes the dRP moiety through the action of an AP lyase (Bennett, et al., 1997). DNA Pol Beta also interacts with XRCC1. DNA Pol Beta is therefore crucial for the inclusion of different components of BER at sites of DNA damage and promoting repair efficiency (Fig. 6). The BER pathway deals with smaller damage to individual bases, such as oxidation, methylation, depurination, and deamination. If the adducts are left unrepaired, they may cause permanent mutations (Boysen & Hecht, 2003). If these mutations are situated at critical sites, including tumor suppressor genes, DNA repair-related genes or oncogenes, they may lead to cellular transformation and the development of tumors. A recent study demonstrates that BER plays an important role in DNA repair in cells exposed to PAHs. Chinese hamster ovary cells (CHO) deficient in the BER pathway were found to be more sensitive to damage induced by DBPDE, as measured by frequency of chromosomal aberrations (Meschini, et al., 2010). Polymorphisms in proteins of the BER pathway are associated with an increase in DNA damage. One of these proteins, XRCC1, was discovered to have four functional polymorphisms: T-77C, Arg194Trp, Arg280His and Arg399Gln, associated with alteration in repair capacity of DNA damage induced by PAH adducts (Ji, et al., 2010).

4.3 Homologous recombination (HR)

Homologous recombination (HR) is a DNA metabolic process found in all forms of life that provides high-fidelity, template-dependent repair or tolerance of complex DNA damage including DNA gaps, DNA double-stranded breaks (DSBs), and DNA interstrand crosslinks (ICLs). The primary function of HR is to search for homology and DNA strand invasion through the Rad51-ssDNA presynaptic filament by positioning the invading 3′-end on a template duplex DNA to initiate repair synthesis. This mechanism participates in DNA repair induced by three specific PAHs: 1-nitrosopyrene (1-NOP), N-acetoxy-2-acetylaminofluorene (N-AcO-AAF), and 4-nitroquinoline 1-oxide (4-NQO). These PAHs were compared for their ability to cause intrachromosomal homologous recombination between two identical genes stably integrated into a genome of a mouse cell. In each case a dose-dependent increase in recombination frequency with differences in the efficiency of each compound was observed (Bhattacharyya, et al., 1989). Polymorphisms in the proteins related to the HR seem to be associated with a protective effect against PAH exposure.

One of these proteins, XRCC3, participates in homologous recombination repair of DNA double strand breaks and cross-links. This factor is a member of a family of Rad-51-related proteins. According to Shen, et al. (2003), it plays a protective role against bladder cancer for the XRCC3 codon 241 polymorphism, a higher risk in smokers. Considering that tobacco smoke has a high concentration of PAHs, this finding suggests that HR is related to some extent in the repair of damaged DNA induced by PAH exposure. Moreover, in an *in vitro* study using CHO cells deficient in the HR pathway, these cells were more sensitive to PAH exposure suggesting that this mechanism plays an important role in DNA repair (Meschini, et al., 2010).

4.4 Translesion synthesis (TLS)

To avoid cell death that may occur as a result of arrested DNA replication at unrepaired lesions cells have a mechanism, referred to as translesion synthesis (TLS), which allows them to overcome replication blockage from DNA damage. Once the lesion is generated in the DNA, the replication machine stalls, followed by either lesion repair or bypass by specialized polymerases (DNA polymerase IV or V, from the Y Polymerase family). Polymerase switching is mediated by, among other factors, the protein PCNA. TLS polymerases often have low fidelity; however, they are highly efficient, inserting the correct nucleotides at specific sites of damage. This process has been studied using the TLS performed by *Sulfolobus solfataricus* DNA polymerase Dpo4. The analysis of an oligonucleotide primer-extended and its dA−PAH adducts, using a liquid chromatography (LC)−mass spectrometry (MS)/MS, revealed this process in-depth including other proteins that may be involved (Zang, et al., 2006). The structure and nature, among other properties, of TLS polymerases is related to their fidelity and efficiency (Rechkoblit, et al., 2002). For a complete review of this process and the role of PAH adducts we recommend a review of Eoff et al. (2010).

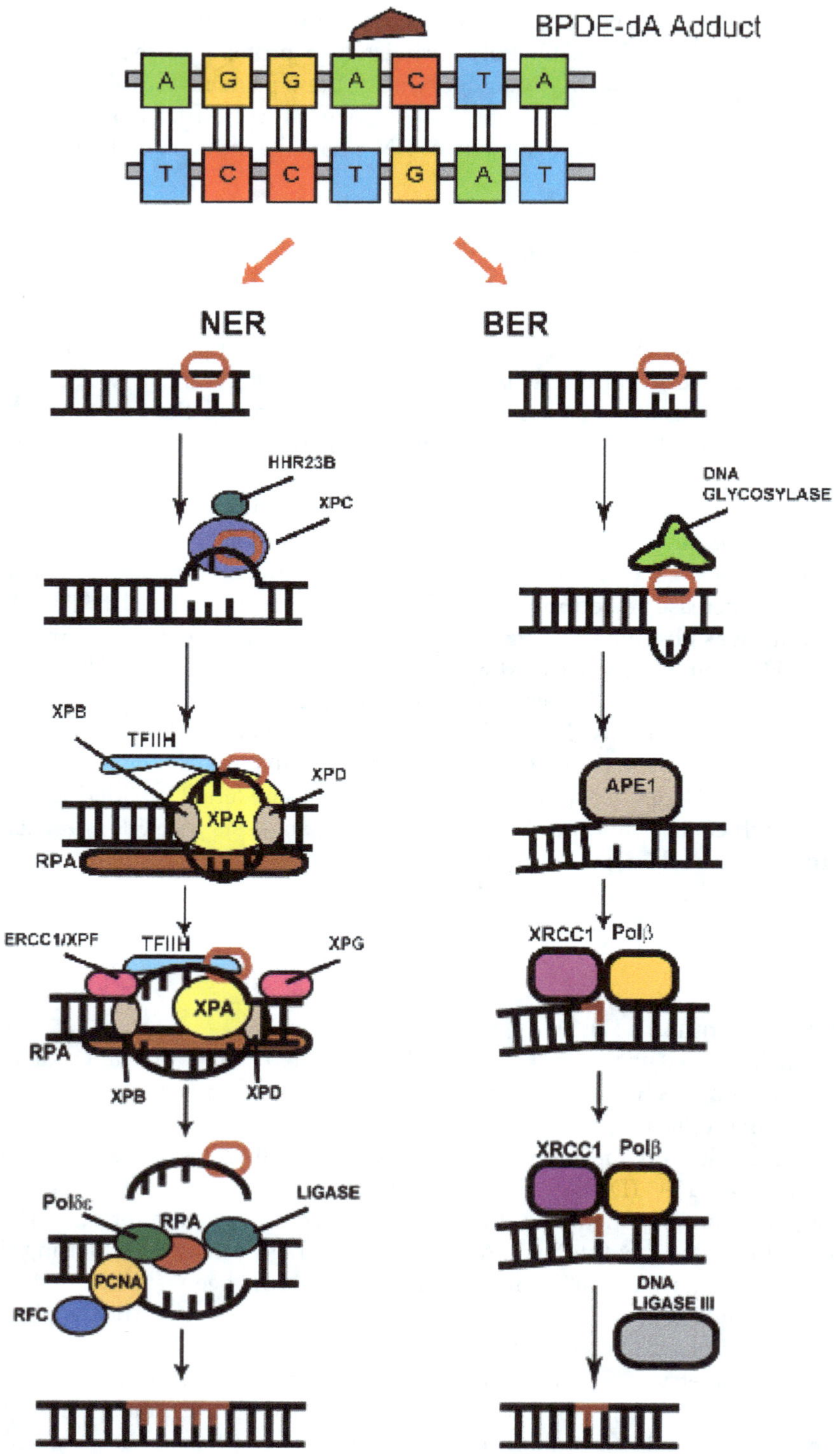

Fig. 6. Common mechanisms of DNA repair from PAH exposure and adduct formation: nucleotide excision repair (NER) and base excision repair (BER).

4.5 Mismatch repair (MMR)

The MMR system is responsible for the post-replicative repair of mismatches and small single stranded DNA loops, and is essential to the prevention of recombination between homologous DNA sequences. Although MMR repair in eukaryotic cells is not fully understood, studies of this mechanism in bacteria have contributed considerably to our understanding of this pathway. MMR is dependent on three highly conserved proteins: MutS, MutL, and MutH. In eukaryotes, homologous proteins as PCNA, RPA, HMGB1, RFC, and ligase I participate and coordinate the MMR process. Eukaryotic cells that are deficient in MMR have a 10-1,000-fold increase in mutation rates (Kunkel & Erie, 2005). In another study, MMR deficient mice showed an increase in PAH-induced lymphoma compared to controls (Zienolddiny, et al., 2006). MMR corrects strand-specific base mispairs and small loop structures. Furthermore, this mechanism recognizes smaller base analoges as mispairs that are participating in oxidative DNA damage repair. Cells deficient in the hMLH1 protein (essential for MMR initiation) have a reduced repair activity when exposed to anthracene (Desler, et al., 2009). This result indicates that MMR has a probable role in DNA repair response resulting from PAH exposure.

4.6 Other repair mechanisms

Further studies are necessary to confirm two other possible mechanisms involved in DNA repair following PAH exposure: non-homologous end joining (NHEJ) and transcription coupled repair (TCR). NHEJ appears to participate in DNA repair after PAH exposure. A recent report described that the V3-3 CHO cell line (NHEJ-deficient), showed a statistically significant dose-dependent enhancement during induced sister chromatid exchanges under PAH exposure. This result indicates that this process is important in DNA repair (Meschini, et al., 2010).

Some adducts perform alterations to the transcription process. The current model for TCR is dependent on the stalling of RNA pol II. Some PAHs such as BPDE and B[c]PhDE produce adducts repaired by TCR, while other studies indicate that PAHs such as B[g]Ch-DE and DB[a,l]P-DE also produce adducts. The efficiency and rate for repairing DNA depends of intrinsic adduct properties (Zhong, et al., 2010). For a complete review of this process we suggest consulting Scicchitano (2005).

5. Methods for detection of DNA damage

DNA damage associated with PAH exposure is mainly assessed by measuring the number of adducts formed. Several methods, such as ^{32}P-postlabelling or immunochemical analysis with specific antibodies, have been applied extensively. However, the arrival of new molecular techniques and innovations in previously well-established biochemical methods, have increased the possibility of the early detection of DNA damage. Polymorphisms and gene expression analysis are helping to determine susceptibility of individuals and populations. Use of mass spectrometry and high performance liquid chromatography (HPLC) with increased sensitivity is another common tool to evaluate and quantify adduct formation. A brief description of the available methods to detect DNA damage is listed in Table 2.

On the other hand, some studies have proposed using molecules included in natural compounds to reduce DNA damage induced by PAHs (Chan, et al., 2003). Green tea consumption may reduce the risk of lung cancer by several hypothesized mechanisms including scavenging oxidative radicals (Bonner, et al., 2005). In previous studies, the role of green tea polyphenols has been associated with protective effects against tumor induction in mice to which PAHs were topically applied (Wang, et al., 1989). Resveratrol (Leung, et al., 2009) and Genistain (Leung, et al., 2009) reduced DNA oxidative damage and adduct formation induced by 7,12-dimethylbenz[*a*]anthracene in MCF-10A cells.

Strategies for detection of PAH exposure	Target molecule or experimental technique	Advantages	Disadvantages	Examples
Metabolites detection and quantitation	Metabolites as a result of exposure detected by chromatography	Sensitive methods and multiple biological sources	Unstable metabolites	1-hydroxypyrene
Adduct detection	Radiolabeled compounds	High sensitive to stable adducts	It may not be possible to detect unstable adducts	DNA adducts
	Mass spectrometry	High sensitivity and selectivity	Suitable just for isotopes	
	^{32}P-Postlabeling assay	High sensitivity to low concentrations, detection of different structures	Interference due endogen adducts	
	Immunoassays	Very high sensitivity	Hard to obtain and validate antibodies	
Primary compound detection	PAH molecules	Indicators of exposure	Some compounds are volatile	Pyrene
Polymorphism analysis	Genotyping	Susceptibility markers	Few studies on populations	CYP1A1 polymorphisms
Gene expression	Molecular biology methods	Changes in gene expression of some genes are related with PAH exposure	Expensive and highly skilled techniques	CYP1B1 expression

Table 2. Methods to detect DNA damage caused by PAH exposure.

These studies offer novel alternatives for the prevention of further DNA damage caused by PAH exposure. Additionally, mechanisms of damage and repair are revealed through understanding the interactions and pathways involved when these molecules come into contact.

Both methods of detection and prevention of DNA damage are candidates for becoming new molecular alternatives for therapy and diagnosis of PAH-exposed individuals, and new tools in environmental biomonitoring.

6. Conclusions

Worldwide, the population is, to some extent, exposed to PAHs. Of primary concern are the carcinogenic, teratogenic and mutagenic properties exhibited by some PAHs. The occurrence of cancer and other diseases associated with PAH exposure has increased in recent decades. As we discussed in this chapter, the major mechanisms of carcinogenesis induced by these compounds are the interaction of PAHs with DNA to form adducts and the generation of reactive oxygen species. Both activities result in DNA damage and mutagenesis in important sites of the genome. Maintenance of genome integrity is critically dependent on efficient repair of DNA lesions by specific DNA repair mechanisms. In addition, the metabolism of PAHs is related with the ability of cells to prevent damage. Polymorphisms in DNA repair or xenobiotic metabolism-related genes are therefore associated with PAH-induced carcinogenesis. For this reason, understanding the metabolic pathways, biochemical transformations and interactions of PAHs with DNA will help to develop better strategies for risk analysis in exposed individuals. Some studies have shown that several natural compounds could help to reduce DNA damage caused by PAH exposure.

These findings offer the possibility for the development of novel drugs that help in the treatment of diseases related to PAH exposure. The analysis of specific polymorphisms of DNA repair genes will help to determine susceptibility in defined populations and the development of new biomarkers and diagnostic tools. Moreover, the study of DNA damage induced by these compounds has included other environmentally important species, such as fish, shrimp and worms. These studies are important in the development of biomarkers for biomonitoring and environmental assessment.

7. Acknowledgments

This work was supported by CONACyT Mexico (60463) to AA and CONACyT (104316) to BM.

8. References

Ali, D., Verma, A., Mujtaba, F., Dwivedi, A., Hans, R. K.& Ray, R. S. (2011). UVB-induced apoptosis and DNA damaging potential of chrysene via reactive oxygen species in human keratinocytes. Toxicol Lett, Vol. 204, No.2-3, (Jul 28), pp. 199-207, 1879-3169 (Electronic) 0378-4274 (Linking)

An, J., Yin, L., Shang, Y., Zhong, Y., Zhang, X., Wu, M., Yu, Z., Sheng, G., Fu, J. & Huang, Y. (2011). The combined effects of BDE47 and BaP on oxidatively generated DNA damage in L02 cells and the possible molecular mechanism. *Mutation Research/Genetic Toxicology and Environmental Mutagenesis*, Vol. In Press, Corrected Proof, pp.

ATSDR. (1996). ToxFAQs™ for Polycyclic Aromatic Hydrocarbons (PAHs), In: Agency for Toxic Substances and Disease Registry, 16.01.2011, Available from http://www.atsdr.cdc.gov/toxfaqs/tf.asp?id=121&tid=25

Bansal, S. K., Zaleski, J.& Gessner, T. (1981). Glucuronidation of oxygenated benzo(a)pyrene derivatives by UDP-glucuronyltransferase of nuclear envelope. *Biochemical and Biophysical Research Communications*, Vol. 98, No.1, pp. 131-139,

Bennett, R. A., Wilson, D. M., 3rd, Wong, D. & Demple, B. (1997). Interaction of human apurinic endonuclease and DNA polymerase beta in the base excision repair pathway. *Proceedings of the National Academy of Sciences of the U S A*, Vol. 94, No.14, (Jul 8), pp. 7166-7169, 0027-8424 (Print) 0027-8424 (Linking)

Bhattacharyya, N. P., Maher, V. M.& McCormick, J. J. (1989). Ability of structurally related polycyclic aromatic carcinogens to induce homologous recombination between duplicated chromosomal sequences in mouse L cells. *Mutation Research/Fundamental and Molecular Mechanisms of Mutagenesis*, Vol. 211, No.2, pp. 205-214,

Binkova, B., Chvatalova, I., Lnenickova, Z., Milcova, A., Tulupova, E., Farmer, P. B.& Sram, R. J. (2007). PAH-DNA adducts in environmentally exposed population in relation to metabolic and DNA repair gene polymorphisms. *Mutation Research/Fundamental and Molecular Mechanisms of Mutagenesis*, Vol. 620, No.1-2, pp. 49-61,

Boffetta, P., Jourenkova, N.& Gustavsson, P. (1997). Cancer risk from occupational and environmental exposure to polycyclic aromatic hydrocarbons. *Cancer Causes Control*, Vol. 8, No.3, (May), pp. 444-472, 0957-5243 (Print) 0957-5243 (Linking)

Bolognesi, C., Parrini, M., Aiello, C.& Rossi, L. (1991). DNA damage induced by 7,12-dimethylbenz[a]anthracene in the liver and the mammary gland of rats exposed to polycyclic aromatic hydrocarbon enzyme inducers during perinatal life. *Mutagenesis*, Vol. 6, No.2, (Mar), pp. 113-116, 0267-8357 (Print) 0267-8357 (Linking)

Bonner, M. R., Rothman, N., Mumford, J. L., He, X., Shen, M., Welch, R., Yeager, M., Chanock, S., Caporaso, N.& Lan, Q. (2005). Green tea consumption, genetic susceptibility, PAH-rich smoky coal, and the risk of lung cancer. Mutat Res, Vol. 582, No.1-2, (Apr 4), pp. 53-60, 0027-5107 (Print) 0027-5107 (Linking)

Boysen, G.& Hecht, S. S. (2003). Analysis of DNA and protein adducts of benzo[a]pyrene in human tissues using structure-specific methods. *Mutation Research/Reviews in Mutation Research*, Vol. 543, No.1, pp. 17-30,

Braithwaite, E., Wu, X.& Wang, Z. (1998). Repair of DNA lesions induced by polycyclic aromatic hydrocarbons in human cell-free extracts: involvement of two excision repair mechanisms in vitro. *Carcinogenesis*, Vol. 19, No.7, (Jul), pp. 1239-1246, 0143-3334 (Print) 0143-3334 (Linking)

Briede, J. J., Godschalk, R. W., Emans, M. T., De Kok, T. M., Van Agen, E., Van Maanen, J., Van Schooten, F. J.& Kleinjans, J. C. (2004). In vitro and in vivo studies on oxygen free radical and DNA adduct formation in rat lung and liver during benzo[a]pyrene metabolism. *Free Radicals Research*, Vol. 38, No.9, (Sep), pp. 995-1002, 1071-5762 (Print)1029-2470 (Linking)

Buterin, T., Hess, M. T., Luneva, N., Geacintov, N. E., Amin, S., Kroth, H., Seidel, A.& Naegeli, H. (2000). Unrepaired fjord region polycyclic aromatic hydrocarbon-DNA adducts in ras codon 61 mutational hot spots. *Cancer Research*, Vol. 60, No.7, (Apr 1), pp. 1849-1856, 0008-5472 (Print) 0008-5472 (Linking)

Castorena-Torres, F., Bermudez de Leon, M., Cisneros, B., Zapata-Perez, O., Salinas, J. E.& Albores, A. (2008). Changes in gene expression induced by polycyclic aromatic hydrocarbons in the human cell lines HepG2 and A549. *Toxicology In Vitro*, Vol. 22, No.2, (Mar), pp. 411-421, 0887-2333 (Print)

Chan, H. Y., Wang, H., Tsang, D. S., Chen, Z. Y.& Leung, L. K. (2003). Screening of chemopreventive tea polyphenols against PAH genotoxicity in breast cancer cells by a XRE-luciferase reporter construct. *Nutrition and Cancer*, Vol. 46, No.1, pp. 93-100, 0163-5581 (Print) 0163-5581 (Linking)

Chatgilialoglu, C.& O'Neill, P. (2001). Free radicals associated with DNA damage. *Experimental Gerontology*, Vol. 36, No.9, (Sep), pp. 1459-1471, 0531-5565 (Print) 0531-5565 (Linking)

Chou, H. C., Ozawa, S., Fu, P. P., Lang, N. P.& Kadlubar, F. F. (1998). Metabolic activation of methyl-hydroxylated derivatives of 7,12-dimethylbenz[a]anthracene by human liver dehydroepiandrosterone-steroid sulfotransferase. *Carcinogenesis*, Vol. 19, No.6, (Jun), pp. 1071-1076, 0143-3334 (Print) 0143-3334 (Linking)

Desler, C., Johannessen, C.& Rasmussen, L. J. (2009). Repair of DNA damage induced by anthanthrene, a polycyclic aromatic hydrocarbon (PAH) without bay or fjord regions. *Chemico-Biological Interactions*, Vol. 177, No.3, (Feb 12), pp. 212-217, 1872-7786 (Electronic) 0009-2797 (Linking)

Dickey, C., Santella, R. M., Hattis, D., Tang, D., Hsu, Y., Cooper, T., Young, T. L.& Perera, F. P. (1997). Variability in PAH-DNA adduct measurements in peripheral mononuclear cells: implications for quantitative cancer risk assessment. *Risk Analysis*, Vol. 17, No.5, (Oct), pp. 649-656, 0272-4332 (Print) 0272-4332 (Linking)

Eoff, R. L., Egli, M.& Guengerich, P. (2010).Impact of Chemical Adducts on Translesion Synthesis in Replicative and Bypass DNA Polymerases From Structure to Function. In: *The Chemical Biology of DNA damage* Wiley-VCH Verlag GmbH & Co. KGaA, 9783527630110,

EPA. (2009). List of Priority Chemicals, In: United States Environmental Protection Agency Web Site, 03.02.2011, Available from http://www.epa.gov/osw/hazard/wastemin/priority.htm

Fetzer, J. C.& Biggs, W. R. (1994). A Review of the Large Polycyclic Aromatic Hydrocarbons. *Polycyclic aromatic compounds*, Vol. 4, No.1, pp. 3 - 17, 1040-6638 March 18, 2011

Geacintov, N. E., Cosman, M., Hingerty, B. E., Amin, S., Broyde, S.& Patel, D. J. (1997). NMR Solution Structures of Stereoisomeric Covalent Polycyclic Aromatic Carcinogen-DNA Adducts: Principles, Patterns, and Diversity. *Chemical Research in Toxicology*, Vol. 10, No.2, pp. 111-146,

Gray, D. L., Warshawsky, D., Xue, W., Nines, R., Wang, Y., Yao, R.& Stoner, G. D. (2001). The effects of a binary mixture of benzo(a)pyrene and 7H-dibenzo(c,g)carbazole on lung tumors and K-ras oncogene mutations in strain A/J mice. *Experimental Lung Research*, Vol. 27, No.3, (Apr-May), pp. 245-253, 0190-2148 (Print) 0190-2148 (Linking)

Gu, A., Ji, G., Zhu, P., Zhou, Y., Fu, G., Xia, Y., Song, L., Wang, S. & Wang, X. (2010). Nucleotide excision repair polymorphisms, polycyclic aromatic hydrocarbon exposure, and their effects on sperm deoxyribonucleic acid damage and male factor infertility. *Fertility and Sterility*, Vol. 94, No.7, pp. 2620-2625.e2625,

Guengerich, F. P. (2000). Metabolism of chemical carcinogens. *Carcinogenesis*, Vol. 21, No.3, (Mar), pp. 345-351, 0143-3334 (Print) 0143-3334 (Linking)

Hsu, G. W., Huang, X., Luneva, N. P., Geacintov, N. E.& Beese, L. S. (2005). Structure of a high fidelity DNA polymerase bound to a benzo[a]pyrene adduct that blocks replication. *Journal of Biological Chemistry*, Vol. 280, No.5, (Feb 4), pp. 3764-3770, 0021-9258 (Print) 0021-9258 (Linking)

Hu, J. J., Hall, M. C., Grossman, L., Hedayati, M., McCullough, D. L., Lohman, K.& Case, L. D. (2004). Deficient nucleotide excision repair capacity enhances human prostate cancer risk. Cancer Res, Vol. 64, No.3, (Feb 1), pp. 1197-1201, 0008-5472 (Print) 0008-5472 (Linking)

IARC. (2010). IARC monographs on the evaluation of carcinogenic risks to humans., In: International Agency for Research in Cancer Web site, 22.02.2011, Available from http://monographs.iarc.fr/ENG/Classification/index.php

Ichiba, M., Hagmar, L., Rannug, A., Hogstedt, B., Alexandrie, A. K., Carstensen, U.& Hemminki, K. (1994). Aromatic DNA adducts, micronuclei and genetic polymorphism for CYP1A1 and GST1 in chimney sweeps. *Carcinogenesis*, Vol. 15, No.7, (Jul), pp. 1347-1352, 0143-3334 (Print) 0143-3334 (Linking)

Ji, G., Gu, A., Zhou, Y., Shi, X., Xia, Y., Long, Y., Song, L., Wang, S.& Wang, X. (2010). Interactions between Exposure to Environmental Polycyclic Aromatic Hydrocarbons and DNA Repair Gene Polymorphisms on Bulky DNA Adducts in Human Sperm. *PLoS ONE*, Vol. 5, No.10, pp. e13145,

Jongeneelen, F. J. (2001). Benchmark guideline for urinary 1-hydroxypyrene as biomarker of occupational exposure to polycyclic aromatic hydrocarbons. *Annals of Occupationa Hygiene*, Vol. 45, No.1, (Jan), pp. 3-13, 0003-4878 (Print) 0003-4878 (Linking)

Karami, S., Boffetta, P., Brennan, P., Stewart, P. A., Zaridze, D., Matveev, V., Janout, V., Kollarova, H., Bencko, V., Navratilova, M., Szeszenia-Dabrowska, N., Mates, D., Gromiec, J. P., Sobotka, R., Chow, W.-H., Rothman, N.& Moore, L. E. (2011). Renal Cancer Risk and Occupational Exposure to Polycyclic Aromatic Hydrocarbons and Plastics. *Journal of Occupational & Environmental Medicine*, Vol. 53, No.2, pp. 218-223 1076-2752

Kim, J. H., Stansbury, K. H., Walker, N. J., Trush, M. A., Strickland, P. T.& Sutter, T. R. (1998). Metabolism of benzo[a]pyrene and benzo[a]pyrene-7,8-diol by human cytochrome P450 1B1. *Carcinogenesis*, Vol. 19, No.10, (Oct), pp. 1847-1853, 0143-3334 (Print) 0143-3334 (Linking)

Kunkel, T. A.& Erie, D. A. (2005). DNA mismatch repair. *Annual Review of Biochemistry*, Vol. 74, pp. 681-710, 0066-4154 (Print) 0066-4154 (Linking)

Lagerqvist, A., Hakansson, D., Frank, H., Seidel, A.& Jenssen, D. (2011). Structural requirements for mutation formation from polycyclic aromatic hydrocarbon dihydrodiol epoxides in their interaction with food chemopreventive compounds. *Food and Chemical Toxicology*, Vol. 49, No.4, (Apr), pp. 879-886, 1873-6351 (Electronic) 0278-6915 (Linking)

Leung, H. Y., Yung, L. H., Poon, C. H., Shi, G., Lu, A. L.& Leung, L. K. (2009). Genistein protects against polycyclic aromatic hydrocarbon-induced oxidative DNA damage in non-cancerous breast cells MCF-10A. *British Journal of Nutrition*, Vol. 101, No.2, (Jan), pp. 257-262, 1475-2662 (Electronic) 0007-1145 (Linking)

Leung, H. Y., Yung, L. H., Shi, G., Lu, A. L.& Leung, L. K. (2009). The red wine polyphenol resveratrol reduces polycyclic aromatic hydrocarbon-induced DNA damage in MCF-10A cells. *British Journal of Nutrition*, Vol. 102, No.10, (Nov), pp. 1462-1468, 1475-2662 (Electronic) 0007-1145 (Linking)

Lin, C. H., Huang, X., Kolbanovskii, A., Hingerty, B. E., Amin, S., Broyde, S., Geacintov, N. E.& Patel, D. J. (2001). Molecular topology of polycyclic aromatic carcinogens determines DNA adduct conformation: a link to tumorigenic activity. Journal of Molecular Biology, Vol. 306, No.5, pp. 1059-1080,

Ling, H., Sayer, J. M., Plosky, B. S., Yagi, H., Boudsocq, F., Woodgate, R., Jerina, D. M.& Yang, W. (2004). Crystal structure of a benzo[a]pyrene diol epoxide adduct in a ternary complex with a DNA polymerase. *Proceedings of the National Academy of Sciences of the U S A*, Vol. 101, No.8, (Feb 24), pp. 2265-2269, 0027-8424 (Print) 0027-8424 (Linking)

Meschini, R., Berni, A., Marotta, E., Filippi, S., Fiore, M., Mancinelli, P., Natarajan, A. T.& Palitti, F. (2010). DNA repair mechanisms involved in the removal of DBPDE-induced lesions leading to chromosomal alterations in CHO cells. *Cytogenetics and Genome Research*, Vol. 128, No.1-3, pp. 124-130, 1424-859X (Electronic) 1424-8581 (Linking)

Monzo, M., Moreno, I., Navarro, A., Ibeas, R., Artells, R., Gel, B., Martinez, F., Moreno, J., Hernandez, R.& Navarro-Vigo, M. (2007). Single nucleotide polymorphisms in nucleotide excision repair genes XPA, XPD, XPG and ERCC1 in advanced colorectal cancer patients treated with first-line oxaliplatin/fluoropyrimidine. *Oncology*, Vol. 72, No.5-6, pp. 364-370, 1423-0232 (Electronic) 0030-2414 (Linking)

Mordukhovich, I., Rossner, P., Jr., Terry, M. B., Santella, R., Zhang, Y. J., Hibshoosh, H., Memeo, L., Mansukhani, M., Long, C. M., Garbowski, G., Agrawal, M., Gaudet, M. M., Steck, S. E., Sagiv, S. K., Eng, S. M., Teitelbaum, S. L., Neugut, A. I., Conway-Dorsey, K.& Gammon, M. D. (2010). Associations between polycyclic aromatic hydrocarbon-related exposures and p53 mutations in breast tumors. *Environmental Health Perspectives*, Vol. 118, No.4, (Apr), pp. 511-518, 1552-9924 (Electronic) 0091-6765 (Linking)

NIST. (2010). NIST chemical kinetics model database., In: National Institute of Standards and Tecnonology database, 03.03.2011, Available from http://kinetics.nist.gov/CKMech/SpeciesSearch.jsp#Help PAH Class

Obolenskaya, M. Y., Teplyuk, N. M., Divi, R. L., Poirier, M. C., Filimonova, N. B., Zadrozna, M.& Pasanen, M. J. (2010). Human placental glutathione S-transferase activity and polycyclic aromatic hydrocarbon DNA adducts as biomarkers for environmental oxidative stress in placentas from pregnant women living in radioactivity- and chemically-polluted regions. *Toxicology Letters*, Vol. 196, No.2, pp. 80-86,

Piipari, R., Savela, K., Nurminen, T., Hukkanen, J., Raunio, H., Hakkola, J., Mantyla, T., Beaune, P., Edwards, R. J., Boobis, A. R.& Anttila, S. (2000). Expression of CYP1A1, CYP1B1 and CYP3A, and polycyclic aromatic hydrocarbon-DNA adduct formation in bronchoalveolar macrophages of smokers and non-smokers. *International Journal of Cancer*, Vol. 86, No.5, (Jun 1), pp. 610-616, 0020-7136 (Print) 0020-7136 (Linking)

Quinn, A. M., Harvey, R. G.& Penning, T. M. (2008). Oxidation of PAH trans-Dihydrodiols by Human Aldo-Keto Reductase AKR1B10. *Chemical Research in Toxicology*, Vol. 21, No.11, pp. 2207-2215,

Quinn, A. M.& Penning, T. M. (2006). Oxidation of PAH trans-dihydrodiols by human aldo-keto reductase (AKR) 1B isoforms: A new AKR subfamily implicated in PAH activation. *Proceedings of Frontiers in Cancer Prevention Research Conference*, Boston, MA, USA, April 1, 2006

Rechkoblit, O., Zhang, Y., Guo, D., Wang, Z., Amin, S., Krzeminsky, J., Louneva, N.& Geacintov, N. E. (2002). trans-Lesion synthesis past bulky benzo[a]pyrene diol epoxide N2-dG and N6-dA lesions catalyzed by DNA bypass polymerases. *Journal of Biological Chemistry*, Vol. 277, No.34, (Aug 23), pp. 30488-30494, 0021-9258 (Print) 0021-9258 (Linking)

Rojas, M., Cascorbi, I., Alexandrov, K., Kriek, E., Auburtin, G., Mayer, L., Kopp-Schneider, A., Roots, I.& Bartsch, H. (2000). Modulation of benzo[a]pyrene diolepoxide-DNA adduct levels in human white blood cells by CYP1A1, GSTM1 and GSTT1 polymorphism. *Carcinogenesis*, Vol. 21, No.1, (Jan), pp. 35-41, 0143-3334 (Print) 0143-3334 (Linking)

Ross, J. A.& Nesnow, S. (1999). Polycyclic aromatic hydrocarbons: correlations between DNA adducts and ras oncogene mutations. *Mutation Research*, Vol. 424, No.1-2, (Mar 8), pp. 155-166, 0027-5107 (Print) 0027-5107 (Linking)

Santodonato, J. (1997). Review of the estrogenic and antiestrogenic activity of polycyclic aromatic hydrocarbons: relationship to carcinogenicity. *Chemosphere*, Vol. 34, No.4, (Feb), pp. 835-848, 0045-6535 (Print) 0045-6535 (Linking)

Scicchitano, D. A. (2005). Transcription past DNA adducts derived from polycyclic aromatic hydrocarbons. *Mutation Research*, Vol. 577, No.1-2, (Sep 4), pp. 146-154, 0027-5107 (Print) 0027-5107 (Linking)

Shen, J., Desai, M., Agrawal, M., Kennedy, D. O., Senie, R. T., Santella, R. M. & Terry, M. B. (2006). Polymorphisms in nucleotide excision repair genes and DNA repair capacity phenotype in sisters discordant for breast cancer. *Cancer Epidemiology, Biomarkers & Prevention*, Vol. 15, No.9, (Sep), pp. 1614-1619, 1055-9965 (Print) 1055-9965 (Linking)

Shields, P. G., Sugimura, H., Caporaso, N. E., Petruzzelli, S. F., Bowman, E. D., Trump, B. F., Weston, A. & Harris, C. C. (1992). Polycyclic aromatic hydrocarbon-DNA adducts and the CYP1A1 restriction fragment length polymorphism. Environ Health Perspect, Vol. 98, (Nov), pp. 191-194, 0091-6765 (Print) 0091-6765 (Linking)

Shimada, T. (2006). Xenobiotic-metabolizing enzymes involved in activation and detoxification of carcinogenic polycyclic aromatic hydrocarbons. *Drug Metabolic Pharmacokinetics*, Vol. 21, No.4, (Aug), pp. 257-276, 1347-4367 (Print) 1347-4367 (Linking)

Strickland, P. T., Kang, D., Bowman, E. D., Fitzwilliam, A., Downing, T. E., Rothman, N., Groopman, J. D. & Weston, A. (1994). Identification of 1-hydroxypyrene glucuronide as a major pyrene metabolite in human urine by synchronous fluorescence spectroscopy and gas chromatography-mass spectrometry. *Carcinogenesis*, Vol. 15, No.3, (Mar), pp. 483-487, 0143-3334 (Print) 0143-3334 (Linking)

Sundberg, K., Dreij, K., Seidel, A. & Jernström, B. (2002). Glutathione Conjugation and DNA Adduct Formation of Dibenzo[a,l]pyrene and Benzo[a]pyrene Diol Epoxides in V79 Cells Stably Expressing Different Human Glutathione Transferases. *Chemical Research in Toxicology*, Vol. 15, No.2, pp. 170-179,

Tang, D., Rundle, A., Mooney, L., Cho, S., Schnabel, F., Estabrook, A., Kelly, A., Levine, R., Hibshoosh, H.& Perera, F. (2003). Sulfotransferase 1A1 (SULT1A1) Polymorphism, PAH-DNA Adduct Levels in Breast Tissue and Breast Cancer Risk in a Case-Control Study. *Breast Cancer Research and Treatment*, Vol. 78, No.2, pp. 217-222,

Vodicka, P., Kumar, R., Stetina, R., Sanyal, S., Soucek, P., Haufroid, V., Dusinska, M., Kuricova, M., Zamecnikova, M., Musak, L., Buchancova, J., Norppa, H., Hirvonen, A., Vodickova, L., Naccarati, A., Matousu, Z.& Hemminki, K. (2004). Genetic polymorphisms in DNA repair genes and possible links with DNA repair rates, chromosomal aberrations and single-strand breaks in DNA. *Carcinogenesis*, Vol. 25, No.5, (May), pp. 757-763, 0143-3334 (Print) 0143-3334 (Linking)

Wang, Z. Y., Khan, W. A., Bickers, D. R.& Mukhtar, H. (1989). Protection against polycyclic aromatic hydrocarbon-induced skin tumor initiation in mice by green tea polyphenols. Carcinogenesis, Vol. 10, No.2, (Feb), pp. 411-415, 0143-3334 (Print) 0143-3334 (Linking)

Williams, J. A.& Phillips, D. H. (2000). Mammary expression of xenobiotic metabolizing enzymes and their potential role in breast cancer. *Cancer Research*, Vol. 60, No.17, (Sep 1), pp. 4667-4677, 0008-5472 (Print) 0008-5472 (Linking)

Yoon, J. H., Lee, C. S.& Pfeifer, G. P. (2003). Simulated sunlight and benzo[a]pyrene diol epoxide induced mutagenesis in the human p53 gene evaluated by the yeast functional assay: lack of correspondence to tumor mutation spectra. *Carcinogenesis*, Vol. 24, No.1, (Jan), pp. 113-119, 0143-3334 (Print) 0143-3334 (Linking)

Yu, M.-H. (2005).Environmental toxicology: biological and health effects of pollutants (2nd), CRC Press, 156670670X (alk. paper), Boca Raton

Zang, H., Chowdhury, G., Angel, K. C., Harris, T. M.& Guengerich, F. P. (2006). Translesion synthesis across polycyclic aromatic hydrocarbon diol epoxide adducts of deoxyadenosine by Sulfolobus solfataricus DNA polymerase Dpo4. *Chemical Research in Toxicology*, Vol. 19, No.6, (Jun), pp. 859-867, 0893-228X (Print) 0893-228X (Linking)

Zhong, Q., Amin, S., Lazarus, P.& Spratt, T. E. (2010). Differential repair of polycyclic aromatic hydrocarbon DNA adducts from an actively transcribed gene. *DNA Repair (Amsterdam)*, Vol. 9, No.9, (Sep 4), pp. 1011-1016, 1568-7856 (Electronic) 1568-7856 (Linking)

Zienolddiny, S., Ryberg, D., Svendsrud, D. H., Eilertsen, E., Skaug, V., Hewer, A., Phillips, D. H., te Riele, H.& Haugen, A. (2006). Msh2 deficiency increases susceptibility to benzo[a]pyrene-induced lymphomagenesis. *International Journal of Cancer*, Vol. 118, No.11, (Jun 1), pp. 2899-2902, 0020-7136 (Print) 0020-7136 (Linking)

7

The DNA-Damage Response to Ionizing Radiation in Human Lymphocytes

Maddalena Mognato, Mauro Grifalconi, Sabrina Canova, Cristina Girardi and Lucia Celotti
University of Padova, Department of Biology, Italy

1. Introduction

The human genome is constantly subjected to DNA damage derived from endogenous and exogenous sources. Normal cellular metabolism can give raise to DNA damage through free radicals production and replication errors, whereas environmental agents, such as ultraviolet (UV) and ionizing radiation (IR), induce specific types of lesions. DNA damage can ultimately lead to genomic instability and carcinogenesis if not properly addressed, thus an elaborate network of proteins has evolved in cells to maintain genome integrity through a pathway termed the DNA-damage response (DDR). DDR allows DNA damage detection, signal propagation and transduction to a multitude of effector proteins, which promote cell survival and activate cell cycle arrest to allow DNA repair. When cells are unable to properly repair DNA, apoptosis or senescence pathways may be triggered, thus eliminating the possibility of passing on damaged or unrepaired genetic material to its progeny. The ultimate goal of DDR is to protect the integrity of genetic information and its faithful transmission, either to DNA by replication or to mRNA by transcription. Therefore, dysregulation of DDR pathway can contribute to carcinogenesis and developmental defects. Ionizing radiation represents a mutagen agent to which human population is exposed due to environmental, professional or accidental reasons. The biological effects of IR depend on the quality and the dose of radiation and on the cell type. Linear energy transfer (LET) represents the energy lost per unit distance as an ionizing particle travels through a material, and it is used to quantify the effects of IR on biological specimens. High-LET radiation (i.e. alpha-particles, neutrons, protons) are densely IR since they lose the energy throughout a small distance, causing dense ionization along their track with high localized multiple DNA damage. Low-LET radiation, such as X and γ-rays, are sparsely IR since they produce ionizations sparsely along their track and, hence, almost homogeneously within a cell. The biological effect of high-LET radiations are in general much higher than those of low-LET radiations with the same energy. This is because high-LET radiation deposits most of its energy within the volume of one cell and the damage to DNA is therefore larger (Anderson et al., 2002; Brenner & Ward, 1992; Prise et al., 2001). Radiation is potentially harmful to humans, because the ionization it produces can significantly alter the structure of molecules within a living cell.The exposure to ionizing radiation elicits a complex cell response to overcome the dangerous effects of DNA-radiation interaction, such as reactive oxygen species (ROS) production, base oxidation and DNA breaks formation (i.e. single-strand breaks, SSBs and double-strand breaks, DSBs). In particular, DSBs represent the most severe form of damage, since an inefficient or inaccurate repair may lead to cell death or genomic instability (Wyman & Kanaar, 2006). The presence of DSBs leads to a cascade of post-translational modifications of a wide variety of proteins, including phosphorylation, ubiquitinylation, sumoylation, poly(ADP-ribosylation), acetylation and methylation (Huen & Chen, 2010). The early DSB response utilizes phosphorylation-dependent protein–protein interactions to coordinate DNA damage recognition and signal amplification. Following DSB formation the histone H2AX, a histone H2A variant that comprises 10-15% of total cellular H2A in higher eukaryotes, is rapidly phosphorylated on its serine residues 139 (γ–H2AX) (Rogakou et al., 1998) by members of the phosphatidylinositol-3-OH kinase (PI(3)K)-like family, such as ataxia telangiectasia mutated (ATM), DNA-PK and ataxia telangiectasia and Rad3 related (ATR) (Kinner et al., 2008). γ-H2AX formation occurs within minutes after damage, and extends for up to 1-2 megabases from the site of the break in mammalian cells, providing a platform for subsequent DNA repair protein recruitment and amplification at DSBs (Harper & Elledge, 2007). The phosphorylation of H2AX creates a signal recognized by many proteins of the DNA damage response, which are recruited to the sites of DSBs, forming the ionizing radiation-induced foci (IRIF, Lukas et al., 2004). The biological function of IRIF is thought to shelter the broken DNA ends from decay and prevent illegitimate repair processes, to amplify the DNA damage signal and to provide a local concentration of DDR factors relevant for DNA repair and metabolism. Stabilization of DDR factor recruitment to γ-H2AX nucleosomes is achieved through the recruitment of a wide variety of proteins regulating ubiquitylation, sumoylation, acetylation, methylation. The mediator of DNA damage checkpoint 1 (MDC1) is the major protein to localize to the sites of DNA breaks in a γ-H2AX-dependent pathway (Riches et al., 2008; Stucki, 2009) MDC1 has a role in controlling the assembly of multiple repair factors at DNA breaks and in amplifying the DNA damage signal. MDC1 orchestrates the recruitment of IRIF-associated proteins, specifically the MRN complex (MRE11, RAD51, NBS1) and many DNA damage repair proteins, including p53-binding protein 1 (53BP1) and BRCA1 (breast cancer 1). DDR is characterized by the synthesis of ubiquitin conjugates at the sites of damage-induced repair foci (Tanq & Greenberg, 2010). Recently, there has been intense interest regarding the role of ubiquitin and ubiquitin-like molecules in DNA damage repair and signalling, along with its interplay with phosphorylation (Al-Hakim et al., 2010). Protein ubiquitylation has emerged as an important regulatory mechanism that impacts almost every aspect of the DNA damage response, in particular in concentrating DNA repair proteins at the sites of DNA damage. The ubiquitylation cascade involves the activities of at least three enzymes: (i) the ubiquitin-activating enzyme (E1); (ii) the ubiquitin-conjugating enzyme (E2); and (iii) the ubiquitin ligase (E3) (Ciechanover et al.,1982; Hershko et al., 1983). E1 employs ATP to adenylate ubiquitin at its C-terminus, which then forms a thioester bond with the E1 active-site cysteine. The modified ubiquitin is then passed on to the E2 enzyme to form another thioester intermediate (the E2~Ub). Finally, ubiquitin is conjugated to its substrate with the aid of an E3 ubiquitin ligase (Al Hakim et al., 2010). The first E3 ubiquitin ligase that acts in this cascade is RING finger protein 8 (RNF8), which accumulates at DSBs via phospho-dependent interactions between its N-terminal fork head associated (FHA) domain and ATM-phosphorylated TQXF motifs on MDC1 (Huen et al., 2007; Kolas et al., 2007; Mailand et al., 2007). At damaged chromatin, RNF8 cooperates with the E2 conjugating enzyme UBC13 to ubiquitylate histones that likely include H2A and H2AX (Huen, et al., 2007; Mailand et al., 2007, Wu et al., 2008). The ubiquitin ligase RNF8 plays an instrumental role in promoting the maturation of DSB-associated chromatin (Huen et al., 2007; Mailand et al., 2007; Kolas et al., 2007; Wang et al., 2007). Through its direct interaction with MDC1, RNF8 is recruited to DSB sites along with the other factors in the initial wave of protein accumulation at IRIF (Mailand et al., 2007). Here, RNF8 initiates a complex and tightly regulated ubiquitylation cascade of histones H2A and H2AX at the DSB-flanking chromatin, which causes chromatin restructuring (through incompletely understood mechanisms) associated with the generation of binding sites for protein complexes that accumulate downstream of these early factors (Huen et al., 2007; Mailand et al., 2007).The covalent attachment of small ubiquitin-like modifier (SUMO) proteins to specific lysine residues of target proteins, a process termed sumoylation, is a recently discovered protein modification that plays an important role in regulating many diverse cellular processes. Sumoylation is a signalling mechanism which, analogous to and in parallel with ubiquitination, plays an important role in chromatin remodelling at DSB sites. Sumoylation is catalyzed by SUMO-specific E1, E2, E3s and is reversed by a family of Sentrin/SUMO-specific proteases, SENPs. The SUMO E3 ligases PIAS1 and PIAS4 are required for recruitment of proteins BRCA1 and 53BP1 to IRIF, respectively, and both SUMO1 and SUMO2/3 accumulate at IRIF (Galanty et al., 2009; Morris et al., 2009). Moreover, replicating protein A (RPA70) sumoylation facilitates recruitment of RAD51 to the DNA damage foci to initiate DNA repair through homologous recombination (Dou et al., 2010).

2. Cellular effects of ionizing radiation in human lymphocytes

2.1 Surviving fraction, *HPRT* mutant frequency and molecular characterization of mutations in irradiated human lymphocytes

To contribute to the understanding of the DDR pathway following radiation-induced damage, we studied the effects of IR on human peripheral blood lymphocytes (PBL) irradiated *in vitro* with different doses of γ-rays and low-energy protons (0.88 MeV; LET: 28keV/μm). Irradiated PBL were assayed for cell viability, for mutant frequency at the hypoxanthine-guanine phosphoribosyl transferase (*HPRT*) gene, and for molecular characterization of mutations. The *HPRT* gene, which in humans covers 44 kb and encodes a non-essential protein, allows a wide variety of mutations, from point mutation to total gene deletion, to be detected by using the *HPRT* mutation assay. Deletion of DNA segments is the predominant form of radiation damage in cells that survive irradiation and the mechanisms for producing deletion mutations appear to be very complex and dependent on target cell, gene studied, dose, dose-rate and radiation quality (Schwartz et al., 2000). Large deletions are thought to derive from two DNA double strand breaks close enough to interact each other. Thus, deletion frequency should be dependent on radiation dose and dose-rate. All PBL samples, irradiated either with γ-rays or protons, showed a dose-dependent cell survival decrease and a *HPRT* mutant frequency increase. In Table 1 we report the data of survival and *HPRT* mutant frequency in human PBL irradiated with different doses of γ-rays and low-energy protons.

Molecular analyses of *HPRT* mutants were carried out in clones derived from PBL exposed to γ-rays (1-4 Gy) and to low-energy protons (0.5-2Gy), and in non-irradiated clones of the same donors. Among the mutant clones obtained from γ-irradiated PBL, point mutations were the only kind of mutation in 1Gy irradiated clones, whereas deletions were the prevalent mutations among clones irradiated at 4Gy. In contrast, no partial or total deletions of the *HPRT* gene were detected in mutant clones isolated after proton irradiation. Figure 1 shows the percentages of mutation types calculated over the total number of mutations derived from human PBL irradiated with both radiation qualities. The difference of the mutational spectrum between γ-rays and protons probably depends on the nature of IR. Complex gene rearrangements and deletions are assumed to be a specific signature of exposure to high-LET radiation in mammalian cells. Nevertheless, the absence of these kind of mutations in PBL irradiated with protons could be due to their lower survival in comparison with γ-irradiated PBL, as a consequence of the more cytotoxic than mutagenic lesions induced.

	SF (%) ± S.E.	HPRT MF ($x10^{-6}$) ± S.E.
γ-rays		
0.5 Gy	99.5 ± 0	2.8 ± 0
1.0 Gy	83.85 ± 11.36	10.5 ± 3.8
2.0 Gy	44.7 ± 7.36	29.2 ± 3.7
3.0 Gy	13.7 ± 4.56	50.6 ± 17.9
4.0 Gy	6.2 ± 2.4	24.7 ± 11.1
Protons		
0.5 Gy	60.84 ± 7.82	5.33 ± 2.18
1.0 Gy	39.87 ± 6.28	9.25 ± 2.8
1.5 Gy	38.42 ± 11.35	16.72 ± 4.86
2.0 Gy	35.5 ± 0	11.7 ± 1
2.5 Gy	29.9 ± 11.35	5.06 ± 0

Table 1. Surviving fraction (SF) and *HPRT* mutant frequency (± standard error, S.E.) in human PBL irradiated with γ-rays and low-energy protons.

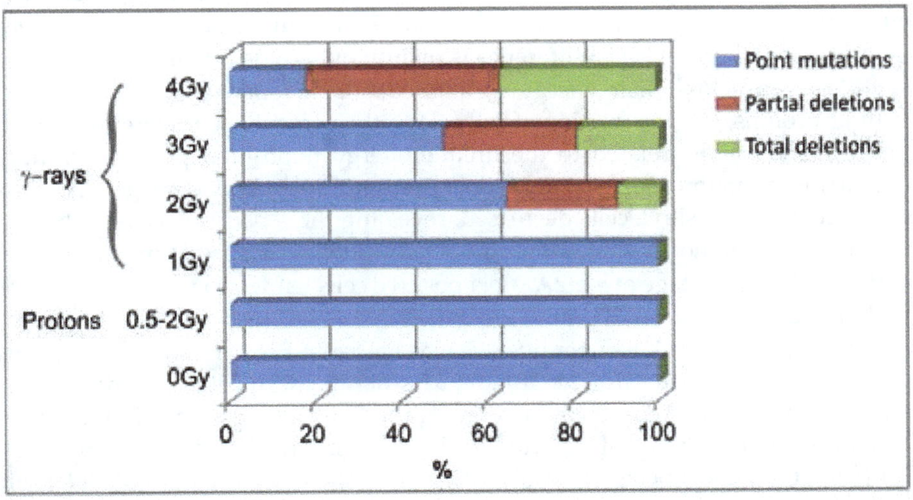

Fig. 1. Characterization of *HPRT* mutant clones derived from PBL irradiated with γ-rays and protons or non-irradiated (0Gy).

2.2 Double strand break repair in irradiated human lymphocytes

To evaluate the repair of DSBs in PBL irradiated with γ-rays or low-energy protons, we analyzed γ-H2AX kinetics through foci formation and disappearance. The presence of nuclear foci was monitored by *in situ* immunofluorescence at different time points after IR. Figure 2 shows the different γ-H2AX foci pattern at 2h after IR with high- and low-LET radiation, reflecting the sparsely and densely nature of IR.

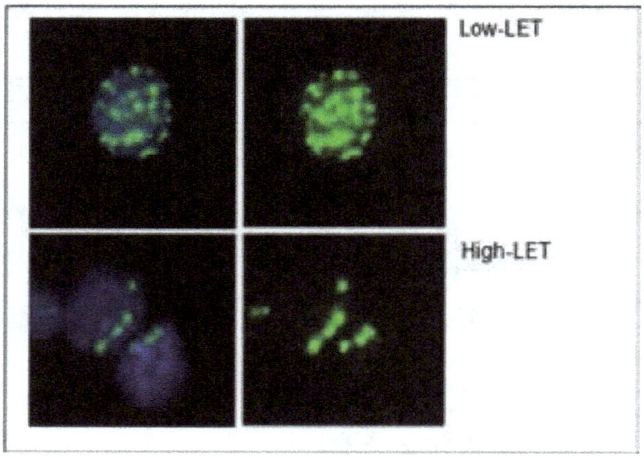

Fig. 2. Visualization by *in situ* immunofluorescence of γ-H2AX foci in human PBL irradiated with γ-rays or low-energy protons. The pattern of γ-H2AX localization within the nucleus is strictly dependent on the quality of radiation. Low-LET radiation, such as γ-rays, hit the cells throughout all directions, and DSBs are sparsely distributed; on the contrary, high-LET radiation such as protons, give raise to clustered DNA damage along tracks.

In irradiated PBL the kinetics of DSB repair was different according to the quality of radiation. In particular, the fraction of foci-positive cells was higher in γ-irradiated than in proton-irradiated lymphocytes at all times, except at 24h after IR. Early after irradiation (30 min and 2h) γ-H2AX foci were present in 80% and 43% of PBL, irradiated respectively with γ-rays and protons (Fig. 3A). This difference is mainly due to the quality of radiation: while sparsely IR as γ-rays lose their energy throughout all directions thus hitting all nuclei, densely IR as protons, hits the fraction of cells along their track. The preferential production of complex aberrations is related to the unique energy deposition patterns produced by densely ionizing radiation, causing highly localized multiple DNA damage. At 6h after IR the percentage of foci-positive cells decreased, revealing the repair capacity of DSBs in both kind of irradiated lymphocytes, although the repair kinetics was faster in γ-irradiated PBL. At 24h after IR the percentage of γ-H2AX foci positive cells tended to reach the value of non-irradiated PBL, either in γ- and in proton-irradiated PBL.

The mean number of γ-H2AX foci per nucleus was higher in PBL irradiated with γ-rays than with protons, at all times after IR (Fig. 3B). In our experiments, most of PBL displayed 10–20 or more γ-H2AX foci/nucleus 30 min after irradiation, giving a maximum yield of 4 foci/Gy, a number similar to that reported for human PBL irradiated with X-rays (about 10 foci/Gy) (Sak et al., 2007; Schertan et al., 2008), but much lower than that determined in human fibroblasts (32.2 foci/Gy) (Hamada et al., 2006). It has been reported that the number of γ-H2AX foci is well consistent with the number of theoretically calculated DSB/Gy of sparsely ionizing radiation (i.e. about 40) (Ward, 1991), if one DSB is contained per focus.

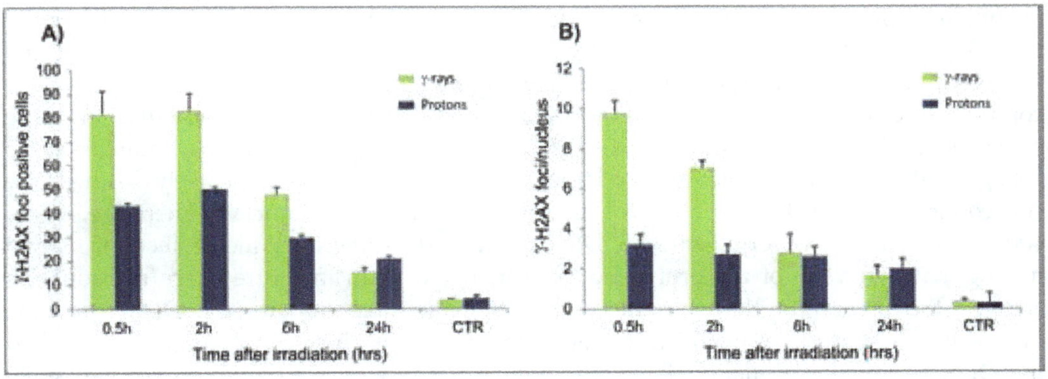

Fig. 3. Kinetics of γ-H2AX foci in PBL irradiated with γ-rays and low energy protons during the time after irradiation. A) Fraction of cells positive for γ-H2AX foci and B) mean number of γ-H2AX foci per nucleus.

The lower number of foci detected in peripheral lymphocytes could depend on the large amount of heterochromatin of resting cells, from which γ-H2AX foci are mostly excluded (Cowell et al., 2007) as well as on the small nuclear volume, where overlapping foci are difficult to detect separately. Thus, in accordance with the observations of Scherthan et al., (2008) we hypothesize that γ-H2AX foci detected very early after irradiation contained more than one DSB; later on, the number of foci decreased and probably each foci contained only one DSB. Furthermore , we found a size increase of γ-H2AX foci in cells irradiated with protons, as compared with gamma irradiations, probably as a consequence of DSBs clusters induced by high-LET radiation. Our results are in accordance with those in melanoma cells exposed to low- and high-LET radiation (Ibañez et al., 2009).

3. Cellular effects of ionizing radiation in human lymphocytes cultured in microgravity condition

The cellular response to ionizing radiation besides on genetic and physiological features of the biological systems, depends also on environmental conditions occurring during DNA repair. Space missions expose humans to an exogenous environment not encountered within our biosphere, in particular the contemporary presence of radiation and a condition of weightlessness called microgravity (10^{-4}–10^{-6}g). One of the important aspects of risk estimation during space flights, is whether the effects of radiation on astronauts are influenced by microgravity. The combination of microgravity and ionizing radiation has been demonstrated to have a synergistic action on human cells, both *in vivo* and *in vitro*. The effects of space environment experienced by astronauts include loss of calcium and minerals from bone, decreased skeletal muscle mass and depressed immune function (Longnecker et al., 2004). *Ex vivo* astronaut studies, in-flight cell cultures, and ground models of microgravity studies, have consistently demonstrated inhibition of lymphocyte proliferation and suppressed or altered cytokine secretion (Lewis et al., 1998; Grimm et al., 2002). Among the biological effects of the reduced gravity in human cell cultures, were described apoptosis induction, cytoskeletal alteration, cell growth inhibition and increased frequency of chromosome aberrations (Lewis et al., 1998; Grimm et al., 2002; Cubano et al., 2000; Sytkowski et al., 2001; Mosesso et al., 2001; Durante et al., 2003). Gene expression analyses on human cells grown in microgravity during space flights or in modeled microgravity (MMG) on Earth, report changes among genes involved in apoptosis induction, cell adhesion, cytoskeletal features and cell differentiation, even if large differences in culture conditions, cell types and methods to simulate microgravity were adopted in those experiments (Hammond et al., 2000; Lewis et al., 2001, Torigoe et al., 2001, Infanger et al., 2007). While the genotoxic effects of ionizing radiation have been intensely studied, the consequence of the reduced gravity together with radiation is still unclear. Therefore, it is of special importance to verify whether DDR is affected by the combined effects of IR and microgravity, in view of the prolonged permanence of man in future space missions. To analyze the possibility that a reduced gravitational force impairs the DDR pathway, increasing the risk of the exposure to conditions occurring during spaceflight, we studied the DDR to ionizing radiation in human PBL incubated in MMG and in parallel static conditions. Microgravity was simulated by culturing PBL in the Rotating Wall Vessel bioreactor (Synthecon, Cellon, Fig. 4) placed inside a humidified incubator, vertically rotating at 23 rpm.

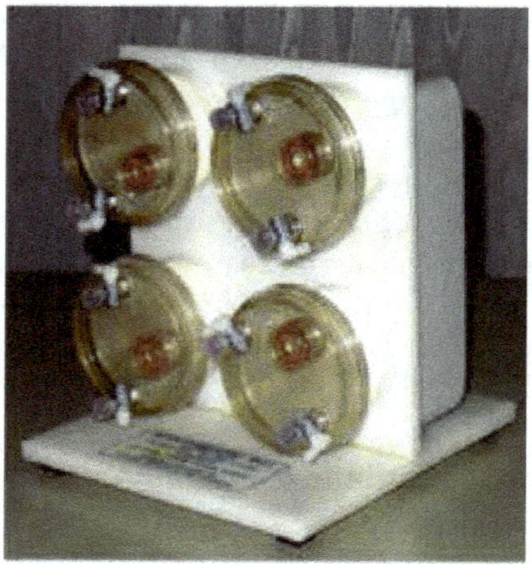

Fig. 4. Rotating Wall Vessel Bioreactor (Synthecon).

The Rotating Wall Vessel was developed at the NASA Johnson Space Center (Houston, TX) to simulate, as accurately as possible, culture conditions predicted to occur during experiments in space. In the rotating system, the gravity is balanced by equal and opposite mechanical forces (centrifugal, Coriolis and shear components), and the gravitational vector is reduced to about 10^{-2} g. In these conditions, single cells are nearly always in suspension, rotating quasi-stationary with the fluid, in a low-shear culture environment (Unsworth 1998, Maccarone et al., 2003). Ground based (1 g) PBL cultures, both irradiated and non-irradiated, were kept at the same cell density in flasks inside a humidified incubator for 24 h.

3.1 The DNA-damage response of human peripheral lymphocytes cultured in microgravity after γ-irradiation

The DNA-damage response was investigated in human PBL irradiated *in vitro* with different doses of gamma rays and incubated for 24 h in 1 g or in modeled microgravity (MMG). While cell survival was only slight affected by MMG, the *HPRT* mutant frequency significantly increased in PBL incubated in MMG after irradiation compared with those maintained in 1 g. Given the increase of *HPRT* mutants in MMG, we investigated whether the reduced gravity affected the progression of the rejoining of double strand breaks (DSBs) in human PBL irradiated with γ-rays and incubated in MMG or in 1g. The kinetics of γ-H2AX foci was monitored during the repair incubation, showing that DSBs rejoining was slower in MMG than in 1g at 6 and 24 h after irradiation. In addition, the mean number of γ-H2AX foci per nucleus was significantly higher in MMG than in 1g at the same time-points (Fig. 5).

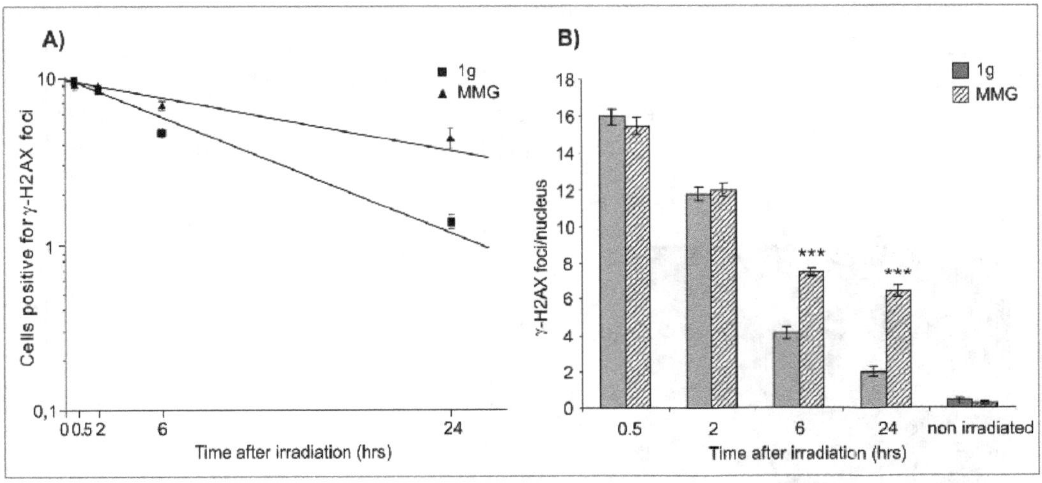

Fig. 5. Kinetics of γ-H2AX foci in PBL irradiated with 5Gy of γ-rays and incubated in 1g or MMG during the repair time. A) Fraction of PBL positive for γ-H2AX foci. B) Mean number of γ-H2AX foci/nucleus (****P*<0.001, *t*-test).

To verify whether the disappearance of γ-H2AX foci correlated with the rejoining of double strand breaks, we subjected irradiated lymphocytes to a non-radioactive PFGE assay (Gradzka et al., 2005). The fraction of DNA released (FR) from the plug after PFGE was considered a measure of DSB level. The kinetics of DSB removal in lymphocytes irradiated and incubated in 1g exhibits a typical fast initial component and a decreasing rate at longer repair intervals, in accordance with data from other authors (Stenerlow et al., 2000; Gradzka et al., 2005). Both the methods we used to quantify DNA fragmentation, reported a lower rate of DSB rejoining in lymphocytes incubated in MMG compared to those in 1g, in agreement with the kinetics of γ-H2AX foci. Our results provide evidences that MMG incubation during DNA repair delayed the rate of radiation-induced DSB rejoining, and increased, as a consequence, the genotoxic effects of ionizing radiation.

We then assessed whether MMG incubation affected IR-induced apoptosis. Human lymphocytes, irradiated and non-irradiated, were scored for the presence of fragmented nuclei and apoptotic bodies. Apoptotic index (A.I.) increased with time after irradiation and at 24 h it was significantly higher in PBL incubated in MMG compared to those in 1g (19.3% vs. 13.7% respectively, $P < 0.001$). Since DSBs can be induced, besides radiation, also by DNA fragmentation during early apoptosis, we measured caspase-3 activation at the same time-points by the cleavage of the peptide substrate DEVD-AFC. Caspase-3 activation was only slightly higher in PBL maintained in MMG than in 1g, in contrast to the high persistence of foci-positive cells ($P < 0.01$), and foci number/nucleus ($P < 0.001$), suggesting that the level of H2AX phosphorylation was principally correlated to a delayed DSB resolution rather than apoptosis induction.

We then tested for the possibility that MMG incubation affects DNA damage response by altering the recruitment of the signaling proteins, 53BP1, NBS1-p343 and ATM-p1981, which co-localize with γ-H2AX foci to DSB sites (Fig. 6A). After irradiation ~90% of cells became foci-positive for the three proteins in both gravity conditions (not shown). In contrast to γ-H2AX, the fraction of foci-positive cells persisted high up to 24 h after irradiation in 1g and no differences between the two culture conditions were detected. The number of foci/nucleus significantly decreased during post-irradiation incubation from 14-16 foci/nucleus at 30 min to 4-5 foci/nucleus at 24 h (Fig. 6B), without differences between samples in 1g and MMG. The discrepancies with the kinetics of γ-H2AX foci suggest that these proteins could represent the remaining scaffold structure used for DSB repair that persisted after the repair has been completed (Markova et al., 2007, van Veelen et al., 2005).

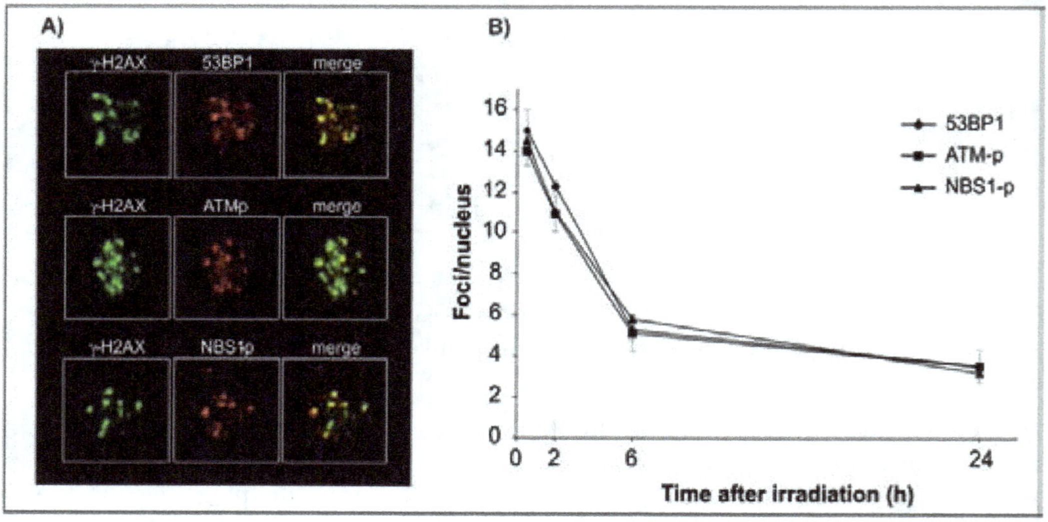

Fig. 6. Kinetics of 53BP1, ATM-p1981, NBS1-p343 foci in PBL irradiated with γ-rays and incubated in 1g. A) Co-localization with γ-H2AX foci to form the ionizing radiation-induced foci (IRIF). B) Mean number of foci per nucleus.

3.2 The DNA-damage response of human tumoral lymphocytes cultured in microgravity after γ-irradiation

We analyzed the DNA damage response to radiation also in human tumoral lymphocytes (TK6 cells, lymphoblastoid B cells) irradiated with γ-rays (1, 2, 4 Gy) and incubated in 1g or in MMG during the repair time. In irradiated TK6 cells, we observed a higher survival in MMG than in 1g, and the difference was significant at 4Gy. In addition, in cells maintained in MMG rather than in 1g after γ-irradiation, higher frequency of HPRT mutants was observed at all irradiation doses, particularly at 4Gy (Figure 7A). Remarkably, at this dose, mutant frequency may often be underestimated, since cells with many and severe mutations are unable to repair DNA damage and die. Instead, in TK6 cells cultured in MMG after irradiation, mutant frequency increased with doses up to 4Gy (Figure 7A). The frequency of micronucleated cells was measured in both gravity conditions after irradiation. At the end of post-irradiation incubation (24 h time-point), the percentage of micronuclei (MN) was significantly higher in both non-irradiated and in irradiated cells incubated in MMG compared with 1g (Fig.7B). Eighteen hours later (42 h from irradiation), the percentage of MN in cultures incubated in MMG was higher than in 1g only at 2Gy γ-ray dose. At 48 h time-point, MN frequencies observed in 1g or MMG were comparable. As expected, MN significantly increased after irradiation in both gravity conditions with respect to non-irradiated cells; a significant difference was still observed at 48 h after irradiation at both 1 and 2Gy. The significant increase of micronucleated cells in MMG suggested that MMG itself was able to induce chromosome damage.

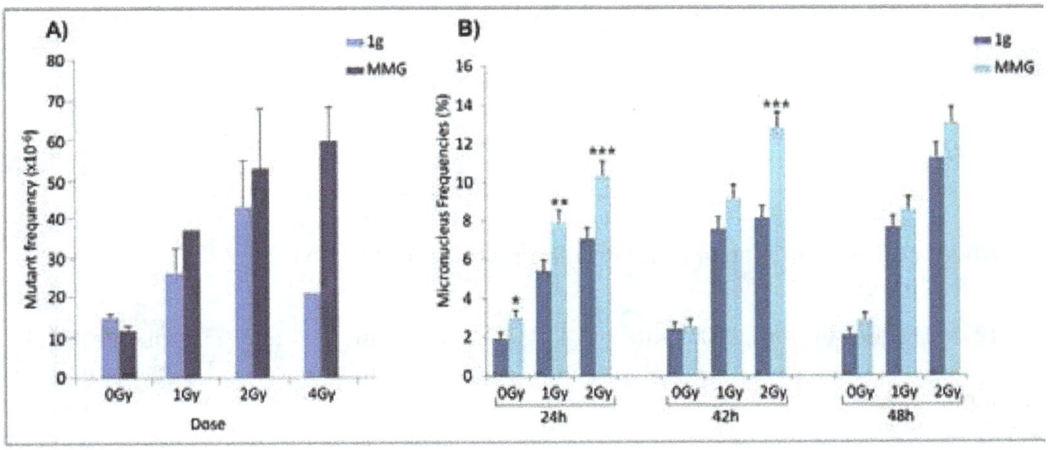

Fig. 7. A) Mutant frequency at the HPRT locus of irradiated and non-irradiated TK6 cells incubated for 24h in 1g or in modeled microgravity. B) Micronucleus frequencies (%) in irradiated and non-irradiated TK6 cells incubated in 1g of MMG for the first 24h after irradiation and then cultured in 1g up to 48 h. *P<0.05; **P<0.01; ***P<0.001 (G test).

The effect of MMG incubation on cell cycle alteration induced by γ−ray exposure was assessed by flow cytometry analysis. Figure 8 shows the cell cycle distribution of TK6 cells at various time-points from irradiation and incubation in MMG or 1g by representative DNA histograms. γ-ray irradiation induced an increase in G2/M-phase cells and a reduction in S-phase cells, both in TK6 maintained in 1g and MMG after irradiation. At the end of MMG or 1g incubation (24 h time-point), the percentages of cells in G1-phase were higher in cultures irradiated with 2-4 Gy and incubated in MMG compared with cells maintained in 1g. Moreover, the G2/M block after irradiation was less evident in MMG than in 1g condition. Also radiation-induced apoptosis was affected in TK6 cells by MMG incubation. Induction of apoptosis was significantly lower in irradiated TK6 cells incubated in MMG compared with cells irradiated with the same dose and incubated in 1g. The differences were more pronounced in cells analyzed at long post-incubation times (72 h time-point).

The observed decrease of apoptotic response in MMG incubated cultures could allow severely damaged cells, which in 1g condition should be eliminated by selection, to survive, with negative consequences on genomic integrity. Alterations in cell response to ionizing radiation due to MMG incubation during the DNA repair period may be caused by the reduced activity of some proteins, which play a crucial role in damage signaling. Previous data have shown that absence or reduction of gravity can alter gene expression (Walther et

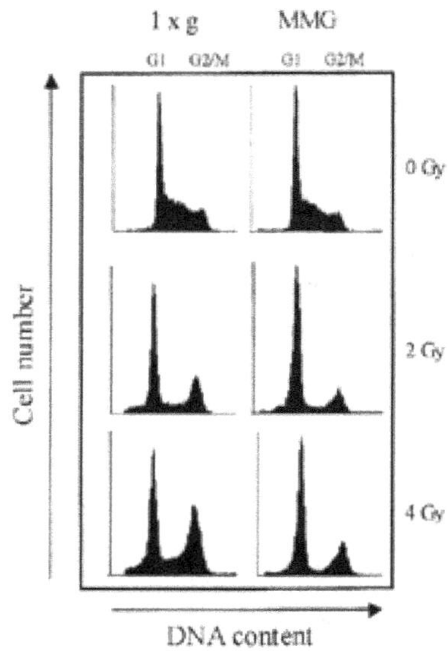

Fig. 8. Cell cycle distribution of irradiated and non-irradiated TK6 cells at the end of 24h incubation in 1g or in MMG.

al., 1998; Hughes-Fulford 2001; Kita et al., 2000), which in turn may explain the results reported here. It remains to be determined if one upstream or several downstream genes belonging to the pathway of the radiation response are involved in the effects induced by MMG incubation.

3.3 Gene expression changes in human lymphocytes cultured in microgravity during the DNA-damage response to radiation

Gene expression changes represent an early bio-indicator of radiation exposure. Given the increase of *HPRT* mutants observed in human lymphocytes incubated in modeled microgravity, we investigated whether this gravity condition can alter the transcription of 14 genes representative of the main DNA repair pathways. The genes analyzed are representative of the major DNA repair pathways: four genes (*Ku70, Ku80, DNA-ligase IV, XRCC4*) are involved in non-homologous end joining processes (NHEJ), three genes (*BRCA1, BRCA2, RAD51*) in homologous recombination (HR), four genes (*XRCC1, PCNA,GADD45A, p21Cip1/Waf1*) in base excision repair (BER) and two genes (*DDB2, XPC*) in nucleotide excision repair (NER). *DNA-ligase I*, involved in both BER and NER repair pathways, was analyzed too. Analyses were carried out in three pools of three donor, each by quantitative real time PCR. Results show that almost all BER and NER genes were up-regulated in irradiated PBL, whereas the expression of HR and NHEJ genes was only slightly or not affected by radiation (Fig.9). Incubation in modeled microgravity after irradiation did not significantly change the expression of genes involved in DNA repair, suggesting that transcriptional impairment was not responsible for the increase of mutant frequency observed in irradiated cells incubated in microgravity in comparison to the static 1 g condition. These findings in agreement with previous studies on gene expression of non-irradiated space flown and RWV cultured cells, showing that DNA repair genes were unaffected by low-gravity whereas intracellular signaling, growth regulatory, cytoskeletal and tumor suppressor genes were altered (Lewis et al., 2001; Hammond et al., 2000; Pardo et al., 2005).

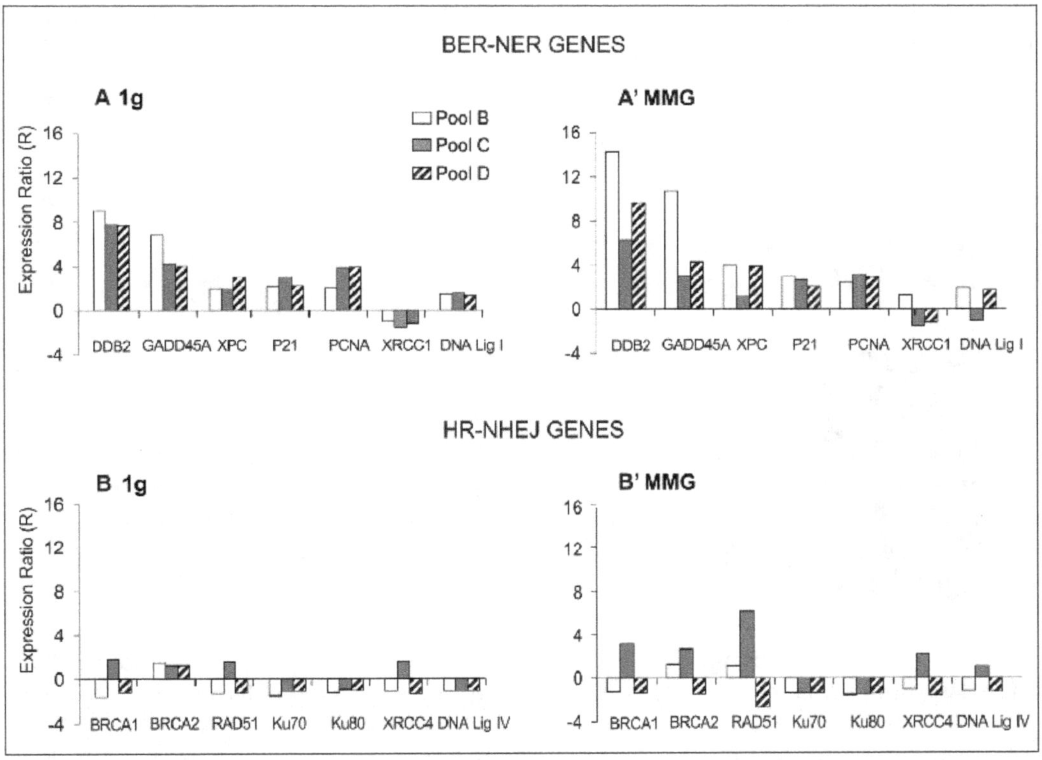

Fig. 9. Expression ratios in PBL of pools B–D incubated in 1 g and modeled microgravity after X-irradiation. (A) *R* values of BER and NER genes in 1g; (A) *R* values of BER and NER in MMG; (B) *R* values of HR and NHEJ genes in 1g; (B) *R* values of HR and NHEJ genes in MMG.

Recently, a new class of important gene modulators has been discovered: microRNAs. They are a large family of small non-coding RNAs of 18-24 nucleotides that negatively regulate gene expression levels by binding to microRNA-binding elements in the 3′ untranslated-region (3′UTR) of target mRNAs thereby triggering decreased protein translation mainly through mRNA degradation (Guo et al., 2010). A single miRNA may have broad effects on gene expression networks, such as regulating cell lineage specificity, cellular functions or stress response. By considering the complexity of the DNA-damage response (DDR), addressed to maintain genome integrity through cell cycle arrest, DNA repair and/or apoptosis, it is expected that miRNAs have an important role in this cellular process. Whilst miRNA-mediated DDR has been studied after UV radiation and hypoxic stress (Pothof et al., 2009; Crosby et al., 2009) that of radiation combined with microgravity has not been studied yet and should give important information about risk assessment in space environment. MicroRNAs profiling were carried out by using the platform "Human miRNA Microarray kit (V2)" (Agilent), according to the Agilent miRNA protocol. For mRNA expression profile we used the "Whole Human Genome Oligo Microarray" (Agilent), consisting of ~41.000 (60-mer) oligonucleotide probes, which span conserved exons across the transcripts of the targeted full-length genes. Identification of differentially expressed genes and miRNAs was performed with one and two class Significance Analysis of Microarray (SAM) program (Tusher et al., 2001) with default settings. Figure 10A shows a dendrogram relative to some miRNAs differentially expressed following ionizing radiation in human PBL.

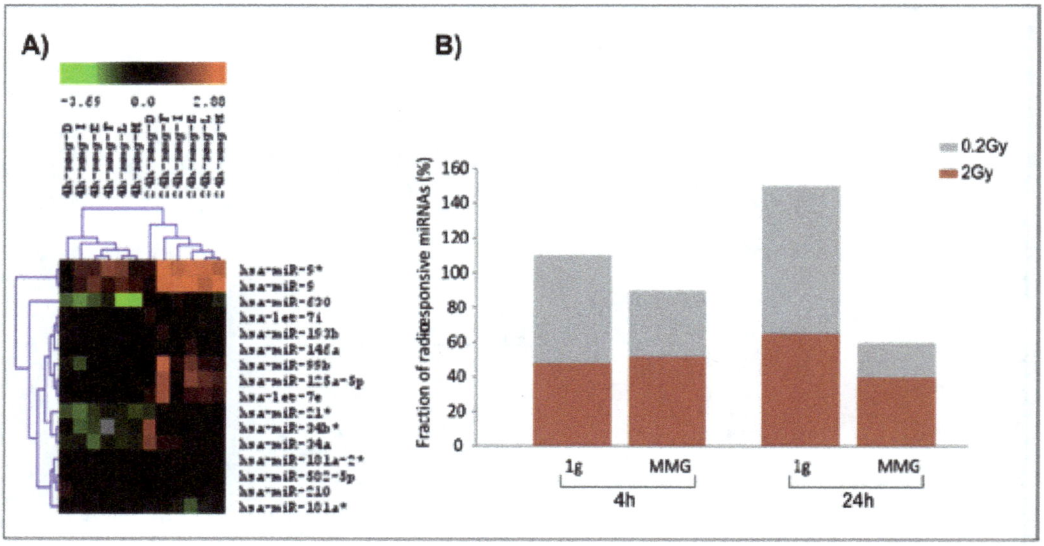

Fig. 10. A) Dendrogram showing several miRNAs differentially expressed in human PBL at 4 and 24h after irradiation with 0.2Gy. Range of expression value is determined as the log2 ratio of irradiated/non-irradiated sample. Down-regulated and up-regulated miRNAs correspond to green and red boxes, respectively. B) Fraction of radio-responsive miRNAs (%) in human PBL irradiated with 0.2 and 2Gy and incubated for 4 and 24h- in 1g or in modeled microgravity (MMG).

MiRNA expression profile was carried out at 4h and 24h after irradiation with 0.2Gy and 2Gy and incubation in 1g and MMG and compared to that of non-irradiated PBL maintained in parallel conditions. Results showed that in both gravity conditions the miRNA expression profile was dose-specific, as indicated by the low percentage of common miRNA responsive to both doses; moreover, the effects of the higher dose predominated at the late time point. Interestingly, MMG tended to decrease the number of radio-responsive miRNAs respect to 1g condition, in particular at 24h after irradiation (Figure 10B).

To predict the target genes of differentially expressed miRNAs we first performed a computational analyses using PITA algorithm available on line (Kertesz et al., 2007). However, all available software for target prediction are characterized by a large fraction of false positives, thus to identify the most likely targets, we have integrated mRNA and miRNA expression data, obtained on the same lymphocyte samples, using MAGIA (MiRNA And Genes Integrated Analysis) web tool (Sales et al., 2010). We used a non-parametric index (Spearman correlation coefficient), the most indicated statistical coefficient for a small number of measures, to estimate the degree of anti-correlation (e.g. up-regulated miRNA and corresponding down-regulated mRNA target) between any putative pairs of miRNA and mRNA (Xin et al., 2009; Wang and Li 2009). The anti-correlated transcripts were then classified according to DAVID (Database for Annotation, Visualization and Integrated Discovery) web tool (Huang et al. 2009), to determine which Gene Ontology (GO) terms were significantly enriched in our set of genes. Results of G0 analysis of anti-correlated genes showed that in MMG-incubated PBL were not enriched the categories of response to stress, to DNA damage and to apoptosis. miRNA-mRNA anti-correlations of DDR pathway were visualized by using Cytoscape software package (Shannon et al., 2003; Cline et al., 2007) (Figure 11). The results showed that, in most cases, the same mRNA was targeted by different miRNA species according to the different condition of gravity.

Future research is addressed to validate several of the anti-correlations highlighted with our analyses as important in DDR pathway. In particular, we will perform a functional assay to demonstrate the regulatory effect of a particular miRNA on its putative target mRNA. The luciferase assay represents the most efficient approach to evaluate the activity of a miRNA on its anti-correlated mRNA. This assay allows to demonstrate the activity of a miRNA on its anti-correlated mRNA by the quantification of the luminescent signal derived from the luciferase reporter enzyme. Cells are co-transfected with a reporter vector containing the firefly luciferase gene together with the 3'UTR target sequence predicted for that miRNA and the miRNA precursor (pre-miRNA) or inhibitor (anti-miRNA), which respectively mimics and inhibits the endogenous miRNA. The binding of pre-miRNA to the complementary target sequence will cause the repression of luciferase gene expression, whereas the binding of anti-miRNA to the endogenous miRNA will induce the expression of luciferase gene. The quantification of the luminescent signal derived from the luciferase reporter enzyme thus allows to demonstrate the activity of a miRNA on its putative target mRNA. In addition to the luciferase assay, it would be interesting to study the role of selected miRNAs in DDR pathway by a biological approach. Usually, several end points such as cell survival, DNA repair, cell cycle progression and apoptosis induction are analyzed in cells over-or under-expressing the miRNA of interest.

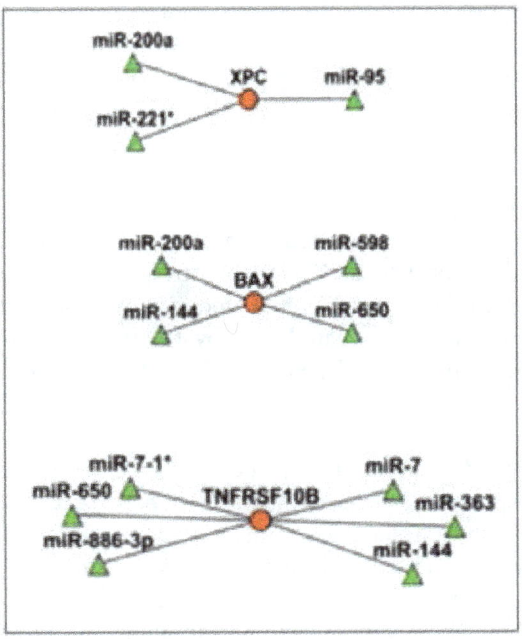

Fig. 11. Example of visualization of inversely correlated miRNA-mRNA relationships in irradiated human PBL. Circles represent transcripts and triangles miRNAs, shown with the color corresponding to the expression value.

4. The DNA-damage response of human lymphocytes to indirect effect of ionizing radiation

In addition the cellular effects arising as a direct response to ionizing radiation, in the last decade it has been suggested that extranuclear or extracellular targets can contribute to the genetic damage in non-irradiated (bystander) cells. The bystander effect (BE) is the biological response of non-irradiated cells induced by contact with irradiated cells. The contact with bystander factors may occur by direct cell–cell interaction or be mediated by the fluid surrounding the cells. It has been reported that the BE causes cell death, cell cycle arrest, apoptosis, changes in gene expression, and increases micronucleus induction, chromosomal aberrations, mutation frequency, and DNA damage in cells neighboring hit cells. In contrast to DNA damage induced by direct irradiation, bystander cell DNA damage is still poorly understood. Many data showed that early events of the radiation induced bystander effect are rapid calcium fluxes and generation of reactive oxygen species in bystander cells. Mitochondria seem to play a central role in bystander signaling: irradiated cell conditioned media can cause changes of mitochondrial distribution, loss of mitochondrial membrane potential, increases in ROS, and increase in apoptosis among the medium receptor cells, which can be blocked by treatments with antioxidants (Chen et al., 2008). Experiments carried out in hepatoma cell lines provide evidence that the BE can be modulated by the p53 status of irradiated cells and that a p53-dependent release of cytochrome-c from mitochondria may be involved in producing BE (He et al., 2011).

We investigated on the mechanisms of the medium-mediated bystander response induced by low doses of γ-rays in human tumoural lymphocytes (TK6 cells), a cell line growing in suspension, in which gap-junction communications are not involved in transferring bystander signals and only medium-mediated molecules may be responsible for BE induction. Cell cultures were irradiated and the culture medium discarded immediately after irradiation and replaced with a fresh one to eliminate ROS originating during irradiation. Irradiated cells were incubated for 6h in fresh medium, which, at the end of incubation time, is referred as conditioned medium (CM) and used to incubate non-irradiated TK6 cells for different times (2-48 h). In bystander cultures, cell mortality at the fixed incubation times ranged between 24 and 19%, very similar values to that of directly irradiated cells (28 and 20%). The mortality percentages for all incubation times were significantly higher with respect to that of the controls (0Gy and 0Gy CM). The survival fraction of directly 1Gy irradiated or CM incubated cells was determined by the clonogenic assay. The data show that both irradiated and bystander TK6 cells had a lower cloning efficiency than their respective controls. Figure 12 reports the results about cell mortality and survival (given as the ratio of the cloning efficiency of treated vs. untreated control cells) in TK6 cells exposed directly to IR or to CM. Apoptosis induction was tested by the presence of fragmented nuclei and apoptotic bodies at 2, 24 and 48h after 1Gy irradiation or CM incubation. The apoptotic index (A.I.) ranged between 7 and 9 % in irradiated cells and between 6 and 7.5 % in bystander cells, and was significantly higher than the relative controls at all times (Figure 13). The induction of apoptosis was also analyzed by the activation of caspase-3, the principal effector caspase, assayed by the cleavage of the peptide substrate DEVD-AFC, at 1, 2, 24 and 48h after irradiation or CM incubation. In bystander cells caspase-3 activation increased from 1.4- to 2.7-fold during the 48h of CM incubation, suggesting that bystander apoptosis increases after 48h. Bystander apoptosis in TK6 cells was sensitive to the inhibitor of caspase-8, the Z-IETD-fmk, added during CM treatment or

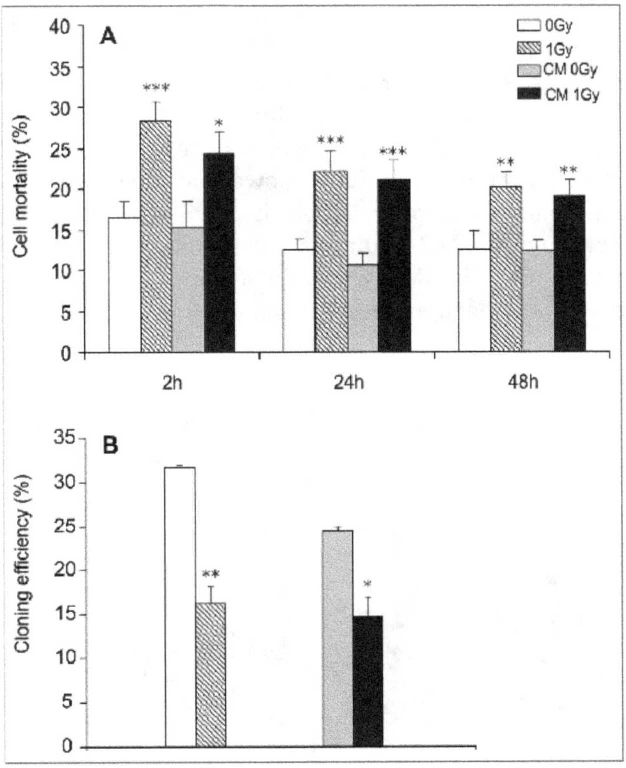

Fig. 12. Cell mortality determined by Trypan blue staining (A) and cloning efficiency (B) in non-irradiated control cells (0Gy), in irradiated cells (1Gy), in cells incubated with conditioned medium from non-irradiated cells (CM 0Gy) and in cells incubated with conditioned medium from irradiated cells (CM 1Gy). Results are the means of 3-5 independent experiments ± S.E. (*P< 0.05, **P<0.01, ***P<0.001, t test).

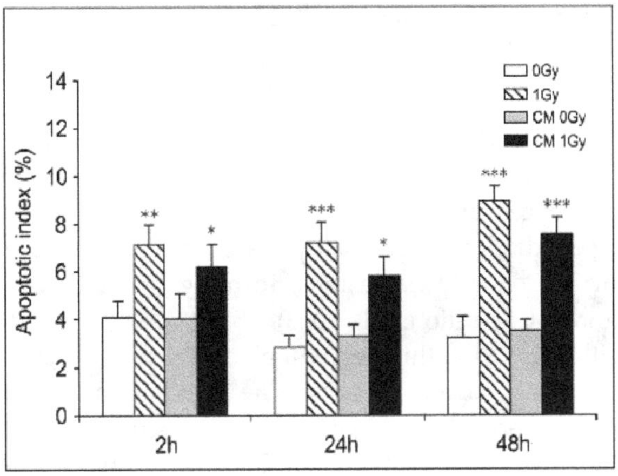

Fig. 13. Apoptotic index (A) in irradiated and bystander cells. Results are the means ± S.E. of 5-8 independent experiments. Significant differences were observed in 1Gy and CM 1Gy vs 0Gy and CM 0Gy, respectively (*P<0.05, **P<0.01, ***P<0.001, t test).

post-irradiation incubation. The presence of the inhibitor significantly decreased the induction of apoptosis to the control level, but it did not significantly decrease the level of apoptosis in either irradiated or non-irradiated controls (Figure 14). These results suggest that caspase-8 activation is triggered by signaling molecules present in the conditioned medium. The addition of the ROS scavenger Cu-Zn superoxide dismutase and N-acetylcysteine to the conditioned medium allowed to investigate the involvement of oxidative stress in inducing bystander apoptosis. ROS scavengers did not significantly decrease the apoptotic index in CM cultures; by treating non-irradiated TK6 cells with medium irradiated without cells (IM), we evaluated the contribute of ROS produced by irradiation in inducing bystander apoptosis.

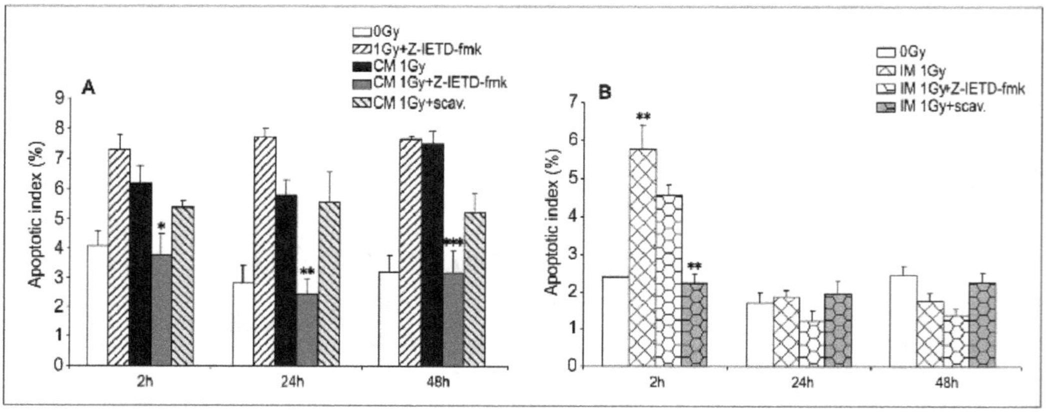

Fig. 14. Apoptotic index in irradiated cells (1Gy), in irradiated cells incubated with caspase-8 inhibitor (1Gy + Z-IETD-fmk), in bystander cells incubated with caspase-8 inhibitor (CM 1Gy + Z-IETD-fmk), and with ROS scavengers SOD and NAC (CM 1Gy + scav.). Results are the means of 3-5 independent experiments ± S.E. Significant differences were observed in CM 1Gy vs CM 1Gy + Z-IETD-fmk at all times. **B**. Apoptotic index in cells incubated with irradiated medium (IM 1Gy), with irradiated medium in the presence of caspase-8 inhibitor (IM 1Gy + Z-IETD-fmk), and ROS scavengers (IM 1Gy + scav.). The values are the means of 3 independent experiments ± S.E. Significant differences were observed at 2 h of incubation with IM 1 Gy vs IM 1Gy + Z-IETD-fmk (*P<0.05, **P<0.01, ***P<0.001, t-test).

IM incubation for 2h increased the apoptotic index which was totally inhibited by ROS scavengers and little affected by incubation with the caspase-8 inhibitor, whereas at 24 and 48h no significant differences among samples incubated with IM were observed. DSBs induced by ionizing radiation can easily be detected by the extensive H2AX phosphorylation occurring near DNA lesions, forming foci that co-localize with several repair proteins (Fernandez-Capetillo et al., 2003). 85% of TK6 were γ-H2AX foci positive at 2h after irradiation with 1Gy, then this percentage decreased to the level of non-irradiated cells 24h later, fitting DNA repair kinetics. The incubation of cells with CM for 2h significantly increased the percentage of γ-H2AX foci positive cells (9-11%) but, when the CM was kept in contact with bystander cells for 24h the number of positive cells decreased to control levels, suggesting that DNA lesions induced at the beginning of CM incubation are repaired and no new damage accumulates later. Data from other human cells show that γ-H2AX foci induction in bystander cells persists in time, probably as a consequence of the formation of bystander factors that themselves generate ROS, leading to a self-sustaining system responsible for long-lasting effects (Yang 2005, Sokolov 2005, Kashino 2004, Lyng 2006). In irradiated TK6 cells both 53BP1 and NBS1p343 proteins co-localized with γ-H2AX foci, whereas in bystander cells co-localization was partial or absent (Figure 15).

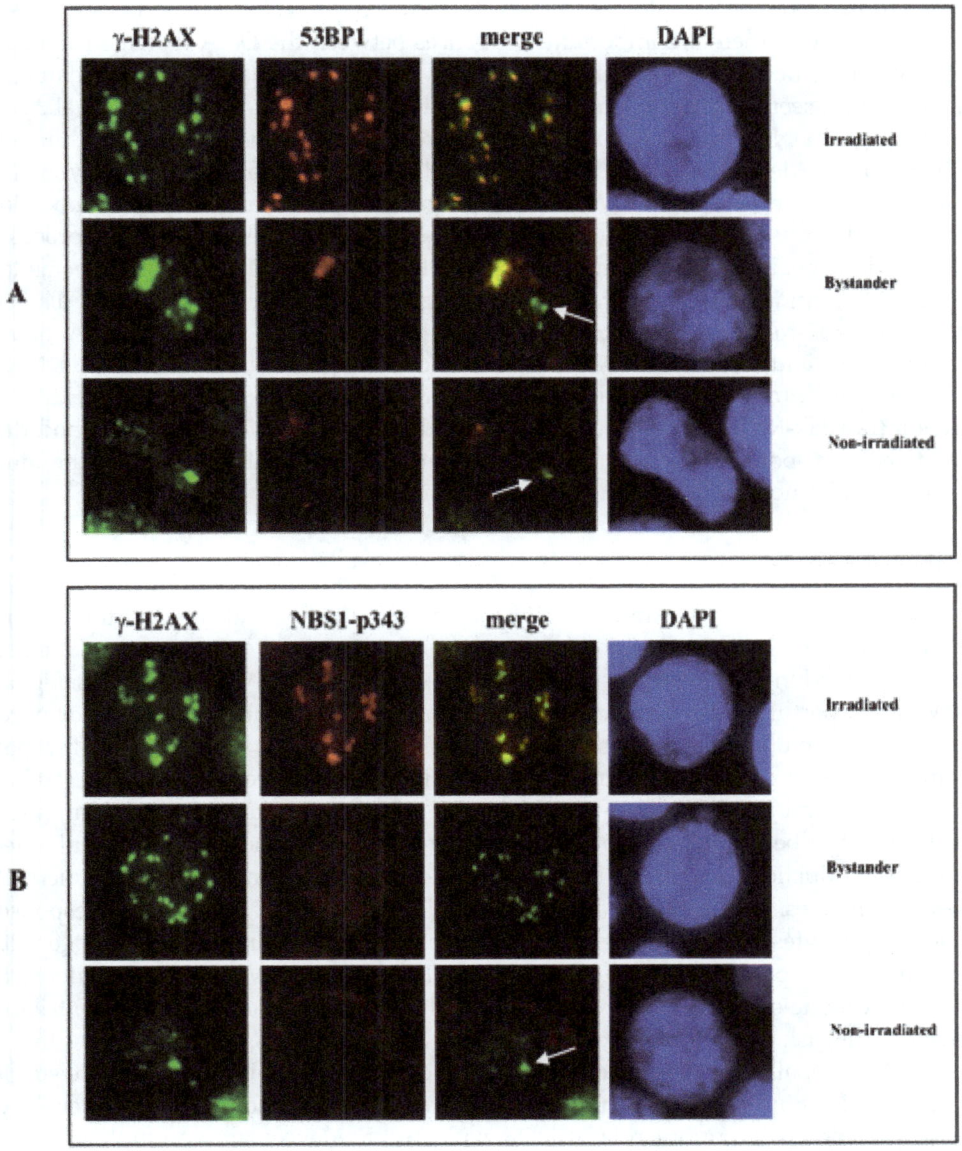

Fig. 15. Non-irradiated, irradiated and bystander TK6 cells were fixed and co-stained with anti- γH2AX (green), anti-53BP1 and anti-NBS1-p343 (red), at 2 h from irradiation or CM incubation. The red and green images were merged and subjected to co-localization analysis. Arrows indicate γH2AX foci without co-localization of 53BP1and NBS1-proteins. Nuclei were counterstained with DAPI.

We suggest that the short-lived ROS released in the medium by irradiated cells are responsible for DNA lesions, unlike double strand breaks, which activate H2AX phosphorylation but do not require the 53BP1 and NBS1p343 proteins to be repaired. It is possible that in our experiments DNA damage induced by CM treatment consisted of a few DSBs, the repair of which requires the recruitment of 53BP1 and NBS1p343 proteins and mainly in other types of DNA lesions, in which repair occurs without these proteins. Recent studies suggest that there are important differences between the DNA damage response in directly irradiated cells and non-targeted cells via bystander signals. The DNA damage in bystander cells seems to persist for a prolonged time (Burdak-Rothkamm et al., 2007), differently from DNA damage induced directly by irradiation which is repaired completely within few hours depending on radiation dose. Studies carried out in p53 wild-type (TK6), p53 null (NH32),and p53 mutant (WTK1) lymphoblastoid cells using siRNA to knockdown DNA PKcs demonstrated the central role of non-homologous end-joining in processing bystander damage, in contrast to the role of homologous recombination which seems to be essential only in inducing sister chromatid exchanges in bystander cells (Zhang et al., 2008). ATM- and Rad3-related (ATR) protein kinases have a central role into DNA damage signaling in bystander cells, with ATM activation occurring downstream of ATR. DNA-PK is not essential in mortality inducing in bystander cells neither for bystander γH2AX foci induction (Burdak-Rothkamm et al., 2007). These differences between bystander and direct DNA damage response offer new potential targets for repair inhibitors, with the aim to protect bystander normal tissues during cancer radiotherapy.

5. Conclusions

The DNA-damage response pathway relies on the recruitment and modification of many different proteins that sense and signal the damage, activate transducer and effector proteins involved in cell cycle arrest, DNA repair and apoptosis. A correct DDR safeguards cells, whereas perturbations/defects in this pathway might contribute to the occurrence or to the acceleration of carcinogenesis. Our results have contributed to highlight cell response of human lymphocytes to DNA damage induced directly or indirectly by ionizing radiation. In particular, novel aspects of low- and high-LET radiation effects on human lymphocytes have been described, such as double strand break repair kinetics, mutational effects, micronuclei induction, apoptosis induction, cell cycle alterations, gene and microRNA expression changes. In addition, we have reported new findings about the cell response of human lymphocytes when ionizing radiation exposure occurred in microgravity, condition which has been experimentally simulated by the Rotating Wall Vessel. The results clearly indicate that modeled microgravity affects the cell response to radiation, thus contributing to increase the risk of radiation exposure during space missions. By considering that the levels of DNA repair genes were not significantly changed in MMG condition, we suppose that perturbations in the cell response to ionizing radiation are due to the altered activity of proteins playing an important role in DDR pathway. Evidences are accumulating on the strict dependence between efficiency in DNA repair and chromatin structural organization (Gontijo et al., 2003, Rübe et al., 2011). The elaborate higher-order organization of chromatin appears to be important in assembling the repair machinery, improving the accessibility of DNA lesions to repair complexes. Modifications of cell structure and perturbations of nuclear architecture induced by microgravity may affect the accessibility in chromatin to DNA repair machinery. The preliminary results obtained from miRNA-mRNA profiling represent new insights about the radio-responsiveness in MMG. They seem promising to clarify the role of miRNAs in DNA-damage response to radiation in microgravity, thus improving the scientific approach towards environmental exposure risk.

The studies on molecular mechanisms of bystander effect could have great implications in evaluating radiation risk of IR exposures, and also have the potential to reassess radiation damage models currently used in radiotherapy. The radiation-induced bystander effect was shown to occur in a number of experimental systems both *in vitro* and *in vivo* and it is supposed to be realized through several pathways of transmission of the stress signal: a direct cellular contact, interaction through gap-junctions and through the culture medium of the irradiated cells. In our experimental system the conditioned medium was the main way by which the irradiated cells communicate their stressed condition to the non-irradiated cells. ROS released by irradiated TK6 cells into the culture medium were short-lived and probably other soluble molecules are necessary to maintain high the level of cell mortality in bystander cells. Recent studies, investigating on the nature of such molecules, suggest that fragments of extracellular genomic DNA, probably released from the apoptotic irradiated cells in the culture medium, are able to induce the bystander effects (Ermakov et al., 2011). Such DNA fragments bind to the Toll-like receptors family, leading to a signaling mechanism whose outcome is the dynamic transformation of the cytoskeleton and alteration in the spatial localization of chromatin portions in the nucleus. Thus, in bystander cells, as for microgravity-incubated lymphocytes, modifications in the nuclear structural organization may affect the assembly of the DNA repair machinery.

6. Acknowledgment

We gratefully acknowledge Dr. Cristiano De Pittà and Dr. Chiara Romualdi of the Department of Biology, University of Padova, for miRNA and mRNA expression profiling and statistical assistance. We acknowledge Dr. Vito Barbieri of the Department of Oncological and Surgical Sciences of Padova's University for cell irradiation with γ-rays and Roberto Cherubini of the INFN, Laboratori Nazionali di Legnaro, Padova, for cell irradiation with low-energy protons.

7. References

Al-Hakim, A.; Escribano-Diaz, C.; Landry, MC.; O'Donnell, L.; Panier, S.; Szilard, RK.; Durocher, D. (2010). The ubiquitous role of ubiquitin in the DNA damage response. *DNA Repair,* Vol. 9, No. 12, pp.1229-40, ISSN 1568-7864.

Anderson, RM.; Marsden, SJ.; Wright, EG.; Kadhim, MA.; Goodhead, DT.; Griffin, CS. (2000). Complex chromosome aberrations in peripheral blood lymphocytes as a potential biomarker of exposure to high-LET alpha-particles. *Int J Radiat Biol,* Vol. 76, pp. 31–42, ISSN 1362-3095.

Anderson, RM.; Stevens, DL.; Goodhead, DT. (2002). M-FISH analysis shows that complex chromosome aberrations induced by alpha -particle tracks are cumulative products of localized rearrangements. *Proc Natl Acad Sci USA.,* Vol. 99, No.19, pp. 12167-72, ISSN 1091-6490.

Brenner, DJ. & Ward, JF. (1992). Constraints on energy deposition and target size of multiply damaged sites associated with DNA double-strand breaks. *Int J Radiat Biol.*, Vol. 61, No. 6, pp. 737-48, ISSN 1362-3095.

Burdak-Rothkamm, S.; Short, S.C.; Folkard, M.; Rothkamm, K.; Prise, K.M. (2007) ATR-dependent radiation-induced gamma H2AX foci in bystander primary human astrocytes and glioma cells. *Oncogene*, Vol. 26, No. 7 (Feb 2007) pp. 993-1002, ISSN 0950-9232.

Chen, S.; Zhao, Y., Han, W.; Zhao, G.; Zhu, L.; Wang, J.; Bao, L.; Jiang, E.; Xu, A.; Hei, TK.; Yu, Z.; Wu, L. (2008) Mitochondria-dependent signalling pathway are involved in the early process of radiation-induced bystander effects. *Br J Cancer*, Vol. 98, No. 11 (Jun 2008) pp. 1839-44, ISSN 0007-0920.

Ciechanover, A.; Elias, S.; Heller, H.; Hershko, A. (1982). "Covalent affinity" purification of ubiquitin-activating enzyme. *J. Biol. Chem.*, 257 (5) 2537–2542. ISSN 0021-9258.

Cline, MS.; Smoot, M.; Cerami, E.; Kuchinsky, A.; Landys, N.; Workman, C.; Christmas, R.; Avila-Campilo, I.; Creech, M.; Gross, B.; Hanspers, K.; Isserlin, R.; Kelley, R.; Killcoyne, S.; Lotia, S.; Maere, S.; Morris, J.; Ono, K.; Pavlovic, V.; Pico, AR.; Vailaya, A.; Wang, PL.; Adler, A.; Conklin, BR.; Hood, L.; Kuiper, M.; Sander, C.; Schmulevich, I.; Schwikowski, B.; Warner, GJ.; Ideker, T.; Bader, GD. (2007). Integration of biological networks and gene expression data using Cytoscape. *Nature Protocols*, Vol. 2, pp. 2366-82, ISSN 1754-2189.

Cowell, I.G.; Sunter, N.J.; Singh, P.B.; Austin, C.A.; Durkacz, B.W.; Tilby, M.J. (2007). gammaH2AX foci form preferentially in euchromatin after ionising-radiation. *PLoS ONE*, Vol. 2, No. 10, ISSN 1932-6203.

Crosby, ME.; Kulshreshtha, R.; Ivan, M.; Glazer, PM. (2009). MicroRNA regulation of DNA repair gene expression in hypoxic stress. *Cancer Research*, Vol. 69, pp. 1221-1229, ISSN 0008-5472.

Cubano, L.A. & Lewis M.L. (2000). Fas/APO-1 protein is increased in spaceflown lymphocytes (Jurkat). *Exp. Gerontol.*, Vol. 35, No. 3, pp. 389–400, ISSN 0531-5565.

Dou, H.; Huang, C.; Singh, M.; Carpenter, PB.; Yeh, ET. (2010). Regulation of DNA repair through deSUMOylation and SUMOylation of replication protein A complex. *Mol Cell.*, Vol. 39, No. 3, pp. 333-45, ISSN 1097-2765.

Durante, M.; Snigiryova, G.; Akaeva E., Bogomazova A., Druzhinin S., Fedorenko B., Greco O., Novitskaya N., Rubanovich A., Shevchenko V., Von Recklinghausen U., Obe G. (2003). Chromosome aberration dosimetry in cosmonauts after single or multiple space flights. *Cytogenet. Genome Res.*, Vol. 103, pp. 40–46, ISSN 1424-8581.

Ermakov A.V., Konkova M.S., Kostyuk S.V., Smirnova T.D., Malinovskaya E.M., Efremova L.V., Veiko N.N.(2011). An extracellular DNA mediated bystander effect produced from low dose irradiated endothelial cells. *Mutat Res.*, (Mar 2011). ISSN 0027-5107.

Galanty, Y.; Belotserkovskaya, R.; Coates, J.; Polo, S.; Miller, KM.; Jackson, SP. (2009). Mammalian SUMO E3-ligases PIAS1 and PIAS4 promote responses to DNA double-strand breaks. *Nature*, Vol. 462, No. 7275, pp. 935-9, ISSN 0028-0836.

Gontijo AM, Green CM, Almouzni G. (2003). Repairing DNA damage in chromatin. *Biochimie.*, Vol. 85, No. 11, pp. 1133-47, ISNN 0300-9084.

Gradzka, I.; Iwanenko, T. (2005). A non-radioactive, PFGE-based assay for low levels of DNA double-strand breaks in mammalian cells. *DNA Repair*, Vol. 4, pp. 1129–1139, ISSN 1568-7864.

Grimm, D., Bauer, J.; Kossmehl, P.; Shakibaei, M.; Schonberger, J.; Pickenhahn, H.; Schulze-Tanzil, G.; Vetter, R.; Eilles, C.; Paul, M.; Cogoli, A. (2002). Simulated microgravity alters differentiation and increases apoptosis in human follicular thyroid carcinoma cells. *FASEB J.*, Vol. 16, pp. 604–606, ISSN 0892-6338.

Guo, H.; Ingolia, NT; Weissman, JS.; Bartel, DP. (2010). Mammalian microRNAs predominantly act to decrease target mRNA levels. *Nature,* Vol. 466, No. 7308, pp. 835–840, ISSN 0028-0836.

Hamada, N.; Schettino, G.; Kashino, G.; Vaid, M.; Suzuki, K.; Kodama, S.; Vojnovic, B.; Folkard, M.; Watanabe, M.; Michael, B.D.; Prise, K.M. (2006). Histone H2AX phosphorylation in normal human cells irradiated with focused ultrasoft X rays: evidence for chromatin movement during repair. *Radiat. Res.,* Vol. 166, pp. 31–38, ISSN 0033-7587.

Hammond, T.G.; Benes, E.; O'Reilly, K.C.; Wolf, D.A.; Linnehan, R.M.; Taher, A.; Kaysen, J.H.; Allen, P.L.; Goodwin, T.J. (2000). Mechanical culture conditions effect gene expression: gravity induced changes on the space shuttle, *Physiol Genom.,* Vol. 3 No. 3, pp. 163–173, ISSN 1094-8341.

Harper, JW. & Elledge SJ. (2007). The DNA damage response: ten years after. *Mol Cell.,* Vol. 28, No. 5, pp.739-45, ISSN 1097-2765.

He, M.; Zhao, M.; Shen, B.; Prise, KM.; Shao, C. (2011). Radiation-induced intercellular signaling mediated by cytochrome-c via a p53-dependent pathway in hepatoma cells. *Oncogene,* Vol. 30, No.16, pp. 1947-55, ISSN 0950-9232.

Hershko, A.; Heller, H.; Elias, S.; Ciechanover, A. (1983). Components of ubiquitin–protein ligase system, Resolution, affinity purification, and role in protein breakdown, *J. Biol. Chem.,* Vol. 258, No. 13, pp. 8206–8214, ISSN 0021-9258.

Huang, DW.; Sherman, BT.; Lempicki, R. (2009). Systematic and integrative analysis of large gene lists using DAVID bioinformatics resources. *Nature Protocols,* Vol. 4, pp. 44-57, ISSN 1754-2189.

Huen, M.S.; Grant, R.; Manke, I.; Minn, K.; Yu, X.; Yaffe, M.B.; Chen, J. (2007). RNF8 transduces the DNA-damage signal via histone ubiquitylation and checkpoint protein assembly, *Cell,* Vol. 131, pp. 901–914, ISSN 0092-8674.

Huen, M.S.Y. & Chen, J. (2010). Assembly of checkpoint and repair machineries at DNA damage sites. *Trends Biochem. Sci.,* Vol. 35, pp. 101-108, ISSN 0968-0004.

Hughes-Fulford, M., (2001). Changes in gene expression and signal transduction in microgravity. *Journal of Gravitational Physiology,* Vol. 8, pp. 1-4.

Ibañez, I.L.; Bracalente, C.; Molinari, B.L.; Palmieri, M.A.; Policastro, L.; Kreiner, A.J.; Burlón, A.A.; Valda, A.; Navalesi, D.; Davidson, J.; Davidson, M.; Vázquez, M.; Ozafrán, M.; Durán, H. (2009). Induction and rejoining of DNA double strand breaks assessed by H2AX phosphorylation in melanoma cells irradiated with proton and lithium beams. *Int J Radiat Oncol Biol Phys.,* Vol. 74, pp. 1226-35, ISSN 0360-3016.

Infanger, M.; Ulbrich, C.; Baatout, S.; Wehland, M.; Kreutz, R.; Bauer, J.; Grosse, J.; Vadrucci, S.; Cogoli, A.; Derradji, H.; Neefs, M.; Küsters, S.; Spain, M.; Paul, M.; Grimm, D. (2007). Modeled gravitational unloading induced downregulation of endothelin-1 in human endothelial cells. *J. Cell. Biochem.,* Vol. 101 pp. 1439–1455, ISSN 0730-2312.

Kashino, G.; Prise, K.M.; Schettino, G.; Folkard, M.; Vojnovic, B.; Michael, B.D.; Suzuki, K.; Kodama, S.; Watanabe, M. (2004). Evidence for induction of DNA double strand breaks in the bystander response to targeted soft X-rays in CHO cells. *Mutat. Res.,* Vol. 556, pp. 209–215, ISSN 0027-5107.

Kertesz, M.; Iovino, N.; Unnerstall, U.; Gaul, U.; Segal, E. (2007). The role of site accessibility in microRNA target recognition. *Nat Genet,* Vol. 39, pp. 1278-84, ISSN 1061-4036.

Kinner, A.; Wu, W.; Staudt, C.; Iliakis, G. (2008). Gamma-H2AX in recognition and signaling of DNA double-strand breaks in the context of chromatin. *Nucleic Acids Res.,* Vol. 36, No.17, pp. 5678-5694, ISSN 0305-1048.

Kita, K.; Moriya, T.; Wu, Y.P.; Sugaya, S.; Takahashi, S.; Nomura, J.; Suzuki, N. (2000). Search for gravity-responsive genes by PCR-based mRNA differential display in human cells. *Journal of gravitational physiology,* Vol. 7, pp. 75-76.

Kolas, N.K.; Chapman, J.R.; Nakada, S.; Ylanko, J.; Chahwan, R.; Sweeney, F.D.; Panier, S.; Mendez, M.; Wildenhain, J.; Thomson, T.M.; Pelletier, L.; Jackson, S.P.; Durocher, D. (2007). Orchestration of the DNA-damage response by the RNF8 ubiquitin ligase. *Science,* Vol. 318, pp. 1637–1640, ISSN 0036-8075.

Lewis, M.L.; Reynolds, J.L.; Cubano, L.A.; Hatton, J.P.; Lawless, B.D.; Piepmeier, E.H. (1998). Spaceflight alters microtubules and increases apoptosis in human lymphocytes (Jurkat). *FASEB J.,* Vol. 12, pp.1007–1018, ISSN 0892-6338.

Lewis, M.L.; Reynolds, J.L.; Cubano, L.A.; Hatton, J.P.; Lawless, B.D.; Piepmeier, E.H. (2001). cDNA microarray reveals altered cytoskeletal gene expression in space-flown leukemic T lymphocytes (Jurkat). *FASEB J.,* Vol. 18, pp. 1783–1785, ISSN 0892-6338.

Longnecker, D.E.; Manning, F.J.; Worth Jr. M.H. (Eds.) (2004). Review of Nasa's Longitudinal Study of Astronaut Health, *National Academies Press,* Washington, DC.

Lukas, J.; Lukas, C.; Bartek, J. (2004). Mammalian cell cycle checkpoints: signalling pathways and their organization in space and time. *DNA Repair,*Vol. 3, No. 8–9, pp. 997–1007, ISSN 1568-7864.

Maccarone, M.; Battista, N.; Meloni, M.; Bari, M.; Galleri, G.; Pippia, P.; Cogoli, A.; Finazzi-Agr`o, A. (2003). Creating conditions similar to those that occur during exposure of cells to microgravity induces apoptosis in human lymphocytes by 5-lipoxygenase mediated mitochondrial uncoupling and cytochrome *c* release. *J. Leukocyte Biol.,* Vol. 73, pp. 472–481, ISSN 0741-5400.

Mailand, N.; Bekker-Jensen, S.; Faustrup, H.; Melander, F.; Bartek, J.; Lukas, C.; Lukas, J. (2007). RNF8 ubiquitylates histones at DNA double-strand breaks and promotes assembly of repair proteins. *Cell,*Vol. 131, pp. 887–900, ISSN 0092-8674.

Markova, E.; Schultz, N.; Belyaev, I.Y. (2007). Kinetics and dose-response of residual 53BP1/γ-H2AX foci: co-localization, relationship with DSB repair and clonogenic survival. *Int. J. Radiat. Biol.*, Vol. 83, pp. 319–329, ISSN 0955-3002.

Morris, J.R. (2010). SUMO in the mammalian response to DNA damage. *Biochem. Soc Trans*, Vol. 38, pp. 92-97, ISSN 0300-5127.

Mosesso, P.; Schuber, M.; Seibt, D.; Schmitz, C.; Fiore, M.; Schinoppi, A.; Penna, S.; Palitti, F. (2001). X-ray-induced aberrations in human lymphocytes in vitro are potentiated under simulated microgravity conditions (Clinostat), *Phys. Med.* XVII (Supplement 1).

Pardo, S.J.; Patel, M.J.; Sykes, M.C.; Platt, M.O.; Boyd, N.L.; Sorescu, G.P.; Xu, M.; van Loon, J.J.; Wang, M.D.; Jo, H. (2005). Simulated microgravity using the random positioning machine inhibits differentiation and alters gene expression profiles of 2T3 rre-osteoblasts. *Am. J. Physiol. Cell Physiol.*, Vol. 288, No.6, pp. 1211–1221, ISSN 0363-6143.

Pothof, J.; Verkaik, N.S.; van IJcken, W.; Wiemer, E.A.; Ta, V.T.; van der Horst, G.T.; Jaspers, N.G.; van Gent, D.C.; Hoeijmakers, J.H.; Persengiev, S.P. (2009). MicroRNA-mediated gene silencing modulates the UV-induced DNA-damage response. *EMBO J*, Vol. 28, pp. 2090-9, ISSN 0261-4189.

Prise, K.M.; Pinto, M.; Newman, H.C.; Michael, B.D. (2001). A review of studies of ionizing radiation-induced double-strand break clustering. *Radiat Res*, Vol. 156, pp. 572–576, ISSN 0033-7587.

Riches, L.C.; Lynch, A.M.; Gooderham, N.J. (2008). Early events in the mammalian response to DNA double-strand breaks. *Mutagenesis*, Vol. 23, No. 5, pp. 331–339, ISSN 0267-8357.

Rogakou, E.P.; Pilch, D.R.; Orr, A.H.; Ivanova, V.S.; Bonner, W.M. (1998). DNA double stranded breaks induce histone H2AX phosphorylation on serine 139, *J. Biol. Chem.*, Vol. 273, pp. 5858–5868, ISSN 0021-9258.

Rübe, C.E.; Lorat, Y.; Shuler, N.; Schanz, S.; Wennemuth, G.; Rübe, C. (2011). DNA repair in the context of chromatin: new molecular insights by the nanoscale detection of DNA repair complexes using transmission electron microscopy. *DNA Repair*, Vol. 10, pp. 427-437, ISSN 1568-7864.

Sales, G.; Coppe, A.; Bisognin, A.; Biasiolo, M.; Bortoluzzi, S.; Romualdi, C. (2010). MAGIA, a web-based tool for MiRNA and Genes Integrated Analysis. *Nucleic Acid Research*, Vol. 38 Suppl: W352-9, ISSN 0305-1048.

Sak, A.; Grehl, S.; Erichsen, P.; Engelhard, M.; Grannaß, A.; Levegrün, S.; Pöttgen, C.; Groneberg, M.; Stuschke, M. (2007). gamma-H2AX foci formation in peripheral blood lymphocytes of tumor patients after local radiotherapy to different sites of the body: dependence on the dose-distribution, irradiated site and time from start of treatment, *Int. J. Radiat. Biol.*, Vol. 83, pp. 639–652, ISSN 0955-3002.

Schwartz, J.L.; Jordan, R.; Sun, J.; Ma, H.; Hsie, A.W. (2000). Dose-dependent changes in the spectrum of mutations induced by ionizing radiations, *Radiat. Res.*, Vol. 153, pp. 312–317, ISSN 0033-7587.

Scherthan, H.; Hieber, L.; Braselmann, H.; Meineke, V.; Zitzelsberger H. (2008). Accumulation of DSBs in gamma-H2AXdomains fuel chromosomal aberrations. *Biochem. Biophys. Res. Commun.*, Vol. 371, pp. 694–697, ISSN 0006-291X.

Shannon, P.; Markiel, A.; Ozier, O.; Baliga, N.S.; Wang, J.T.; Ramage, D.; Amin, N.; Schwikowski, B.; Ideker, T. (2003). Cytoscape: a software environment for integrated models of biomolecular interaction networks. *Genome Research,* Vol. 13, pp. 2498-504, ISSN 1088-9051.

Sokolov, M.V.; Smilenov, L.B.; Hall, E.J.; Panyutin, I.G.; Bonner, W.M.; Sedelnikova, O.A. (2005). Ionizing radiation induces DNA double-strand breaks in bystander primary human fibroblasts. *Oncogene* Vol. 24, pp. 7257–7265, ISSN 0950-9232.

Stucki, M. (2009). Histone H2A.X Tyr142 phosphorylation: a novel sWItCH for apoptosis? *DNA Repair,* Vol. 8, No. 7, pp. 873-6, ISSN 1568-7864.

Sytkowski, A.J. & Davis, K.L. (2001). Erythroid cell growth and differentiation in vitro in the simulated microgravity environment of the Nasa Rotating Wall Vessel Bioreactor. *In Vitro Cell Dev. Biol. Anim.,* Vol. 37, pp. 79–83.

Tanq, J.B. & Greenberg (2010). Connecting the Dots: Interplay Between Ubiquitylation and SUMOylation at DNA Double Strand Breaks. *Genes Cancer,* Vol. 1, No. 7, pp. 787-796.

Torigoe, T.; Ichinohe, T.; Sato, N.; Yano, S. (2001). Analysis of gene expression of lymphocytes in microgravity. *Biol. Sci. Space,* Vol. 15, pp. 306–307.

Tusher, V.G.; Tibshirani, R.; Chu, G. (2001). Diagnosis of multiple cancer types by shrunken centroids of gene expression. *Proc Natl Acad Sci U S A,* Vol. 98, pp. 5116-121, ISSN 1091-6490.

Unsworth, B.R. & Lelkes, P.I. (1998). Growing tissues in microgravity, *Nat. Med.* Vol. 4, pp. 901–907, ISSN 1078-8956.

van Veelen, L.R.; Cervelli, T.; van de Rakt, M.W.M.M.; Theil, A.F.; Essers, J.; Kanaar, R. (2005). Analysis of ionizing radiation-induced foci of DNA damage repair proteins. *Mutat. Res.,* Vol. 574, pp. 22–33, ISSN 0027-5107.

Walther, I.; Pippia, P.; Meloni, M.A.; Turrini, F.; Mannu, F.; Cogoli, A. (1998). Simulated microgravity inhibits the genetic expression of interleukin-2 and its receptor in mitogen-activated T lymphocytes. *FEBS lett., Vol.* 436, pp. 115-118, ISSN 0014-5793.

Ward, J.F. (1991). DNA damage and repair. *Basic Life Sci.,* Vol. 58, pp. 403–415.

Wu, J.; Huen, M.S.; Lu, L.Y.; Ye, L.; Dou, Y.; Ljungman, M.; Chen, J.; Yu, X. (2008). Histone ubiquitination associates with BRCA1-dependent DNA damage response. *Mol. Cell Biol.,* Vol. 29, No. 3, pp. 849–860, ISSN 0270-7306.

Wyman C., & Kanaar, R. (2006). DNA double strand break repair: all's well that ends well. *Annu. Rev. Genet.,* Vol. 40, pp. 363-383, ISSN 0066-4197.

Xin, F.; Li, M.; Balch, C.; Thomson, M.; Fan, M.; Liu, Y.; Hammond, S.M.; Kim, S.; Nephew, K.P. (2009). Computational analysis of microRNA profiles and their target genes suggests significant involvement in breast cancer antiestrogen resistance. *Bioinformatics,* Vol. 25, pp. 430-434, ISSN 1367-4803.

Yang, H.; Asaad, N.; Held, K.D. (2005). Medium-mediated intercellular communication is involved in bystander responses of X-ray-irradiated normal human fibroblasts, *Oncogene* Vol. 24, pp. 2096–2103, ISSN 0950-9232.

Zhang, Y.; Zhou, J.; Held, K.D.; Redmond, R.W.; Prise, K.M.; Liber, H.L. (2008). Deficiencies of double-strand break repair factors and effects on mutagenesis in directly gamma-irradiated and medium-mediated bystander human lymphoblastoid cells. *Radiat. Res.*, Vol. 169, No. 2, pp. 197–206, ISSN 0033-7587.

8

DNA Repair: Lessons from the Evolution of Ionizing-Radiation-Resistant Prokaryotes – Fact and Theory

Haïtham Sghaier
Research Unit UR04CNSTN01 "Medical and Agricultural Applications of Nuclear Techniques", National Center for Nuclear Sciences and Technology (CNSTN), Sidi Thabet Technopark, Sidi Thabet, Tunisia

1. Introduction

At the outset, I believe that the concept of ionizing-radiation (IR) resistance needs to be clarified in a tangible manner for readers of this chapter. I propose the following general definition adopted in a previous paper (Sghaier et al., 2008): An ionizing-radiation-resistant prokaryotes (IRRP) is any vegetative prokaryote that can thrive after exposure to high, acute IR (generally, with a D_{10} value - the dose necessary to effect a 90% reduction in Colony Forming Units - greater than 1 kGy) using efficient physiological, genetic and proteic protection and repair mechanisms to fully amend its DNA DSBs. IR resistance has been observed in a broad range of prokaryotic groups (Kopylov et al., 1993), including hyperthermophilic Archaea (*P. abyssi, P. furiosus, Thermococcus marinus, Thermococcus radiotolerans* and *Thermococcus gammatolerans*) (DiRuggiero et al., 1997; Jolivet et al., 2003a; Jolivet et al., 2003b; Jolivet et al., 2004), halophilic Archaea (*Halobacterium* sp.) (Kottemann et al., 2005), the *Deinococcus-Thermus* group (many *Deinococcus* sp. and *Truepera radiovictrix*) (Albuquerque et al., 2005), Actinobacteria (*Rubrobacter radiotolerans, Rubrobacter xylanophilus* and *Kineococcus radiotolerans*) (Yoshinaka et al., 1973; Ferreira et al., 1999; Phillips et al., 2002; Chen et al., 2004), Proteobacteria (*Methylobacterium radiotolerans* and *Acinetobacter radioresistens*) (Ito and Iizuka, 1971; Nishimura et al., 1994), Cyanobacteria (*Chroococcidiopsis* sp.) (Billi et al., 2000), and Sphingobacteria (*Hymenobacter actinosclerus*) (Collins et al., 2000). However, with the exception of *Deinococcus* and *Pyrococcus*, very little information is available regarding the mechanisms of IR resistance and comparative genomics in the above-mentioned prokaryotes. *D. radiodurans* is the current gold-medallist of IR resistance among prokaryotes with a completely sequenced genome (Liolios et al., 2006; Liolios et al., 2010), and can amend more than 100 DSBs per chromosome, induced by IR, without loss of viability (Moseley, 1983; White et al., 1999). After breaking of its 3.2 Mb genome into 20–30 kb pieces by a high dose of IR, *D. radiodurans* fascinatingly reassembles its genome such that 3 hr later fully restructured nonrearranged chromosomes are present (Galhardo and Rosenberg, 2009). Nine interrelated explanations for the extreme IR resistance of *D. radiodurans* have been proposed: (i) the binding of IrrI (DR0171) to genomic repeat sequences that might prevent exhaustive chromosomal degradation after IR exposure - *irr* for IR resistance - (Udupa et al., 1994), (ii) the

RecA(DR2340)-promoted DNA strand exchangeby quite efficient pathways (Kim and Cox, 2002; Sghaier et al., 2010), (iii) the unusual genomic toroidal morphology (Levin-Zaidman et al., 2003) commented in an another paper (Battista et al., 2003), (iv) the prompt PprI/IrrE(DR0167)-induced DNA repair in response to IR stress - *pprI* for inducer of pleiotropic proteins promoting DNA repair - (Earl et al., 2002; Hua et al., 2003; Lu et al., 2009), (v) the critical role played by PprA (DRA0346) in a presumed IR-induced DNA end-joining repair mechanism - PprA for pleiotropic protein promoting DNA repair A - (Narumi et al., 2004), (vi) the divergent evolutionary route of adaptation to IR resistance in comparison to IR-sensitive prokaryotes (IRSP) (Omelchenko et al., 2005; Makarova et al., 2007; Sghaier et al., 2008) including the acquisition of a putative radiation/desiccation response motif (RDRM) and regulon (RDR) (Makarova et al., 2007; Makarova and Daly, 2011), (vii) the stabilization by "holding proteins" of base pairing between closely opposed strand breaks (Cox and Battista, 2005), (viii) the extended synthesis-dependent strand annealing (ESDSA) process, which involves PolA-accomplished DNA synthesis (completed by crossovers achieved by RecA) (Zahradka et al., 2006), with the participation of Pol III and RadA (Galhardo and Rosenberg, 2009; Slade et al., 2009), and (ix) the protein-centered view of IR toxicity (Daly et al., 2007; Daly, 2010; Daly et al., 2010) based on the Mn(II)-facilitated recovery from IR injury (Daly et al., 2004). Yet, why *D. radiodurans* is an extremely IR-resistant bacterium whereas *Escherichia coli* is not is still an open question. For instance, previous literature (Daly et al., 2004; Daly et al., 2007; Daly, 2010; Daly et al., 2010) have suggested that protein protection from damage by oxidation and IR is what makes *D. radiodurans* IR-resistant compared to IRSP including *E. coli*. If so, it raises the question of whether *E. coli* might be able to amend a genome fragmented by restriction enzymes even though it can not amend severe damage induced by IR (Slade et al., 2009), unless it is mutated (Harris et al., 2009).

Interestingly, *D. radiodurans* and *P. furiosus* are able to efficiently repair DSBs in a similar manner (DiRuggiero et al., 1997). In addition, *D. radiodurans* and *P. abyssi* respond in a similar fashion to DNA damage caused by IR (Jolivet et al., 2003b). DNA replication in *D. radiodurans* is known to cease following irradiation (Dean et al., 1966; Moseley and Copland, 1976), which is comparable to the efficient strategy utilized by *P. abyssi* in response to DNA damage that includes an uncoupling of DNA repair and DNA synthesis (Jolivet et al., 2003b). Another shared feature in irradiated *D. radiodurans* and *P. abyssi* is the transport of damaged DNA that should prevent the accumulation of genetic mistakes (Jolivet et al., 2003b). Further study will be necessary to discover mechanistic commonalities among IRRP.

Presently, one of the most significant conclusions that investigators drew by comparing IRRP with IRSP was that the most resistant cells accumulated about 300 times more Mn and about three times less Fe than the most sensitive cells which contributes to protecting their enzymes and the repair functions they catalyze (Daly et al., 2004; Daly et al., 2007; Daly, 2010; Daly et al., 2010). Interestingly, a recent survey of an Fe-rich site in Tunisia (Tamra mine in Nefza) showed relatively high concentrations of Fe (~9.9%) and Mn (~2242 ppm) with a high environmental radioactivity level (~1.5 microsieverts/hour (μSv/h)) nearby the site. In the United States of America (USA), the Ocean Drilling Program, under contract with the National Science Foundation, has recently surveyed environments representative of a broad range of subsurface conditions found in marine sediments (D'Hondt et al., 2004). Among the most striking features of deeply buried sediments (20-100 meters below the sea floor (mbsf)) are Mn-rich sites with high natural γ-radiation levels (see Figure F14 in http://www-odp.tamu.edu/publications/prelim/201_prel/201PREL.PDF and http://www.ldeo.columbia.edu/BRG/ODP/ODP/LEG_SUMM/201/leg201.html#fig4) (Daly MJ, personal communication, 2006). In this context, anaerobic and hyperthermophilic *Deinococcus* sp. have been isolated from the subsurfaces of hydrothermal vents at depths of 64.8 to 128.9 mbsf, where temperatures range from 76 to 91.4°C (Kimura et al., 2003). This finding supports the possibility of the coexistence within the same ecological niche of *Deinococcus* species and other anaerobic hyperthermophilic archaea.

16 rDNA-based phylogenies place *Deinococcus* very close to hyperthermophiles and the root of the phylogenetic tree, with organisms exhibiting IR resistance forming a scattered group (Woese, 1987; Cox and Battista, 2005). In this context, Cavalier-Smith employed aspects of palaeontology, sequence trees, and the methods of transition analysis and congruence testing to demonstrate that the last universal common ancestor (LUCA) lies within eubacteria; specifically, among negibacteria of the superphylum Eobacteria (Hadobacteria and Chlorobacteria) (Cavalier-Smith, 2006). Several important characters indicate that Hadobacteria, including the genus *Deinococcus*, are more primitive than other phyla, with the exception of Chlorobacteria (Cavalier-Smith, 2006). As far as the dispersed phylogenetic clades of IRRP are concerned, the idea of Cox and Battista (Cox and Battista, 2005) concerning convergent evolution remains possible, but it needs further explanation as to how IR-resistant lineages became similar to each other. An immediate question is whether horizontal gene transfer was involved in the convergent evolution of some pivotal genes essential for IR resistance in IRRP. If so, several different evolutionary scenarios are possible: either the genetic gain consisted of a few relatively large DNA fragments, or the genetic gain included individual genes one-by-one. Additionally, the theory of convergent evolution requires that IRRP responded in a similar fashion to DNA damage caused by IR (DSBs) through adaptation to identical environments under the same driving forces. More interestingly, Cox and Battista raised the possibility that IR resistance could be a vestige of DNA repair systems that were present in ancestral species, and has been retained in those organisms that continue to require this phenotype (Cox and Battista, 2005). Their explanation asserts that most descendents "lost" the ancestor's ability to cope with DNA damage and predicts that the molecular mechanisms of IR resistance should be similar among IR-resistant species. Given new insights from pertinent organisms, novel comparative analytical tools, and extensive phylogenetic endeavours, it should soon be possible to test current and future hypotheses concerning the origin of IRRP (see (Omelchenko et al., 2005; Makarova et al., 2007; Sghaier et al., 2007; Makarova and Daly, 2011) and references therein).

Presently, besides many genome projects of IRRP in progress (*e.g. Acinetobacter radioresistens*), many completely sequenced IR-resistant genomes are available on public genome databases (*e.g. Deinococcus proteolyticus* MRP (Liolios et al., 2010)) or were published very recently (*e.g. Deinococcus maricopensis* DSM21211 (Pukall et al., 2011)). However, completely sequenced IR-resistant genomes (Liolios et al., 2010), with published information regarding their IR resistance, are relatively limited in number and restricted in genera: *Deinococcus deserti* VCD115 (de Groot et al., 2005; de Groot et al., 2009; Baudet et al., 2010), *Deinococcus geothermalis* DSM 11300 (Makarova et al., 2007), *D. radiodurans* R_1 (White et al., 1999), two species of *Halobacterium* (*H. salinarum* R1 (Pfeiffer et al., 2008) and *Halobacterium* sp. NRC-1 (Ng et al., 2000)) (Ng et al., 2008), *Kineococcus radiotolerans* SRS30216 (Bagwell et al., 2008), *Rubrobacter xylanophilus* DSM 9941, *Methylobacterium radiotolerans* JCM 2831 (Liolios et al., 2010), three species of *Pyrococcus* (*P. abyssi* GE5 (Cohen et al., 2003), *P. furiosus* DSM 3638 (Maeder et al., 1999), and *P. horikoshii* OT3 (Kawarabayasi et al., 1998)), *Thermococcus gammatolerans* EJ3

(Jolivet et al., 2003a; Liolios et al., 2010), and *Truepera radiovictrix* DSM 17093 (Ivanova et al., 2011). In concordance with previous literature (Koonin, 2003), genes shared by the above-mentioned members of prokaryotic IR-resistant taxa based on TaxPlot available through the NCBI database (Sayers et al., 2011) suggest that the hypothesis of a common ancestor is quantitatively tenable. Qualitatively (Ouzounis et al., 2006), and in contrast to other phenotypes such as those characterized by (hyper)thermophily or pathogenecity, IR resistance does not have characteristic large genetic traits (mutagenesis cassettes, genomic islets (< 10 kilobase pairs (kb)) or fitness islands (> 10 kb), *etc.*) that are either correlated to IR resistance, specific to IRRP, or absent in IRSP. Hallmark genes correlated to IR resistance could be classified into four major evolutionary families on the basis of their mode of contribution to DNA repair (directly through interactions with DNA or indirectly by interactions without DNA) and their prokaryotic distribution:

- Family 1: Composed of genes assuming fundamental and direct functions related to DNA replication and repair (*e.g. polA, recA*) (Kim and Cox, 2002; Zahradka et al., 2006). Members of this family, or their orthologs, are present in all previously studied IRRP (Ouzounis et al., 2006; Sghaier et al., 2008). For instance, RecA protein is quintessential for the fidelity of repair of IR-induced DNA breaks and, consequently, for genome stability in *D. radiodurans* (Repar et al., 2010). In addition, the RecA mutant is among the most IR-sensitive mutants found in *D. radiodurans* (Moseley and Copland, 1975).
- Family 2: Containing genes that contribute directly to IR resistance (*e.g.* DNA nonhomologous end-joining complex) (Weller et al., 2002). Genes of this family are present in several IR-resistant lineages (Aravind and Koonin, 2001).
- Family 3: Comprising genes that contribute indirectly to IR resistance (*e.g.* superoxide dismutase, catalase) (Markillie et al., 1999). These genes are shared by some IRRP (Klotz and Loewen, 2003).
- Family 4: Containing genus- or species-specific genes that contribute directly or indirectly to IR resistance (*e.g. pprI* and *pprA* in *Deinococcus*) (Hua et al., 2003; Narumi et al., 2004). Interestingly, genes of this family enhance DNA repair abilities (Narumi et al., 2004) and regulation mechanisms through check points (Hua et al., 2003).

Previous work by Zahradka *et al.* revealed the relevant two-stage DNA repair process involving PolA and RecA DNA repair enzymes during recovery of *D. radiodurans* from IR (Zahradka et al., 2006). Moreover, the key steps and enzymes involved in ESDSA were identified (Galhardo and Rosenberg, 2009; Slade et al., 2009). Particularly, *polA* and *recA* homologs, belonging to Family 1 (see above), are found among all IRRP. Therefore, the proposal of an ancestral ESDSA repair process (Zahradka et al., 2006) is plausible from a comparative genomics perspective. Since ancestral proteins are reconstructable (Thornton, 2004), the above data suggest that ESDSA might shed light through complementation assays on the IR sensitivity or IR resistance of any node in a phylogenetic tree of PolA or RecA. For instance, a resurrected ancestral PolA protein might be used to complement IR-sensitive cells that are deficient in PolA and for which the wild-type is IR-resistant. The PolA-RecA-mediated repair process possesses the following important characteristics:

1. Functionally, its proteins (PolA and RecA) are important for IR resistance (DiRuggiero et al., 1997; Cox and Battista, 2005; Zahradka et al., 2006; Galhardo and Rosenberg, 2009; Slade et al., 2009; Repar et al., 2010).
2. Phylogenetically, it is a ubiquitous repair mechanism, and it is traced back to LUCA (DiRuggiero et al., 1999; Koonin, 2003; Ouzounis et al., 2006).

3. Evolutionarily, its informational proteins have not been subject to lateral gene transfer (Jain et al., 1999; Koonin, 2003; Ouzounis et al., 2006; Cohen et al., 2011).

The first stage of the two-stage DNA repair process involves a PolA-dependent ESDSA mechanism (Zahradka et al., 2006). This stage mainly requires a functional PolA enzyme and at least two genome copies that are broken at different positions. Knowing that IR-sensitive *D. radiodurans polA* mutants are fully complemented by expression of the *polA* gene from the relatively IR-sensitive *E. coli* (Gutman et al., 1994), and that many IRSP are polyploid (Daly and Minton, 1995), it is legitimate to propose that the first stage of the two-stage DNA repair process could be functional in IRSP. However, the possibility that some deinococcal hypothetical protein(s) or orphan(s) facilitates DNA synthesis by 'any' functional PolA must be seriously considered. This preparation of chromosomal fragments by hypothetical protein(s), albeit not demonstrated, might explain the delay of 1.5 hours in DNA synthesis in the wild-type (Zahradka et al., 2006) and is consistent with the presence of many species-specific proteins in *D. radiodurans*.

The second stage of the two-stage DNA repair process involves RecA-dependent crossovers in *D. radiodurans* (Zahradka et al., 2006), belonging to Mn-accumulating bacteria (Daly et al., 2004). In general, (1) ionic strength affects RecA binding preferential affinity to DNA in relation to single-stranded DNA or double-stranded DNA (Cazenave et al., 1983), and (2) Mn ions have possible effects on DNA structure (stabilization of the helix, neutralization of the negative charge of the phosphate backbone, prevention of DNA renaturation, *etc.*) (Polyanichko et al., 2004). Thus, it is legitimate at this point to assume that the *in vivo* affinity for DNA of 'any' RecA within *D. radiodurans* will differ from its *in vivo* affinity for DNA within an IR-sensitive cell like *E. coli*. Until more research is done, investigators presently agree that repair of DNA DSBs mediated by *recA*-like genes is an extremely active and distinct repair mechanism in *Deinococcus* and *Pyrococcus* (DiRuggiero et al., 1997; Kim and Cox, 2002; Zahradka et al., 2006; Sghaier et al., 2010).

Experimental support for the theory of an ancestral ESDSA repair process is needed. Having been discovered in *D. radiodurans* (Zahradka et al., 2006), an essential attribute of ESDSA is that its presence should also be testable experimentally in IR-resistant archaea.

A consideration of the evolution of IRRP in terms of phenotypic consequences representing genetic change would provide answers on how these organisms evolved. For example, comparative genomic surveys revealed that the radiation-desiccation resistance phenotype of *D. radiodurans* might have gradually evolved via cross-species gene transfer (Omelchenko et al., 2005). One aspect of this theory does seem correct: in contrast to *Pyrococcus*, *Deinococcus* clearly escaped with other Terrabacteria from a state of genetic shrinkage to "genetic gamble" in response to stress during land colonization (Battistuzzi et al., 2004). In this context, the "desiccation adaptation hypothesis" (Mattimore and Battista, 1996) suggests that the IR resistance of *D. radiodurans* is a consequence of its adaptation to desiccation. However, there is no genome-wide data or any experimental data to suggest that desiccation tolerance is antecedent to IR resistance. If this hypothesis is wrong, evolution of IRRP can be misinterpreted profoundly in numerous ways. Briefly, the data presented by Mattimore and Battista (Mattimore and Battista, 1996) only implied a strong positive correlation between these two phenotypes. In fact, a co-author of the "desiccation adaptation hypothesis" showed that inactivation of DRB0118, a constitutively expressed protein, greatly sensitizes *D. radiodurans* to desiccation, but not to IR (Battista et al., 2001). In addition, the ill-founded "desiccation adaptation hypothesis" (Mattimore and Battista, 1996) fails to explain the extreme IR resistance observed in several members of the domain

Archaea (*e.g. Pyrococcus, Thermococcus*). A recent *in vitro* investigation (Beblo et al., 2011) led to a definitive refutation of the "desiccation adaptation hypothesis" (Mattimore and Battista, 1996) and to an implicit vindication of the "radiation adaptation hypothesis" (Sghaier et al., 2007). In brief, it was demonstrated that desiccation-tolerant as well as desiccation-intolerant (hyper-) thermophilic archaea survived comparably high doses of IR (Beblo et al., 2011). In so far as other mechanisms of IR resistance are concerned, it is not surprising that the *Deinococcus* lineage does not share with *Pyrococcus* its five transcripts (DR0423, *ddrA*; DR0070, *ddrB*; DR0003, *ddrC*; DR0326, *ddrD*; DRA0346, *pprA*), most likely evolving in response to IR and desiccation (Tanaka et al., 2004). This network of five transcripts is *Deinococcus* lineage-specific. Similarly, a putative DNA-repair gene cluster of five conserved hypothetical genes in *P. furiosus* (PF0639, PF0640, PF0641, PF0642, PF0643), specifically induced by exposure to IR and probably involved in translesion synthesis, seems to be unique to thermophilic archaea and bacteria (Williams et al., 2007). Does this mean that this putative cluster is important for thermophily? The answer is probably no. One could highlight the fact that the mechanism that protects the DNA against thermal degradation does not prevent the formation of DNA breaks during irradiation (Gerard et al., 2001).

A corollary to all these analyses is the notion that there is a multiplicity of evolutionary and functional processes associated with IR resistance (Omelchenko et al., 2005; Makarova et al., 2007; Sghaier et al., 2007; Daly, 2010; Makarova and Daly, 2011; Slade and Radman, 2011). However, this integrative appraisal does not exclude the possibility of common processes among IRRP. Future analyses might consider more experimental and genomic data from a variety of IRRP in order to determine whether they possess a set of genes that would refute either the concept of convergent evolution or the idea of a common ancestor.

2. Acknowledgements

This work was performed under the auspices of the Tunisian National Center for Nuclear Sciences and Technology (CNSTN). Special thanks to Dr. Issay Narumi from Japan Atomic Energy Agency (JAEA) for previous discussions that improved an initial draft.

3. References

Albuquerque, L., Simoes, C., Nobre, M.F., Pino, N.M., Battista, J.R., Silva, M.T. et al. (2005) *Truepera radiovictrix* gen. nov., sp. nov., a new radiation resistant species and the proposal of *Trueperaceae* fam. nov. *FEMS Microbiol Lett* 247: 161-169.

Aravind, L., and Koonin, E.V. (2001) Prokaryotic homologs of the eukaryotic DNA-end-binding protein Ku, novel domains in the Ku protein and prediction of a prokaryotic double-strand break repair system. *Genome Res* 11: 1365-1374.

Bagwell, C.E., Bhat, S., Hawkins, G.M., Smith, B.W., Biswas, T., Hoover, T.R. et al. (2008) Survival in nuclear waste, extreme resistance, and potential applications gleaned from the genome sequence of *Kineococcus radiotolerans* SRS30216. *PLoS One* 3: e3878.

Battista, J.R., Park, M.J., and McLemore, A.E. (2001) Inactivation of two homologues of proteins presumed to be involved in the desiccation tolerance of plants sensitizes *Deinococcus radiodurans* R1 to desiccation. *Cryobiology* 43: 133-139.

Battista, J.R., Cox, M.M., Daly, M.J., Narumi, I., Radman, M., and Sommer, S. (2003) The structure of *D. radiodurans*. *Science* 302: 567-568; author reply 567-568.

Battistuzzi, F.U., Feijao, A., and Hedges, S.B. (2004) A genomic timescale of prokaryote evolution: insights into the origin of methanogenesis, phototrophy, and the colonization of land. *BMC Evol Biol* 4: 44.

Baudet, M., Ortet, P., Gaillard, J.C., Fernandez, B., Guerin, P., Enjalbal, C. et al. (2010) Proteomics-based refinement of *Deinococcus deserti* genome annotation reveals an unwonted use of non-canonical translation initiation codons. *Mol Cell Proteomics* 9: 415-426.

Beblo K, Douki T, Schmalz G, Rachel R, Wirth R, Huber H, Reitz G, Rettberg P. (2011) Survival of thermophilic and hyperthermophilic microorganisms after exposure to UV-C, ionizing radiation and desiccation. *Arch Microbiol* [Epub ahead of print]

Billi, D., Friedmann, E.I., Hofer, K.G., Caiola, M.G., and Ocampo-Friedmann, R. (2000) Ionizing-radiation resistance in the desiccation-tolerant cyanobacterium *Chroococcidiopsis*. *Appl Environ Microbiol* 66: 1489-1492.

Cavalier-Smith, T. (2006) Rooting the tree of life by transition analyses. *Biol Direct* 1: 19.

Cazenave, C., Toulme, J.J., and Helene, C. (1983) Binding of RecA protein to single-stranded nucleic acids: spectroscopic studies using fluorescent polynucleotides. *EMBO J* 2: 2247-2251.

Chen, M.Y., Wu, S.H., Lin, G.H., Lu, C.P., Lin, Y.T., Chang, W.C., and Tsay, S.S. (2004) Rubrobacter taiwanensis sp. nov., a novel thermophilic, radiation-resistant species isolated from hot springs. *Int J Syst Evol Microbiol* 54: 1849-1855.

Cohen, G.N., Barbe, V., Flament, D., Galperin, M., Heilig, R., Lecompte, O. et al. (2003) An integrated analysis of the genome of the hyperthermophilic archaeon *Pyrococcus abyssi*. *Mol Microbiol* 47: 1495-1512.

Cohen, O., Gophna, U., and Pupko, T. (2011) The complexity hypothesis revisited: connectivity rather than function constitutes a barrier to horizontal gene transfer. *Mol Biol Evol* 28: 1481-1489.

Collins, M.D., Hutson, R.A., Grant, I.R., and Patterson, M.F. (2000) Phylogenetic characterization of a novel radiation-resistant bacterium from irradiated pork: description of *Hymenobacter actinosclerus* sp. nov. *Int J Syst Evol Microbiol* 50 Pt 2: 731-734.

Cox, M.M., and Battista, J.R. (2005) *Deinococcus radiodurans* - the consummate survivor. *Nat Rev Microbiol* 3: 882-892.

D'Hondt, S., Jorgensen, B.B., Miller, D.J., Batzke, A., Blake, R., Cragg, B.A. et al. (2004) Distributions of microbial activities in deep subseafloor sediments. *Science* 306: 2216-2221.

Daly, M.J. (2010) *Deinococcus radiodurans*: Revising the Molecular Basis for Radiation Effects on Cells. In *Extremophiles Handbook*. Horikoshi, K. (ed): Springer Japan KK, pp. 1-16.

Daly, M.J., and Minton, K.W. (1995) Interchromosomal recombination in the extremely radioresistant bacterium *Deinococcus radiodurans*. *J Bacteriol* 177: 5495-5505.

Daly, M.J., Gaidamakova, E.K., Matrosova, V.Y., Kiang, J.G., Fukumoto, R., Lee, D.Y. et al. (2010) Small-molecule antioxidant proteome-shields in *Deinococcus radiodurans*. *PLoS One* 5: e12570.

Daly, M.J., Gaidamakova, E.K., Matrosova, V.Y., Vasilenko, A., Zhai, M., Leapman, R.D. et al. (2007) Protein oxidation implicated as the primary determinant of bacterial radioresistance. *PLoS Biol* 5: e92.

Daly, M.J., Gaidamakova, E.K., Matrosova, V.Y., Vasilenko, A., Zhai, M., Venkateswaran, A. et al. (2004) Accumulation of Mn(II) in *Deinococcus radiodurans* facilitates gamma-radiation resistance. *Science* 306: 1025-1028.

de Groot, A., Chapon, V., Servant, P., Christen, R., Saux, M.F., Sommer, S., and Heulin, T. (2005) *Deinococcus deserti* sp. nov., a gamma-radiation-tolerant bacterium isolated from the Sahara Desert. *Int J Syst Evol Microbiol* 55: 2441-2446.

de Groot, A., Dulermo, R., Ortet, P., Blanchard, L., Guerin, P., Fernandez, B. et al. (2009) Alliance of proteomics and genomics to unravel the specificities of Sahara bacterium *Deinococcus deserti*. *PLoS Genet* 5: e1000434.

Dean, C.J., Feldschreiber, P., and Lett, J.T. (1966) Repair of x-ray damage to the deoxyribonucleic acid in *Micrococcus radiodurans*. *Nature* 209: 49-52.

DiRuggiero, J., Brown, J.R., Bogert, A.P., and Robb, F.T. (1999) DNA repair systems in archaea: mementos from the last universal common ancestor? *J Mol Evol* 49: 474-484.

DiRuggiero, J., Santangelo, N., Nackerdien, Z., Ravel, J., and Robb, F.T. (1997) Repair of extensive ionizing-radiation DNA damage at 95 degrees C in the hyperthermophilic archaeon *Pyrococcus furiosus*. *J Bacteriol* 179: 4643-4645.

Earl, A.M., Mohundro, M.M., Mian, I.S., and Battista, J.R. (2002) The IrrE protein of *Deinococcus radiodurans* R1 is a novel regulator of *recA* expression. *J Bacteriol* 184: 6216-6224.

Ferreira, A.C., Nobre, M.F., Moore, E., Rainey, F.A., Battista, J.R., and da Costa, M.S. (1999) Characterization and radiation resistance of new isolates of *Rubrobacter radiotolerans* and *Rubrobacter xylanophilus*. *Extremophiles* 3: 235-238.

Galhardo, R.S., and Rosenberg, S.M. (2009) Extreme genome repair. *Cell* 136: 998-1000.

Gerard, E., Jolivet, E., Prieur, D., and Forterre, P. (2001) DNA protection mechanisms are not involved in the radioresistance of the hyperthermophilic archaea *Pyrococcus abyssi* and *P. furiosus*. *Mol Genet Genomics* 266: 72-78.

Gutman, P.D., Fuchs, P., and Minton, K.W. (1994) Restoration of the DNA damage resistance of *Deinococcus radiodurans* DNA polymerase mutants by *Escherichia coli* DNA polymerase I and Klenow fragment. *Mutat Res* 314: 87-97.

Harris, D.R., Pollock, S.V., Wood, E.A., Goiffon, R.J., Klingele, A.J., Cabot, E.L. et al. (2009) Directed evolution of ionizing radiation resistance in *Escherichia coli*. *J Bacteriol* 191: 5240-5252.

Hua, Y., Narumi, I., Gao, G., Tian, B., Satoh, K., Kitayama, S., and Shen, B. (2003) PprI: a general switch responsible for extreme radioresistance of *Deinococcus radiodurans*. *Biochem Biophys Res Commun* 306: 354-360.

Ito, H., and Iizuka, H. (1971) Taxonomic studies on a radio-resistant *Pseudomonas*. Part XII. Studies on the microorganisms of cereal grain. *Agric Biol Chem* 35: 1566-1571.

Ivanova, N., Rohde, C., Munk, C., Nolan, M., Lucas, S., Del Rio, T.G. et al. (2011) Complete genome sequence of *Truepera radiovictrix* type strain (RQ-24). *Stand Genomic Sci* 4: 91-99.

Jain, R., Rivera, M.C., and Lake, J.A. (1999) Horizontal gene transfer among genomes: the complexity hypothesis. *Proc Natl Acad Sci U S A* 96: 3801-3806.

Jolivet, E., L'Haridon, S., Corre, E., Forterre, P., and Prieur, D. (2003a) *Thermococcus gammatolerans* sp. nov., a hyperthermophilic archaeon from a deep-sea hydrothermal vent that resists ionizing radiation. *Int J Syst Evol Microbiol* 53: 847-851.

Jolivet, E., Corre, E., L'Haridon, S., Forterre, P., and Prieur, D. (2004) *Thermococcus marinus* sp. nov. and *Thermococcus radiotolerans* sp. nov., two hyperthermophilic archaea from deep-sea hydrothermal vents that resist ionizing radiation. *Extremophiles* 8: 219-227.

Jolivet, E., Matsunaga, F., Ishino, Y., Forterre, P., Prieur, D., and Myllykallio, H. (2003b) Physiological responses of the hyperthermophilic archaeon "*Pyrococcus abyssi*" to DNA damage caused by ionizing radiation. *J Bacteriol* 185: 3958-3961.

Kawarabayasi, Y., Sawada, M., Horikawa, H., Haikawa, Y., Hino, Y., Yamamoto, S. et al. (1998) Complete sequence and gene organization of the genome of a hyper-thermophilic archaebacterium, *Pyrococcus horikoshii* OT3. *DNA Res* 5: 55-76.

Kim, J.I., and Cox, M.M. (2002) The RecA proteins of *Deinococcus radiodurans* and *Escherichia coli* promote DNA strand exchange via inverse pathways. *Proc Natl Acad Sci U S A* 99: 7917-7921.

Kimura, H., Asada, R., Masta, A., and Naganuma, T. (2003) Distribution of microorganisms in the subsurface of the manus basin hydrothermal vent field in Papua New Guinea. *Appl Environ Microbiol* 69: 644-648.

Klotz, M.G., and Loewen, P.C. (2003) The molecular evolution of catalatic hydroperoxidases: evidence for multiple lateral transfer of genes between prokaryota and from bacteria into eukaryota. *Mol Biol Evol* 20: 1098-1112.

Koonin, E.V. (2003) Comparative genomics, minimal gene-sets and the last universal common ancestor. *Nat Rev Microbiol* 1: 127-136.

Kopylov, V.M., Bonch-Osmolovskaya, E.A., Svetlichnyi, V.A., Miroshnicheko, M.L., and Skobin, V.S. (1993) Gamma-irradiation resistance and UV sensitivity of extremely thermophilic archaebacteria and eubacteria. *Mikrobiologiya* 62: 90-95.

Kottemann, M., Kish, A., Iloanusi, C., Bjork, S., and DiRuggiero, J. (2005) Physiological responses of the halophilic archaeon *Halobacterium* sp. strain NRC1 to desiccation and gamma irradiation. *Extremophiles* 9: 219-227.

Levin-Zaidman, S., Englander, J., Shimoni, E., Sharma, A.K., Minton, K.W., and Minsky, A. (2003) Ringlike structure of the *Deinococcus radiodurans* genome: a key to radioresistance? *Science* 299: 254-256.

Liolios, K., Tavernarakis, N., Hugenholtz, P., and Kyrpides, N.C. (2006) The Genomes On Line Database (GOLD) v.2: a monitor of genome projects worldwide. *Nucleic Acids Res* 34: D332-334.

Liolios, K., Chen, I.M., Mavromatis, K., Tavernarakis, N., Hugenholtz, P., Markowitz, V.M., and Kyrpides, N.C. (2010) The Genomes On Line Database (GOLD) in 2009: status of genomic and metagenomic projects and their associated metadata. *Nucleic Acids Res* 38: D346-354.

Lu, H., Gao, G., Xu, G., Fan, L., Yin, L., Shen, B., and Hua, Y. (2009) *Deinococcus radiodurans* PprI switches on DNA damage response and cellular survival networks after radiation damage. *Mol Cell Proteomics* 8: 481-494.

Maeder, D.L., Weiss, R.B., Dunn, D.M., Cherry, J.L., Gonzalez, J.M., DiRuggiero, J., and Robb, F.T. (1999) Divergence of the hyperthermophilic archaea *Pyrococcus furiosus* and *P. horikoshii* inferred from complete genomic sequences. *Genetics* 152: 1299-1305.

Makarova, K.S., and Daly, M.J. (2011) Comparative Genomics of Stress Response Systems in *Deinococcus* Bacteria. In *Bacterial Stress Responses*. Storz, G., and Hengge, R. (eds). Washington, DC: ASM Press, pp. 445-457.

Makarova, K.S., Omelchenko, M.V., Gaidamakova, E.K., Matrosova, V.Y., Vasilenko, A., Zhai, M. et al. (2007) *Deinococcus geothermalis*: the pool of extreme radiation resistance genes shrinks. *PLoS One* 2: e955.

Markillie, L.M., Varnum, S.M., Hradecky, P., and Wong, K.K. (1999) Targeted mutagenesis by duplication insertion in the radioresistant bacterium *Deinococcus radiodurans*: radiation sensitivities of catalase (*katA*) and superoxide dismutase (*sodA*) mutants. *J Bacteriol* 181: 666-669.

Mattimore, V., and Battista, J.R. (1996) Radioresistance of *Deinococcus radiodurans*: functions necessary to survive ionizing radiation are also necessary to survive prolonged desiccation. *J Bacteriol* 178: 633-637.

Moseley, B.E., and Copland, H.J. (1975) Isolation and properties of a recombination-deficient mutant of *Micrococcus radiodurans*. *J Bacteriol* 121: 422-428.

Moseley, B.E., and Copland, H.J. (1976) The rate of recombination repair and its relationship to the radiation-induced delay in DNA synthesis in *Micrococcus radiodurans*. *J Gen Microbiol* 93: 251-258.

Moseley, B.E.B. (1983) Photobiology and radiobiology of *Micrococcus* (*Deinococcus*) *radiodurans*. *Photochem Photobiol Rev* 7: 223-274.

Narumi, I., Satoh, K., Cui, S., Funayama, T., Kitayama, S., and Watanabe, H. (2004) PprA: a novel protein from *Deinococcus radiodurans* that stimulates DNA ligation. *Mol Microbiol* 54: 278-285.

Ng, W.V., Berquist, B.R., Coker, J.A., Capes, M., Wu, T.H., DasSarma, P., and DasSarma, S. (2008) Genome sequences of *Halobacterium* species. *Genomics* 91: 548-552; author reply 553-544.

Ng, W.V., Kennedy, S.P., Mahairas, G.G., Berquist, B., Pan, M., Shukla, H.D. et al. (2000) Genome sequence of *Halobacterium* species NRC-1. *Proc Natl Acad Sci U S A* 97: 12176-12181.

Nishimura, Y., Uchida, K., Tanaka, K., Ino, T., and Ito, H. (1994) Radiation sensitivities of *Acinetobacter* strains isolated from clinical sources. *J Basic Microbiol* 34: 357-360.

Omelchenko, M.V., Wolf, Y.I., Gaidamakova, E.K., Matrosova, V.Y., Vasilenko, A., Zhai, M. et al. (2005) Comparative genomics of *Thermus thermophilus* and *Deinococcus radiodurans*: divergent routes of adaptation to thermophily and radiation resistance. *BMC Evol Biol* 5: 57.

Ouzounis, C.A., Kunin, V., Darzentas, N., and Goldovsky, L. (2006) A minimal estimate for the gene content of the last universal common ancestor--exobiology from a terrestrial perspective. *Res Microbiol* 157: 57-68.

Pfeiffer, F., Schuster, S.C., Broicher, A., Falb, M., Palm, P., Rodewald, K. et al. (2008) Evolution in the laboratory: the genome of *Halobacterium salinarum* strain R1 compared to that of strain NRC-1. *Genomics* 91: 335-346.

Phillips, R.W., Wiegel, J., Berry, C.J., Fliermans, C., Peacock, A.D., White, D.C., and Shimkets, L.J. (2002) *Kineococcus radiotolerans* sp. nov., a radiation-resistant, gram-positive bacterium. *Int J Syst Evol Microbiol* 52: 933-938.

Polyanichko, A.M., Andrushchenko, V.V., Chikhirzhina, E.V., Vorob'ev, V.I., and Wieser, H. (2004) The effect of manganese(II) on DNA structure: electronic and vibrational circular dichroism studies. *Nucleic Acids Res* 32: 989-996.

Pukall R, Zeytun A, Lucas S, Lapidus A, Hammon N, Deshpande S, Nolan M, Cheng JF, Pitluck S, Liolios K, Pagani I, Mikhailova N, Ivanova N, Mavromatis K, Pati A, Tapia R, Han C, Goodwin L, Chen A, Palaniappan K, Land M, Hauser L, Chang YJ, Jeffries CD, Brambilla EM, Rohde M, Göker M, Detter JC, Woyke T, Bristow J, Eisen JA, Markowitz V, Hugenholtz P, Kyrpides NC, Klenk HP. (2011) Complete genome sequence of *Deinococcus maricopensis* type strain (LB-34). *Stand Genomic Sci* 4(2):163-172.

Repar, J., Cvjetan, S., Slade, D., Radman, M., Zahradka, D., and Zahradka, K. (2010) RecA protein assures fidelity of DNA repair and genome stability in *Deinococcus radiodurans*. *DNA Repair (Amst)* 9: 1151-1161.

Sayers, E.W., Barrett, T., Benson, D.A., Bolton, E., Bryant, S.H., Canese, K. et al. (2011) Database resources of the National Center for Biotechnology Information. *Nucleic Acids Res* 39: D38-51.

Sghaier, H., Ghedira, K., Benkahla, A., and Barkallah, I. (2008) Basal DNA repair machinery is subject to positive selection in ionizing-radiation-resistant bacteria. *BMC Genomics* 9: 297.

Sghaier, H., Satoh, K., Ohba, H., and Narumi, I. (2010) Assessing the role of RecA protein in the radioresistant bacterium *Deinococcus geothermalis*. *African Journal of Biochemistry Research* 4: 111-118.

Sghaier, H., Narumi, I., Satoh, K., Ohba, H., and Mitomo, H. (2007) Problems with the current deinococcal hypothesis: an alternative theory. *Theory Biosci* 126: 43-45.

Slade, D., and Radman, M. (2011) Oxidative stress resistance in *Deinococcus radiodurans*. *Microbiol Mol Biol Rev* 75: 133-191.

Slade, D., Lindner, A.B., Paul, G., and Radman, M. (2009) Recombination and replication in DNA repair of heavily irradiated *Deinococcus radiodurans*. *Cell* 136: 1044-1055.

Tanaka, M., Earl, A.M., Howell, H.A., Park, M.J., Eisen, J.A., Peterson, S.N., and Battista, J.R. (2004) Analysis of *Deinococcus radiodurans*'s transcriptional response to ionizing radiation and desiccation reveals novel proteins that contribute to extreme radioresistance. *Genetics* 168: 21-33.

Thornton, J.W. (2004) Resurrecting ancient genes: experimental analysis of extinct molecules. *Nat Rev Genet* 5: 366-375.

Udupa, K.S., O'Cain, P.A., Mattimore, V., and Battista, J.R. (1994) Novel ionizing radiation-sensitive mutants of *Deinococcus radiodurans*. *J Bacteriol* 176: 7439-7446.

Weller, G.R., Kysela, B., Roy, R., Tonkin, L.M., Scanlan, E., Della, M. et al. (2002) Identification of a DNA nonhomologous end-joining complex in bacteria. *Science* 297: 1686-1689.

White, O., Eisen, J.A., Heidelberg, J.F., Hickey, E.K., Peterson, J.D., Dodson, R.J. et al. (1999) Genome sequence of the radioresistant bacterium *Deinococcus radiodurans* R1. *Science* 286: 1571-1577.

Williams, E., Lowe, T.M., Savas, J., and DiRuggiero, J. (2007) Microarray analysis of the hyperthermophilic archaeon *Pyrococcus furiosus* exposed to gamma irradiation. *Extremophiles* 11: 19-29.

Woese, C.R. (1987) Bacterial evolution. *Microbiol Rev* 51: 221-271.

Yoshinaka, T., Yano, K., and Yamaguchi, H. (1973) Isolation of highly radioresistant bacterium, *Arthrobacter radiotolerans* nov. sp. *Agric Biol Chem* 37: 2269-2275.

Zahradka, K., Slade, D., Bailone, A., Sommer, S., Averbeck, D., Petranovic, M. et al. (2006) Reassembly of shattered chromosomes in *Deinococcus radiodurans*. *Nature* 443: 569-573.

9

DNA Helix Destabilization by Alkylating Agents: From Covalent Bonding to DNA Repair

Gaëlle Lenglet, Sabine Depauw, Denise Mendy-Belaiche and Marie-Hélène David-Cordonnier
INSERM, Jean-Pierre Aubert Research Center (JPARC), Team 4 Molecular and Cellular Targeting for Cancer Treatment and University of Lille-Grand Nord, Institut pour la Recherche sur le Cancer de Lille, Place de Verdun, Lille France

1. Introduction

Preservation of the integrity of the DNA, carrier of heritage information, is crucial for cell survival. Altered genetic information could lead to major perturbations in cell organization, function and proliferation of cancer cells. Because cancer cells are highly proliferative with high number of replication, DNA was the first clinically used anti-cancer therapeutic target with the drugs directly (intercalators/alkylating drugs) or indirectly (micro-tubules, topoisomerases inhibitors, modifiers of histone acetylation...) targeting DNA. Despite the actual development of targeted chemotherapies (against membrane receptors, kinases, the proteasome,…), direct DNA targeting drugs still represent a major part of the actual anti-cancer pharmacopeia in terms of total prescriptions and efficacy. Compounds mainly bind DNA in three different ways: non-covalent (fitting in major or minor grooves), intercalation between two successive base pairs, or covalent bonding to a base, and generally lead to a stabilization of the DNA double helix. Only a few number from intercalating and alkylating families destabilizes the DNA helix. Cytotoxic effects of alkylating agents (used/developed for chemotherapy or from carcinogens) are strongly attenuated by the cellular DNA repair processes. Optimal use of DNA alkylating drugs in therapy requires a clear understanding of their DNA repair processes. Similarly, knowing how cells cope with the carcinogens-induced DNA damages is of major interest regarding health in our actual society, so prompt to use chemical compounds insufficiently studied for long term toxicities and sometimes eventually identified as carcinogens (food and industries). DNA repair processes infer with both those Yin and Yang aspects of alkylating compounds using different machineries: base excision repair (BER); nucleotide excision repair (NER: long/short-patch, transcription-coupled/global genome); mismatch repair (MMR); homologous recombination (HR) or non-homologous end-joining (NHEJ). Fanconi anemia (FA) repair acts as a coordinator of those repair pathways (Moldovan & D'Andrea, 2009). Since there are yet various complete reviews on DNA repair processes in the literature, the present review will focus on the repair process of DNA destabilizing compounds.

2. DNA destabilizing compounds

Stability of DNA double helix is mainly due to reversible non-covalent hydrogen bonds between Watson-Crick base-pairs. Local or global denaturation (melting or breathing) of the double-stranded DNA (dsDNA) helix is dispensable for different cellular processes: DNA replication, transcription and repair (Choi et al., 2004; Schneider et al., 2001). DNA melting is affected by sequence (AT- or GC-rich portions, some successive base pairs arrangements) and their specific tilt, roll, twist effects (Benham, 1996; Dornberger et al., 1999; Krueger et al., 2006), the formation of local hairpins, 3D structures at terminal regions of the DNA helix (Putnam et al., 1981) or internal portions of B- to Z-DNA transition (Harvey, 1983). Such locally opened sites are good substrates for, or are generated by, some cellular proteins: DNA helicases (Betterton & Julicher, 2005), single strand binding proteins (SSBP) such as replication protein A (RPA) (Wold, 1997), UP1 and myeloma helix-destabilizing protein (Herrick & Alberts, 1976; Planck & Wilson, 1980), GAPDH-related protein P8 (Karpel & Burchard, 1981), High Mobility Group (HMG) proteins (Butler et al., 1985), c-Abl kinase (David-Cordonnier et al., 1998, 1999), HIV-1 nucleocapsid protein (Narayanan et al., 2006), prion protein (Bera et al., 2007), NF-κB transcription factor (Mura & McCammon, 2008) and UHRF-1 protein (Arita et al., 2008). Besides large DNA opening, small modifications such as base flipping locally perturb DNA stability (Hornby & Ford, 1998) during mismatches or repair proteins interaction from NER (Cao et al., 2004), BER (Bellamy et al., 2007; Tubbs et al., 2007) or DNA methylases/demethylases (Sundheim et al., 2008).
Besides naturally occurring DNA breathing, unzipping is induced by clinically used or potential anti-tumor compounds. The vast majority of DNA-interacting compounds stabilize the DNA double helix; only a very few of them displays the pecular ability to destabilize DNA helix. In this latter group, most belong to DNA intercalating or alkylating families.

2.1 DNA intercalators as helix destabilizing agents

2.1.1 Mono-intercalators

Historically, the first DNA intercalating compound evidencing DNA destabilization properties was acridine orange (Figure 1), a well-known dsDNA intercalating compound and a strong single-stranded DNA (ssDNA) binder. It emitted green fluorescence emission from dsDNA binding and red luminescence from ssDNA interaction. Acridine orange enhances the global helix stability but exerts local denaturation of DNA (Kapuscinski & Darzynkiewicz, 1983; 1984; Darzynkiewicz et al, 1983). Ellipticine and adriamycin (Figure 1) also induce local unzipping of the DNA and bind ssDNA (Zunino et al., 1972), in contrast with ethidium bromide (BET), highly specific to dsDNA and stabilizing DNA. Intercalation of acridine orange, ellipticine and adriamycin progressively unzip the DNA helix preferentially in heterochromatin, ribosomes and polysomes (Darzynkiewicz et al., 1983).

2.1.2 Bis-intercalators

Bisacridine A (BisA) (Figure 1) is a DNA unwinding bis-intercalator deriving from acridine orange by cyclization of two acridine planar chromophores using polyammonium bridges. Initially designed to interact with ss- rather than ds-DNA (Teulade-Fichou et al., 1995), BisA shifts duplexes DNA toward hairpins and destabilizes dsDNA (Slama-Schwok et al., 1997).

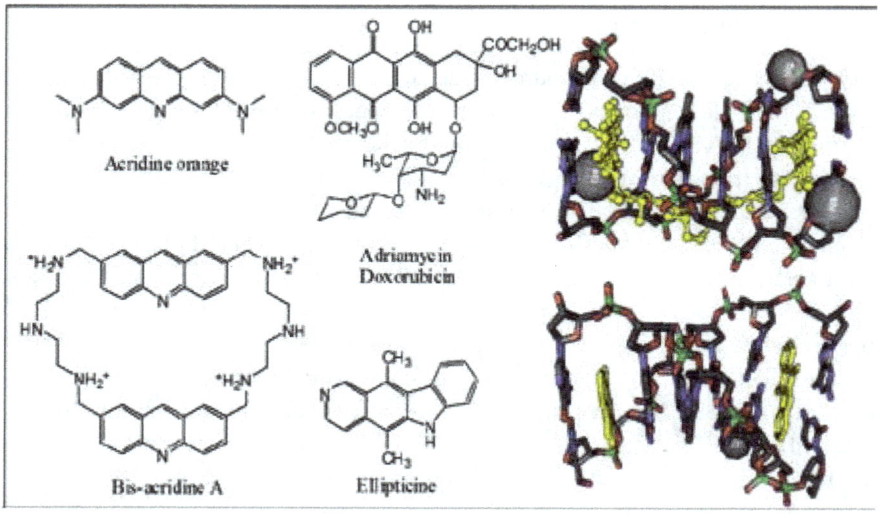

Fig. 1. DNA intercalators that destabilize the DNA helix: structures and 3D orientation of morpholino-doxorubicin (Top, [mmdbId:52942]) or ellipticine (Bottom, [mmdbId:52189]).

2.2 DNA alkylators as helix destabilizing agents

Some DNA alkylating drugs could also locally destabilize DNA double helix. Some of those are used/developed as anticancer drugs such as cisplatin and metal-derivatives, or more recently the benzoacronycine derivative S23906-1. They contrast with most DNA alkylating agents used or not in chemotherapy that stabilize DNA helix (for instance mitomycin C, dinuclear platinum, nitrogen mustards or ecteinascidine 743) (Basu et al., 1993; David-Cordonnier et al., 2005; Fridman et al., 2003; Kasparkova et al., 1999). Electrophilic alkylating drugs react at nucleophilic positions of G-C or A-T bp with preferential targets: N^7 position of dG or dA and O^6 position of dG in the major groove, N^3 positions of dG or dA and exocyclic NH_2 group on C^2 of dG (also called N^2) in the minor groove (Figure 2).

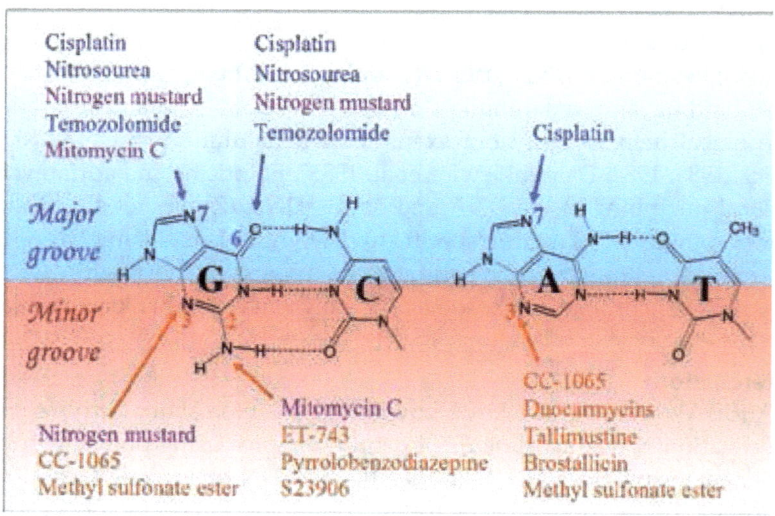

Fig. 2. Position of the reactive sites of some DNA alkylators on G-C or A-T base pairs.

2.2.1 Cisplatin and other transition-metal antitumor agents as DNA destabilizing drugs

Fortuitously discovered in 1965, cisplatin (or *cis*-diaminedichloridoplatinum(II) is used in clinic since 1978 and is still frequently administrated in combinatory chemotherapies as one of the most effective anticancer drugs against solid tumors (Figure 3). Cisplatin forms inter- and intra-strand crosslinks as well as monovalent adducts. Those lesions occur primarily though covalent bonding to the N^7 atom of guanines. The most common lesions are intra-strand crosslink at the 5′-GG (65%) or 5′-AG (25%) dinucleotides and inter-strand crosslinks (5-8%). This latter lesion is more frequent using transplatin (12%), *trans*-$PtCl_2(NH_3)$(quinoline) and *trans*-$PtCl_2(NH_3)$(thiazole) derivatives (up to 30%) (Figure 3). Cisplatin-induced intra-strand crosslinks at GpG base-pairs result in a strong DNA helix bending toward the major groove with an angle of 55-78° associated with DNA distortion, resulting in a destabilization of the Watson-Crick base pairing and local denaturation of the DNA helix (bending at 45° and unwinding by $79^{+}/.4°$) (Bellon, 1991; Malinge et al., 1994; Todd & Lippard, 2010). In platinated-GpG intra-strand crosslinks, the distortion varies and depends on the sequence context, with up to a 7 bp distortion for 1,3-intrastrand crosslinks within a TGTGT sequence (Kasparkova et al., 2008a). Such destabilization was found to be enthalpic, but not entropic, in origin. Similarly, when occurring at 5′-TGGT site, cisplatin adducts decrease the melting temperature of the DNA by more than 10°C which is much higher than that induced on 5′-CGGT and 5′-AGGC sequences (~6°C) (Malina et al., 2007).
Such effects are not observed with transplatin which does not change the transition entropy or enthalpy and, consequently, does not destabilize the DNA helix (Kasparkova et al., 2008a). Third-generation platinum antitumor derivative oxaliplatin (Figure 3) induces greater DNA bending, unwinding and helix destabilization than cisplatin, whereas JM118 (Figure 3) induces DNA destabilization profiles similar to that of cisplatin (Kostrhunova et al., 2010). JM118 is the major metabolite of satraplatin (JM216), the first orally administered platinum drug that also evidenced promising therapeutic activities in prostate cancer. JM118 induces a DNA bending with an angle of 28° toward the major groove, an angle smaller than that obtained with cisplatin for the same sequence (34°) (Kostrhunova et al., 2010).
Besides the nature of the platinated drug, the surrounding DNA sequence is also of major importance for helix stability. Indeed, monofunctional platinum adducts at 5′-TGC triplet induces major DNA destabilization (Brabec et al., 1992) but none at 5′-AGT or 5′-TGA triplet (Schwartz et al., 1989). DNA is not the unique nucleic acid destabilized by platinated derivatives as evidenced using *cis*-$[PtCl(NH_3)_2(OH_2)]^+$, *cis*-$[PtCl(NH_3)(c\text{-}C_6H_{11}NH_2)(OH_2)]^+$ and *trans*-$[PtCl(NH_3)(\text{quinoline})(OH_2)]^+$ (Figure 3) which not only destabilize ds-DNA but also ds-RNA (ΔTm of -11°C and -5°C, respectively) (Hägerlöf et al., 2006).
Besides platinum derivatives, ruthenium compounds were developed as anti-cancer drugs. NAMI-A was the first ruthenium derivative that entered phase I clinical trials in 1999 as an anti-metastatic drug (Bergamo et al., 2002), followed by KP1019 (FFC14A) in 2003 (Hartinger et al., 2008). Two gallium compounds, gallium maltolate and KP46 (FFC11), also entered phase I clinical trials in 2003 (Lum et al., 2003). As for cisplatin, ruthenium derivatives evidenced DNA destabilization properties. This is particularly well described for Ru-CYM ($[(\eta 6\text{-}\pi\text{-cymene})Ru(II)(en)\text{-}(Cl)]^+$ and Ru-BIP, Ru-DHA or Ru-THA as biphenyl, dihydroanthracene or tetrahydroanthracene derivatives, respectively (Figure 3). Such organometallic ruthenium(II) arene complexes were rationally designed for chemotherapy with the idea that changing platinum for ruthenium would provide additional coordination sites in the octahedral complexes to modify the oxidation rate and change ligand affinity

and binding kinetics (C.X. Zhang & Lippard, 2003). From this series, Ru-CYM presents the highest DNA helix destabilization activity, together with the smaller unwinding angle in supercoiled plasmid DNA (7° *vs.* 14° for Ru-BIP, Ru-DHA and Ru-THA), in correlation with its lack of intercalation and the formation of monoadducts at N^7-dG (Nováková et al., 2009). New Ru-derivatives monodentate-Ru(II) and $[Ru(terpy)(4,4'\text{-}(COLysCONH_2)_2bpy)Cl]^{3+}$ also destabilize DNA (Nováková et al., 2010; Triantafillidi et al., 2011). For gallium-complexed compounds, interaction of trivalent Ga-cations with calf-thymus DNA resulted in major helix destabilization with perturbations at A-T base pairs sites (R. Ahmad et al. 1996).

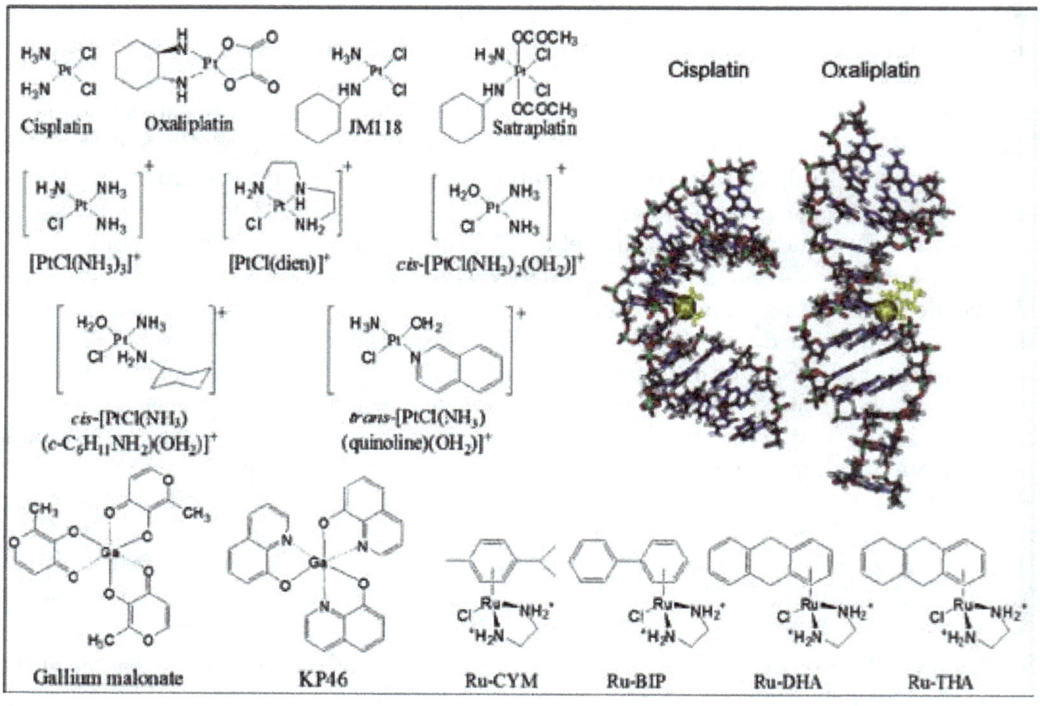

Fig. 3. Structure of cisplatin and other transition-metal agents as DNA destabilizing drugs and 3D orientation [mmdbId:47796] (cisplatin) and [mmdbId:69361] (oxaliplatin).

2.2.2 Carcinogens as DNA destabilizing agents

DNA interaction of carcinogen, adduct formation and their repair processes are widely studied using carcinogens from environmental and tobacco smoke. Some of them have the ability to destabilize the DNA helix: BPDE ((+/-)-*anti*-benzo[*a*]pyrene-7,8-dihydrodiol-9,10-epoxide) and 4-OHEN (4-hydroxyequilenin-O-quinone) (Figure 4).

The smoke carcinogen benzo[*a*]pyrene (BaP) is metabolized into several enantiomers of BPDE that covalently bond the exocyclic NH_2 group of guanines to form a bulky adduct in the minor groove of the DNA helix, resulting in its destabilization (Zou & Van Houten, 1999). Due to the orientation of the reactive epoxide group on asymmetric carbons, several enantiomers are produced. The most carcinogenic is 10S(+)-*trans-anti*-BPDE N^2-dG adduct followed by the stereo-isomeric 10R(+)-*cis-anti*-BPDE-N^2-dG adducts. Covalent bonding to DNA is associated with base-displaced intercalation where the bulky adduct prevents the hydrogen bonding of the amino group of guanine with the opposite cytosine. This results in a base-flipping where the (+)-*anti*-B[*a*]P-N^2-dG bulky adduct is located in the minor groove and the opposite cytosine is positioned in the major groove (Cosman et al., 1993). The precise orientation of this highly carcinogenic 10S(+)-*trans-anti*-B[*a*]P-N^2-dG adduct depends on the sequence surrounding the target guanine (Cai et al., 2010). DNA is untwisted at 5′-CGG*C sites where a large bend is induced in the DNA helix, but not at 5′-CG*GC sequences where, conversely, DNA helix is destabilized in its portion orientated 5′ to the lesion (Rodríguez et al., 2007). Such differences result in different protein/DNA recognition and repair activities (see 3.4). Thermal destabilization was also observed using 14R(+)-*trans-anti*-DB[*a,l*]P-N^2-dG adduct (Zheng et al., 2010) or *14S*(-)-*trans-anti*-DB[*a,l*]P-N^6-dA adducts whereas *14R*(+) isomer stabilizes the ds-DNA (Cai et al., 2011).

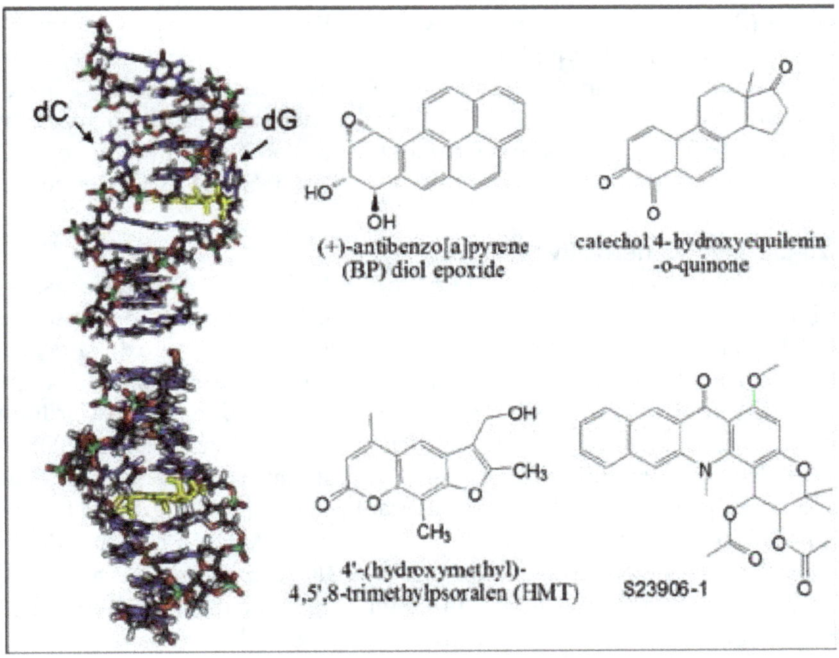

Fig. 4. 3D orientation of (+)-*anti*-BPDE [mmdbId:52106] and the psoralen derivative HMT [mmdbId:52343] and structure of some DNA alkylators that destabilize the DNA helix.

The hormone-derived genotoxic compound, 4-OHEN, derives from equilin and equilenin, two equine oestrogens present in hormone substitution therapies used to prevent the uncomfortable effects of menopauses but are also thought to increase breast cancer incidence in the population of hormonally-treated women (Rossouw et al., 2002). Its ortho-quinone form is cytotoxic and genotoxic (Pisha et al., 2001) through the formation of bulky DNA lesions at dA, dC and dG (but not at T residues) (Kolbanovskiy et al., 2005) which were detected in both cell culture and breast cancer biopsies from patients treated with hormone substitution therapies (Embrechts et al., 2003). 4-OHEN derived from the intermediate catechol 4-hydroxyequilenin which was generated from a rapid conversion of both equilin and equilenin in the organism to four stereo-isomers differently affecting the 3D-structure of the DNA helix (Ding et al., 2007). For adducts on cytosine, the *syn*- or *anti*-conformations of the bulky rings of 4-OHEN point along the major or the minor groove (Ding et al., 2005). Interestingly, alkylation at dA or dC residues is associated with a strong decrease in the melting temperature (Tm) of a 11-bp oligonucleotide, with the magnitude of the negative ΔTm values being lower when the adduct is located at 1 or 2-bp from the end of the 11-bp DNA (-6 to -9°C) then when it is located in its medium part (positions 4 to 8) with up to a -21 to -27°C decrease of Tm. Similarly, the stereoisomeric orientation of the 4-OHEN adduct affects the base-stacking, groove sizes and subsequent distortions and is also crucial for the extent of DNA destabilization (Kolbanovskiy et al., 2005).

2.2.3 Psoralen derivatives

Psoralen is a chemotherapeutic agent known to cause DNA inter-strand crosslinks (ICLs) upon absorption of two photons from UVA irradiation at 365 nm, preferentially at 5'-TA and to a lesser extend at 5'-AT dinucleotides. This activity was the basis for use of psoralen and UVA exposure (PUVA therapy) to treat cutaneous diseases like psoriasis, vitiligo, atopic dermatitis or cutaneous T cell lymphomas. However, such treatment increased the risk of squamous and basal cell carcinomas (Teicher, 1996). Psoralen-induced ICLs are classically used models for DNA repair of ICLs. The psoralen derivative 4'-(hydroxymethyl)-4,5',8-trimethylpsoralen (HMT) (Figure 4) evidenced DNA destabilization by mono-addition of a psoralen residue to both thymines (one on each strand) of 5'-GGGTACCC sequence.

2.2.4 Benzo-acronycine derivatives

Acronycine is a natural alkaloid extracted from the bark of an Australian ash scrub that presented interesting antitumor activities but was poorly soluble and, consequently, too toxic in first clinical trials. The discovery of an unstable acronycine epoxide opened the way to the rational drug design of S23906-1 (Figure 4), that appeared to be a highly active compound (Guilbaud et al., 2001) with an original mode of action (David-Cordonnier 2002; 2005; Depauw et al., 2009) and consequently entered phase I clinical trials in 2006. As for the clinically used drug Ecteinascidine 743 (ET-743, Trabectedin, Yondelis ™ from Pharmamar), S23906-1 alkylates the exocyclic NH_2 group of guanines in the minor groove. But, in contrast with ET-743, S23906-1 does not reinforce the stability of the ds-DNA helix but destabilizes it, generating portions of ss-DNA (David-Cordonnier et al., 2005; Depauw et al., 2009). Various spectral and biochemical approaches convinced with this conclusion. Indeed, classical DNA melting temperature studies evidenced a strong decrease of the Tm values upon alkylation with S23906-1 or other biologically active benzo-acronycine derivatives. Similarly, spectral analysis of the ratio of fluorescence properties of picogreen (a ds- and ss-DNA interacting dye) and BET (a ds-DNA specific dye) evidenced an increase of picogreen *vs.* BET fluorescence which enlightens the generation of single-stranded portions of the DNA upon S23906-1 alkylation. Biochemical approaches like digestion of the alkylated DNA by single-strand specific nuclease S1 and electrophoretic mobility shift assays (EMSAs) confirmed the opening of the DNA. The destabilization was relatively wide since mapping with nuclease S1 evidenced locally opened DNA portions within a 117 bp DNA fragment alkylated by S23906-1 whereas EMSAs, performed with oligonucleotides as long as 24 bp, evidenced fully single-stranded alkylated oligonucleotides in the presence of S23906-1 or derivatives (David-Cordonnier et al., 2005; Depauw et al., 2009).

3. Repair processes for DNA destabilizing lesions

DNA adducts are critical lesions for cell proliferation and survival. Single or multiple DNA repair machineries could be implicated in the removal of these damages, as for example

BER, GG-NER (global genome) or TC-NER (transcription-coupled), MMR, HR or NHEJ. Only few data are published about the consequences of non-covalent DNA destabilizing agents on protein/DNA binding from the repair machineries. These data on BisA function reported that insertion of BisA could flip the mispaired thymine to an extrahelical base subsequently inducing a sterical blockage of DNA glycosylases binding (David, 2003). The present section will therefore focus on alkylating compounds. As examples, we will shortly present the repair processes for the well-studied temolozomide-induced lesions in the major groove and for the DNA stabilizing drug ET-743, as an original minor groove alkylating agents that "poison" the NER machinery to exert its anti-tumor properties, before presenting the current knowledge on DNA repair of DNA destabilizing lesions.

3.1 Repair of temolozomide-induced DNA lesions

Temolozomide (TMZ, Temodar®, Figure 5) is a monofunctional alkylating agent chemically related to dacarbazine. It is active in vitro and in vivo against a wide variety of tumor type and particularly efficient in malignant glioma (Newlands et al., 1997). Contrasting with dacarbazine, TMZ does not require to be activated by enzymatic oxidation, but spontaneously hydrolyses to 5-(3-methyltriazen-l-yl)-imidazole-4-carboximide (MITC) at pH above 7. MITC is then broken down to (*i*) the reactive methyldiazonium cation which next loses the methyl group in the presence of DNA or proteins and (*ii*) the inactive 5-aminoimidazole-4-carboxyamide moiety (AIC) (**1**). TMZ treatment leads to different adducts on the double helix DNA: N^3-methyladenine, N^7-methylguanine and O^6-methylguanine

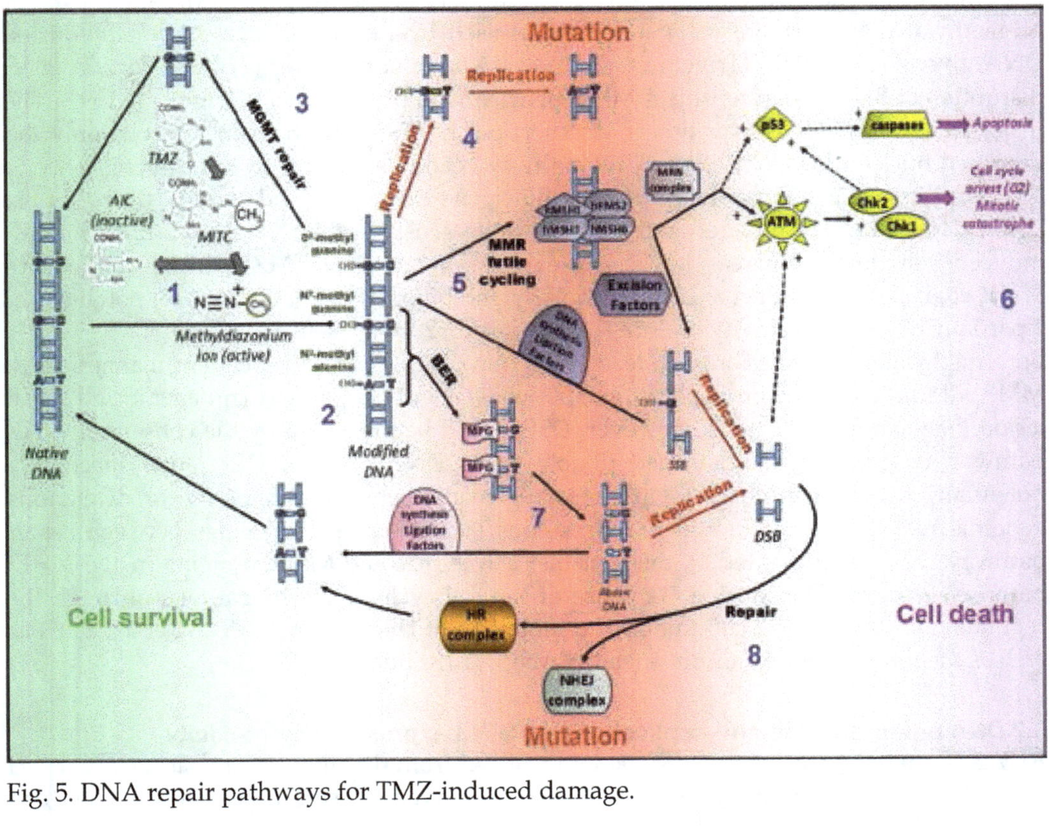

Fig. 5. DNA repair pathways for TMZ-induced damage.

(Newlands et al., 1997) and cell sensitivity to TMZ treatment depends on multiple DNA repair mechanisms (**2**). The major one is the recognition of methyl lesions from O^6 position of guanines by the O^6-methylguanine DNA methyltransferase (MGMT) protein which directly converts the methylated DNA to its normal, undamaged state (**3**). MGMT enzymatic activity is crucial for TMZ resistance in vivo suggesting that MGMT expression may predict the response of patients to TMZ treatment (Everhard et al., 2006; McCormack et al., 2009). However, other repair mechanisms are also implicated since some cell lines with low MGMT expression still evidence significant resistance to TMZ (Fukushima et al., 2009).

When O^6-methyguanine is not repaired by MGMT, it may lead to an O^6-methylguanine:thymine mismatch during DNA replication. The following DNA replication cycle can then pair thymine with adenine in place of the original guanine, thus leading to transition mutations (**4**). However, the cytotoxic property of TMZ is mostly linked to MMR pathway through O^6-methylguanine:thymine mismatch recognition and repair by this system (**5**). MMR is not involved in TMZ chemo-resistance but in TMZ cytotoxicity, associated with cell cycle blockade at G2 checkpoint (Caporali et al., 2004), activation of p53 and ATM, leading to cell death (**6**). The MRN (Mre11/Rad50/Nbs1) complex was evidenced as the earliest sensor of TMZ-induced damage (Mirzoeva et al., 2006). It undergoes a series of conformational changes that activates the protein sensor ATM (ataxia telangiectasia mutated) which, subsequently, activates Chk1 and Chk2 to block cell cycle. TMZ induces p53-mediated apoptosis in MMR-proficient but not in MMR-deficient cells (D'Atri et al., 1998). Thus, deficient MMR is another mechanism for resistance to TMZ (Cahill et al., 2007).

Besides MGMT and MMR, BER is also implicated in TMZ lesion repair. More than 80% of N^7-methylated purines are recognized and excised by the BER enzyme N-methylpurine DNA glycosylase (MPG) (Trivedi et al., 2008; J. Zhang et al., 2010) (**7**). As a consequence, disruption of BER system sensitizes MMR-deficient and proficient cells (Liu et al., 1999). The major MPG-dependent repair occurs via short-patch BER, a mechanism whereby only the damaged nucleotide is excised. So, BER pathway is another contributor of cell resistance to TMZ and its efficacy depends on specific BER gene expression and activity (Fishel et al., 2008). DNApol β or MPG-deficient cells are more sensitive than wild-type cells to TMZ-induced cell death, whereas MPG over-expression increases TMZ-induced cytotoxicity (Tang et al., 2011; Trivedi et al., 2008). Similarly, inhibition of poly(ADP-ribose) polymerase-1 partially restored sensitivity to TMZ (J. Zhang et al., 2010).

Both methylated DNA lesions can lead to SSBs in a DNA repair-dependent manner (BER, MMR). If unrepaired before replication, SSBs convert in DSBs, a more mutagenic and lethal lesion (Newlands et al., 1997). However, DSBs could be processed by the conservative HR pathway to give back undamaged double stand DNA or by NHEJ repair machinery potentially resulting in chromosomal rearrangements between chromatide or deleterious genomic rearrangements as other toxic lesions (**8**). Other inter-crossings between repair pathways are not presented in this scheme: a role of some MMR proteins in the NHEJ pathway to repair DSB during G1 phase of the cell cycle or in HR pathway through the regulation of the early G2 checkpoint and inhibition of DSB repair (Y. Zhang et al., 2009) as well as the implication of Fanconi anemia FANC-D1 (Kondo et al., 2011).

3.2 DNA repair process and implication in ET-743 expressing cytotoxicity

ET-743 is a tetrahydroisoquinoline alkaloid isolated from the tunicate *Ecteinascidia turbinata* which is approved as an orphan drug against advanced soft tissue sarcoma and, in association with doxorubicine, in refractory cisplatin-sensitive ovarian cancers. This DNA minor groove binder (Pommier et al., 1996) bends DNA toward the major groove (Hurley & Zewail-Foote, 2001). ET-743 (Figure 6) is composed of three subunits: A and B are involved in DNA binding at specific sites (David-Cordonnier et al. 2005; García-Nieto et al., 2000; Pommier et al., 1996) and C protrudes out of the double helix thus facilitating the interaction of ET-743 with nuclear proteins such as transcription factors or DNA repair proteins (**1**). The formation of such protein/ET-743-DNA complex prevents the transcription of different genes (Friedman et al., 2002; Jin et al., 2000) and induces a rapid degradation of transcribing RNA polymerase II in TC-NER proficient, but not deficient, cells (Aune et al., 2008).

By contrast with other DNA damaging agents, NER-deficient cell lines are resistant to ET-743, and restoration of NER functions sensitizes cells to the drug. Indeed, the TC-NER complex is trapped during the repair process of ET-743-DNA damage (Damia et al., 2001; Takebayashi et al., 2001) through the formation of a stable XPG/DNA 'cytotoxic complex' (Herrero et al., 2006)(**2**). In a replication-independent manner, the MRN complex is recruited (**3**) and induces DSBs subsequently recognized by DNA-PK from the HR machinery. DNA-PK then phosphorylates H2AX and activates ATM (Damia et al., 2001) and Chk1 to bypass G2/M and S phases checkpoints and promote cell death (Herrero et al., 2006).

Protein recognition of ET-743-DNA adducts also induces the formation of DSBs through replication fork collapse (Soares et al., 2007; Takebayashi et al., 2001)(**4**), as well known for topoisomerase/drug/DNA poisoning complexes. Such DSBs are repaired by HR (acting mainly in G2-M phases) but not by NHEJ (Soares et al., 2007; Tavecchio et al., 2008)(**5**).

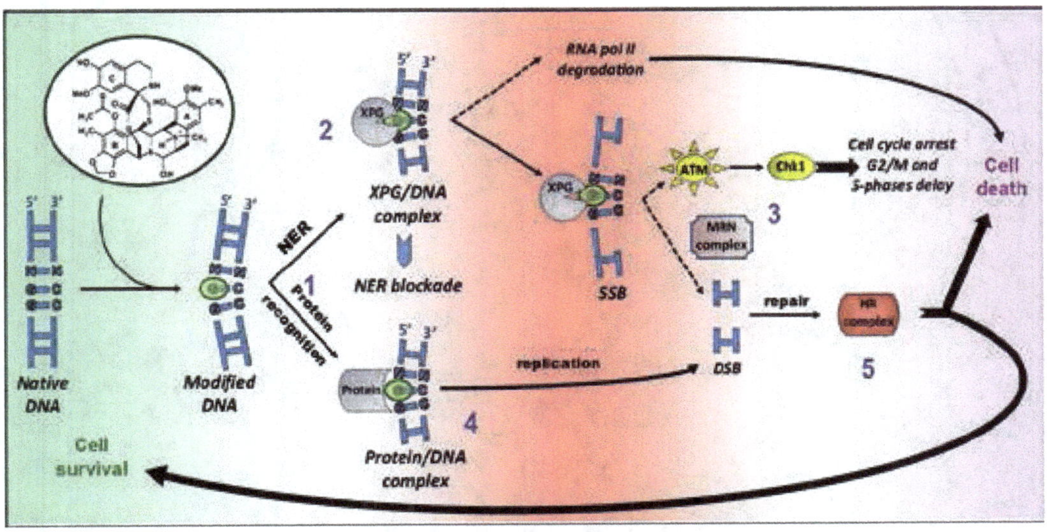

Fig. 6. DNA repair pathways for ET-743-induced DNA damage.

3.3 DNA repair for cisplatin and other transition-metal antitumor agents

Regarding DNA repair, local destabilization of the double helix, base-flipping, DNA bending and poor base-stacking following cisplatin alkylation are determinant for recognition of DNA lesions by repair proteins (C.G. Yang et al., 2009; W. Yang, 2006). Several repair machineries are implicated in metal-drug-induced DNA adduct recognition, removal and cytotoxicity (Basu & Krishnamurthy, 2010; S. Ahmad, 2010). First, NER is an important actor for the removal of both 5′-GG, 5′-AG and 5′-GNG cisplatin intra-strand crosslinks, with a preference for the latter site. The induced-kink, being greater for 5′-GNG than 5′-GG or 5′-AG alkylated sites, seems to be of major relevance for NER recognition (**1**, in Figure 7). Particularly, platinum adducts are recognized by the global genome-NER XPC/hHR23B "sensor complex" (Neher et al., 2010) and XPC expression or polymorphism predicts the response to cisplatin treatment in lung cancers (Lai et al., 2011; L.B. Zhu et al., 2010). Lesions induced by cisplatin, oxaliplatin and JM216 are similarly repaired whereas transplatin-induced lesions, which poorly affect 3D structure of DNA, are poorly repaired by NER.

MMR is also important to remove platinated lesions (**2**). Facilitated by cisplatin-induced kink, MSH2 binding is associated with a 60° angle generated through intercalation of its Phe39 at the lesion site. MSH2/MSH6 complex (Mut-Sα) recognizes cisplatin crosslinks (Castellano-Castillo et al., 2008; Fourrier et al., 2003) but not transplatin mono-adducts from $[Pt(dien)Cl]^{+}$. Translesion bypass is also implicated in cisplatin toxicity. Interestingly, oxaliplatin lesions are more bypassed by DNA polymerases than cisplatin, in relation with their difference in DNA bending/destabilization potencies. Mutants FANC-C and -D of Fanconi anemia pathway also sensitize cells to Pt-drug (Kachnic et al., 2010).

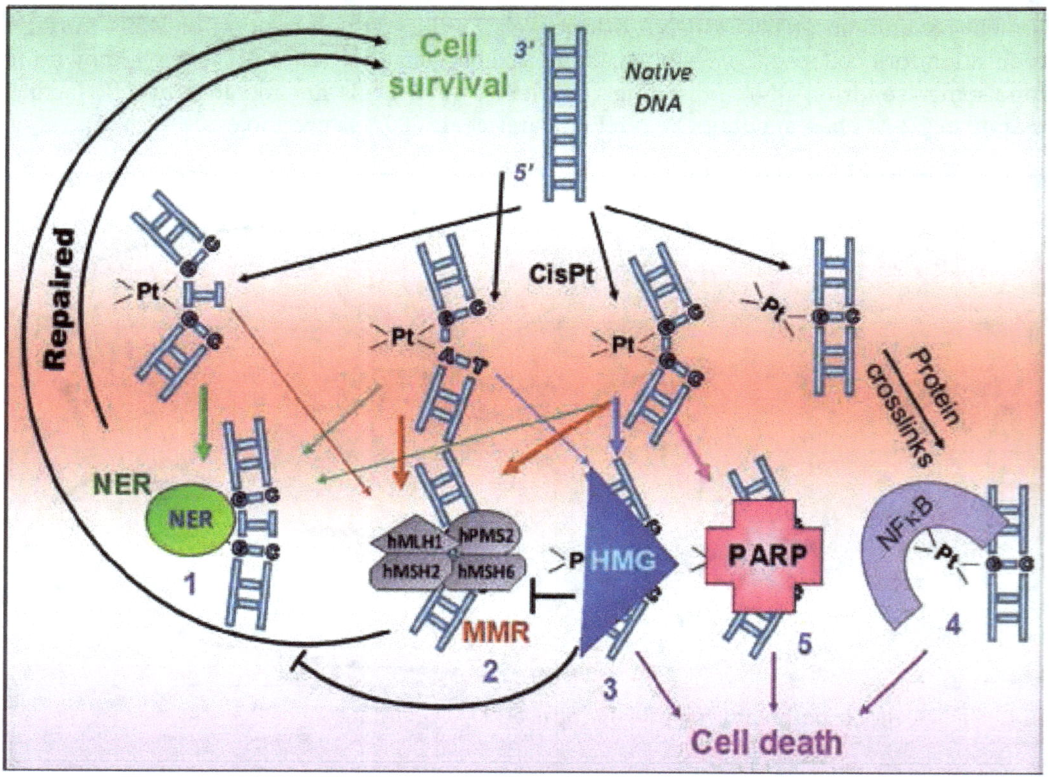

Fig. 7. DNA repair pathways for platinated DNA.

Of major concern, cisplatin adducts are also recognized by HMG proteins (**3**). Similarly to MutS complex recognition, the large induced bend is crucial for this recognition and fits perfectly with the L-shaped structure of HMG DNA binding domain (HMG-box) to reduce the "cost" of DNA bending for HMG-box (Privalov et al., 2009). Insertion of Phe37 between the two platinated guanines in 5′GG dinucleotide stabilizes the binding but is regulated in a redox manner. Indeed, the formation of a disulfure bond between the thiol groups of Cys22 and Cys44 on helix II and III, respectively, of HMG-box infers with the correct planar insertion of Phe37 between the two guanines at crosslink site (Park & Lippard, 2011). Binding of HMG-B1 (and HMG-B2) stabilizes the cisplatin-induced bent and supercoiling of the DNA helix, increases the sensitivity of the cells to cisplatin and shields the platinated adducts from repair by the human DNA excision machinery (J.C. Huang et al., 1994). As a consequence of the degree of kink of the DNA, HMG proteins poorly bind to oxaliplatin adducts which induce relatively small DNA-bending and DNA destabilization (Figure 3), and so poorly protects them from DNA repair (Kasparkova et al., 2008b). This difference correlates with the lower level of DNA lesions in oxaliplatin- versus cisplatin-treated cells. If HMG-B1 and -B2 binding participates in platinated-agent-induced cytotoxicity (Sharma et al., 2009), bent platinated-DNA is also a good substrate for transcription factors from HMG-box family such as SRY, LEF-1 and UBF-1, resulting in the transcriptional changes observed in treated cells (Chvalova et al., 2008; Treiber et al., 1994; Trimmer et al., 1998). For the repair of other platinum derivative-induced DNA damages, JM108 evidenced higher level of protein/DNA cross-links such as DNA-Pt_{II}-NF-κB cross-linked complexes (**4**). Those lesions are less efficiently removed from DNA by the cell repair system (Kostrhunova et al., 2010). Other studies described the binding of PARP-1 protein to cisplatin adduct at 5′-GG and 5′-GNG intra-strand crosslinks on duplex DNA with a preference for 5′-GG platinated site to protect it from DNA repair and thus to increase cytotoxicity (G.Y. Zhu et al., 2010), particularly in MSH3-deficient cells (Takahashi et al., 2011) (**5**). Such side effect of PARP-1 orientates current phase I/II clinical trials using PARP inhibitors (CEP-6800, AZD2281 or ABT-888) as sensitizing agents in combination with cisplatin and carboplatin. A recent paper suggests that PARP is a pharmacological target of platinum- and other metal-based drugs showing PARP inhibition using Pt- (cisplatin), Ru- (RAPTA-T, NAMI-A) or Au- (Auphen, Aubipy) derived drugs (Mendes et al., 2011).

In a general manner, NER process of DNA lesions induced by ruthenium-drug appears to be less efficient than for platinum adducts. Ru-CYM and Ru-THA destabilize the DNA helix via different enthalpic effects and differ in terms of their DNA base-pair intercalation propensities. Comparison of their DNA repair processes has been used as a model for understanding the link between DNA destabilization and repair. Interestingly, Ru-CYM adducts (that destabilize the DNA helix much more than Ru-THA adducts) are excised more efficiently than Ru-THA complex adducts. Such observation is in good agreement with lower binding of RPA helicase to Ru-THA- than to Ru-CYM- adducts (Nováková et al., 2005). Ru-THA is also more cytotoxic than Ru-CYM, suggesting that DNA destabilization plays a major role in the cytotoxicity of these series of compounds.

3.4 DNA repair for the carcinogen BaP (BPDE) and 4-OHEN adducts

In prokaryote, the NER sensor protein UvrB recognizes BPDE/DNA adduct (**1** in Figure 8). Lesion-induced local thermodynamic destabilization and associated nucleotide flipping facilitate this recognition (Jia et al., 2009) with excision efficiencies changing up to a factor of 3 with stereoisomery (i.e. (+) *vs.* (-), *cis- vs. trans*-orientation)(Zou & Van Houten, 1999).

By contrast, the BaP-induced lesions are recognized in eukaryotic higher cells by the NER machinery's "sensor" protein XPC, associated with HR23B to initiate DNA repair (**2**). Weaker recognition by XPC/HR23B complex of the (+)-*trans*-B[*a*]P-N^2-dG adduct, relatively to that of the other conformers, contributes to its higher mutagenic potential (Mocquet et al., 2007). Lesion recognition by XPC requires DNA bending facilitated by local conformational flexibility (Clement et al., 2010) and destabilization of the base-pairing (Brown et al., 2010). Such recognition is driven by Trp690 and Thp733 amino-acids identified as "aromatic sensors" (Maillard et al., 2007). Upon treatment with BaP, human bronchial epithelial 16HBE cells expressed higher levels of the heat shock protein 70 and the NER proteins XPA and XPG, both three proteins co-localizing in the nucleus, suggesting that Hsp70 is also implicated in the DNA repair response to BPDE-DNA adducts (J. Yang et al., 2009). The highly mutagenic (+)-(7R,8S,9S,10R)-7,8-dihydroxy-9,10-epoxy-7,8,9,10-tetrahydro-benzo[*a*]pyrene-DNA lesion leads to different repair processes depending on sequence context, associated with the destabilization potency. Indeed, for an identical BaP-DNA lesion leading to differently orientated bulky lesions, sequence-dependent effect was observed: DNA destabilized at 5′-CG*GC site is more rapidly excised in cell-free human HeLa extracts than DNA bent at 5′-CGG*C site (Rodríguez et al., 2007). As the DNA helix is readily opened upon alkylation, recognition of the lesion by repair protein (including induction of base flipping) is less energetic and, thus, is quicker for DNA already destabilized at 5′-CG*GC site than for duplex DNA bent at 5′-CGG*C site, clearly evidencing the importance of DNA sequence/global structure context for an efficient repair of BPDE-DNA adducts (Yuqin et al., 2009). Moreover, interesting data arise from comparison of the 3D conformation and the NER excision efficiencies for dA adducts formed using the bay region BPDE and the fjord region benzo[*c*]phenanthrene diol epoxide (B[*c*]PhDE) (M. Wu et al., 2002). The bay region of B[*a*]P is more extended, planar and rigid than the B[c]Ph fjord region, being twisted and curved. Consequently, B[*a*]P-dA adducts are associated with greater backbone distortion, unwinding, intercalation potency and

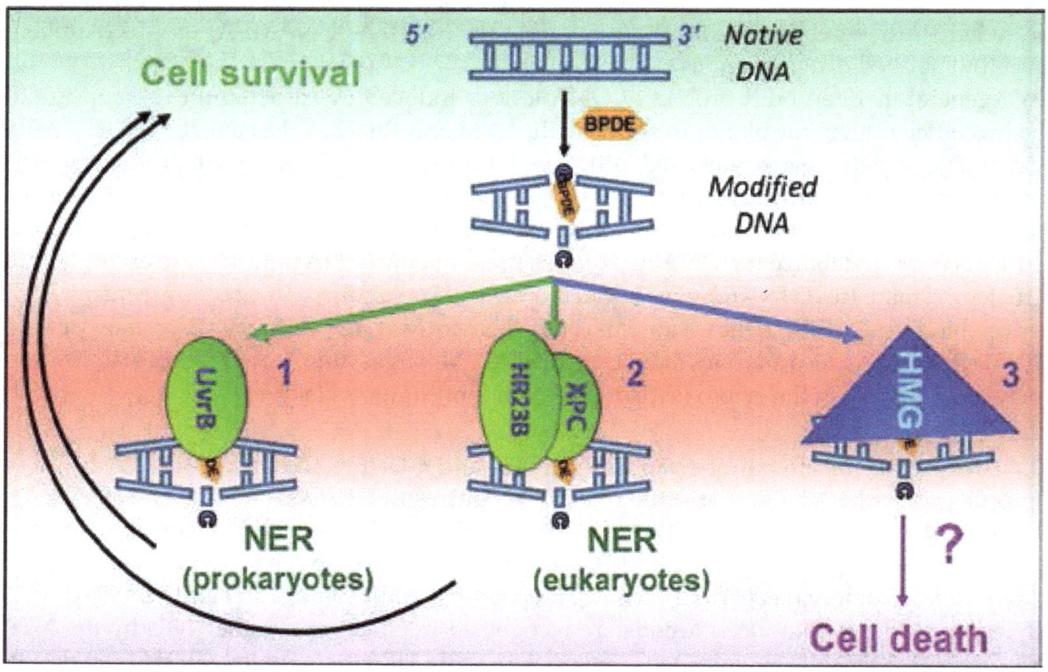

Fig. 8. DNA repair pathways for BPDE-induced DNA damage.

disturbed Watson-Crick hydrogen bonding than B[*c*]Ph-dA adducts, in correlation with stronger excision efficiency by NER machinery. The fjord region B[*c*]Ph-dA adducts being poorly excised lead to more tumorigenic activities. HMG-1 and -2 proteins are also implicated in bulky BPDE-adducts recognition (Lanuszewska & Widlak, 2000) but the consequences on repair or cell death are unknown (**3**). HMG binding might protects adduct recognition by repair proteins as for platinated DNA, but this needs further evaluation.

Excision of bulky 4-OHEN-DNA adducts by NER proteins also depends on both the nature of the alkylated base, its stereo-isomery and the sequence context. For instance, 4-OHEN-dC adducts are more efficiently excised from the DNA than the 4-OHEN-dA adducts (D. Chen et al., 2006). It was reported in male zebrafish that 17a-ethinylestradiol, as a source of 4-OHEN, induces a decrease in NER activity as part of a decrease of the expression level of some NER genes such as XPC, XPA, XPD and XPF, but not of HR23B (Notch et al., 2007).

3.5 DNA repair for psoralen-DNA adducts

DNA alkylation by psoralen can lead to inter-strand crosslinks (ICL) or mono-adducts (MA). Psoralen-ICLs (Figure 9) are eliminated during the replication process, associated with HR (**1**), MMR (**2**) and error-prone translesion DNA polymerases (Dronkert & Kanaar, 2001). NER proteins such as XPC/hHR23B complex and XPA/RPA complexes are also implicated in the repair of psoralen-ICL (Thoma et al., 2005) and could cooperate with MMR to excise the lesions (Zhao et al., 2009). By contrast, thymine-psoralen mono-adducts (**3**) are moderately excised from the DNA by the NER system (Vasquez et al., 2002), because of adduct recognition by HMG-B1 which recruits RPA helicase (**4**) (Lange et al., 2009) or by MMR

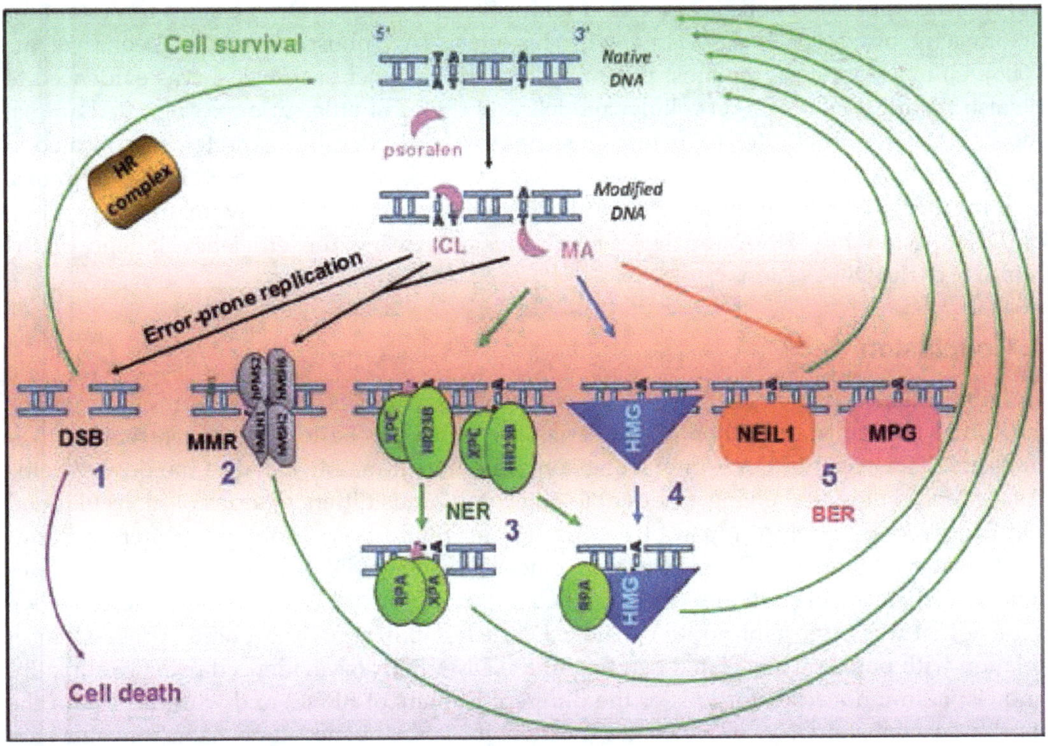

Fig. 9. DNA repair pathways for psoralen-induced DNA damage.

(Q. Wu et al., 2005; 2008). Psoralen monoadducts are good substrates for 3-Methyladenine DNA glycosylase (MPG) (Maor-Shoshani et al., 2008) and the human oxidative DNA glycosylase, NEIL1, which catalyses the β,δ-elimination at AP site, leaving a 3′-P termini at the resulting SSB (**5**) (Couvé-Privat et al., 2007). Fanconi anemia pathway was also implicated in the repair process, in link with NEIL1 stability and NER efficiency (Macé-Aimé et al., 2010).

3.6 DNA repair for benzoacronycine-DNA adducts

S23906-1 alkylates the DNA in the minor groove and induces a strong destabilization of the DNA helix. Two reactive acetate groups are positioned on asymmetric carbons leading to four pure enantiomers: 2 *cis* (1R;2R and 1S;2S) (the *cis*-racemate being S23906-1) and two *trans* (1R;2S and 1S;2R) isomers. Both pure enantiomers react with DNA and destabilize the DNA helix but at different extends. The most potent DNA destabilizing ones (1S;2S and 1S;2R) being those presenting the most active anti-tumour activities in animal models (Depauw et al., 2009). Therefore, the rate of DNA destabilization is different depending on the orientation of the core of the adducts regarding the opened drug/DNA structure, and correlates with different cellular and anti-tumour effects. Such strong destabilisation could affect single-stranded endonuclease and DNA repair activities. There is currently only partial knowledge on the repair of S23906-1 DNA adducts. The NER proteins XPC and CSB are involved in cell sensitivity to S23906-1, associated with both global genome repair and transcription-coupled NER (Rocca et al., 2010). ATR coordination, RPA recognition and Chk1 activation were also implicated in responses to S23906-1 DNA damages (Soares et al., 2011). Process of the lesions is associated with DSB as secondary DNA lesions important for cytotoxicity of S23906-1, associated with histone H2AX phosphorylation (Léonce et al., 2006). Of major interest, the most potent destabilizing isomer of S23906-1 was evidenced to be also the most cytotoxic on cellular models and the most efficient on xenografted animal models (Depauw et al., 2009). Current ongoing research is identifying proteins implicated in S23906-1/DNA adduct recognition and evaluating their impact on S23906-1 cytotoxic activity (personal communication). Locally destabilized DNA could favour the recognition of DNA lesion by "DNA repair sensors" thus increasing the efficiency/kinetic of the removal of the DNA lesion.

4. Conclusion

Destabilization of the DNA helix that is induced by drugs is an important aspect of the antitumor mechanism of action of this series of compounds besides they represent just few droplets in an ocean of DNA-interacting compounds that mainly stabilize the double helix. As evidenced here, stabilizing *vs.* destabilizing compounds differs in terms of molecular and cellular processes: DNA repair, transcription or replication. From the different series (platinum, ruthenium, BPDE, benzoacronycines), the level of DNA destabilization correlates with the efficiency of protein recognition and anti-tumor/cytotoxic activities. Therefore, we believe that it is important not to consider DNA destabilization as a unique process but in relation with potential associated bending of the DNA helix (as evidenced using oxaliplatin- and cisplatin-induced distortions or the different isomers of BPDE) and with the size of the locally destabilized DNA (for instance, portions of DNA opened by benzoacronycines are strongly sensitive to single-strand-specific nucleases). The most recent and ongoing studies on the importance of DNA destabilization on DNA repair processes and induced-cytotoxic activities illustrate the need for an accurate examination of precise mode of binding /bonding to DNA of potential anti-cancer drugs in terms of 3D structure/activity relationships and to clearly evaluate the cellular consequences (cytotoxicity, DNA repair processes).

5. Acknowledgment

We thank the Ligue Nationale Contre le Cancer (Comité du Nord) and the Institut pour la Recherche sur le Cancer de Lille (IRCL) for grants, as well as the Université de Lille 2, the Conseil Régional Nord/Pas-de-Calais and the IRCL for a PhD fellowship to Gaëlle Lenglet.

6. References

Ahmad, R.; Naoui, M.; Neault, J.F.; Diamantoglou, S. & Tajmir-Riahi, H.A. (1996). An FTIR spectroscopic study of calf-thymus DNA complexation with Al(III) and Ga(III) cations. *Journal of Biomolecular Structure & Dynamics*, Vol.13, No.5, (April 1996), pp. 795-802, ISSN 0739-1102

Ahmad, S. (2010). Platinum-DNA interactions and subsequent cellular processes controlling sensitivity to anticancer platinum complexes. *Chemistry & Biodiversity*, Vol.7, No.3, (March 2010), pp. 543-66, ISSN 1612-1880

Arita, K.; Ariyoshi, M.; Tochio, H.; Nakamura, Y. & Shirakawa, M. (2008). Recognition of hemi-methylated DNA by the SRA protein UHRF1 by a base-flipping mechanism. *Nature*, Vol.455, No.7214, (October 2008), pp. 818-21, ISSN 0028-0836

Aune, G.J.; Takagi, K.; Sordet, O.; Guirouilh-Barbat, J.; Antony, S.; Bohr, V.A. & Pommier, Y. (2008). Von Hippel-Lindau-coupled and transcription-coupled nucleotide excision repair-dependent degradation of RNA polymerase II in response to trabectedin. *Clinical Cancer Research*, Vol.14, No.20, (October 2008), pp. 6449-55, ISSN 1078-0432

Basu, A.K.; Hanrahan, C.J.; Malia, S.A.; Kumar, S.; Bizanek, R. & Tomasz, M. (1993). Effect of site-specifically located mitomycin C-DNA monoadducts on in vitro DNA synthesis by DNA polymerases. *Biochemistry*, Vol.32, No.18, (May 1993), pp. 4708-18, ISSN 0006-2960

Basu, A. & Krishnamurthy, S. (2010). Cellular responses to Cisplatin-induced DNA damage. *Journal of Nucleic Acids*, (August 2010), pp. 201367, ISSN 2036-7996

Bellamy, S.R.; Krusong, K. & Baldwin, G.S. (2007). A rapid reaction analysis of uracil DNA glycosylase indicates an active mechanism of base flipping. *Nucleic Acids Research*, Vol.35, No.5, (February 2007), pp. 1478-87, ISSN 0305-1048

Bellon, S.F.; Coleman, J.H. & Lippard, S.J. (1991). DNA unwinding produced by site-specific intrastrand cross-links of the antitumor drug *cis*-diamminedichloroplatinum(II). *Biochemistry*, Vol.30, No.32, (August 1991), pp. 8026-35, ISSN 0006-2960

Benham, C.J. (1996). Duplex destabilization in superhelical DNA is predicted to occur at specific transcriptional regulatory regions. *Journal of Molecular Biology*, Vol.255, No.3, (January 1996), pp. 425-34, ISSN 0022-2836

Bera, A.; Roche, A.C. & Nandi, P.K. (2007). Bending and unwinding of nucleic acid by prion protein. *Biochemistry*, Vol.46, No.5, (February 2007), pp. 1320-8, ISSN 0006-2960

Bergamo, A.; Gava, B.; Alessio, E.; Mestroni, G.; Serli, B.; Cocchietto, M.; Zorzet, S. & Sava, G. (2002). Ruthenium-based NAMI-A type complexes with in vivo selective metastasis reduction and in vitro invasion inhibition unrelated to cell cytotoxicity. *International Journal of Oncology*, Vol.21, No.6, (December 2002), pp. 1331-8, ISSN 1019-6439

Betterton, M.D. & Julicher, F. (2005). Opening of nucleic-acid double strands by helicases: active versus passive opening. *Physical Review E: Statistical, Nonlinear, and Soft Matter Physics*, Vol.71, No.1 Pt 1, (January 2005), pp. 011904, ISSN 1550-2376

Brabec, V.; Reedijk, J. & Leng M. (1992). Sequence-dependent distortions induced in DNA by monofunctional platinum(II) binding. *Biochemistry*, Vol.31, No.49, (December 1992), pp. 12397-402, ISSN 0006-2960

Brown, K.L.; Roginskaya, M.; Zou, Y.; Altamirano, A.; Basu, A.K. & Stone, M.P. (2010). Binding of the human nucleotide excision repair proteins XPA and XPC/HR23B to the 5R-thymine glycol lesion and structure of the *cis-(5R;6S)* thymine glycol epimer in the 5'-GTgG-3' sequence: destabilization of two base pairs at the lesion site. *Nucleic Acids Research*, Vol.38, No.2, (January 2010), pp. 428-40, ISSN 0305-1048

Butler, A.P.; Mardian, J.K. & Olins, D.E. (1985). Nonhistone chromosomal protein HMG 1 interactions with DNA. Fluorescence and thermal denaturation studies. *Journal of Biological Chemistry*, Vol.260, No.19, (September 1985), pp. 10613-20, ISSN 0021-9258

Cahill, D.P.; Levine, K.K.; Betensky, R.A.; Codd, P.J.; Romany, C.A.; Reavie, L.B.; Batchelor, T.T.; Futreal, P.A.; Stratton, M.R.; Curry, W.T.; Iafrate, A.J. & Louis, D.N. (2007). Loss of the mismatch repair protein MSH6 in human glioblastomas is associated with tumor progression during temozolomide treatment. *Clinical cancer research*, Vol.13, No.7, (April 2007), pp 2038-45, ISSN 2038-2045

Cai, Y; Patel, DJ; Broyde, S & Geacintov, NE. (2010). Base sequence context effects on nucleotide excision repair. *Journal of Nucleic Acids*. Pii.174252, (August 2010), ISSN 2036-7996

Cai, Y.; Ding, S.; Geacintov, N.E. & Broyde S. (2011). Intercalative conformations of the *14R* (+)- and *14S* (-)-*trans-anti*-DB[*a*;l]P-N^6-dA adducts: Molecular Modeling and MD Simulations. *Chemical Research in Toxicology*, In press, (February 2011), ISSN 0893-228X

Cao, C.; Jiang, Y.L., Stivers, J.T. & Song, F. (2004). Dynamic opening of DNA during the enzymatic search for a damaged base. *Nature Structural & Molecular Biology*, Vol.11, No.12, (December 2004), pp. 1230–36, ISSN 1545-9993

Caporali, S. ; Falcinelli, S.; Starace, G.; Russo, M.T.; Bonmassar, E.; Jiricny, J. & D'Atri, S. (2004). DNA damage induced by temozolomide signals to both ATM and ATR: role of the mismatch repair system. *Molecular Pharmacology*, Vol.66, (September 2004), pp 478 –91, ISSN 0026-895X

Castellano-Castillo, M.; Kostrhunova, H.; Marini, V.; Kasparkova, J.; Sadler, P.J; Malinge, J.M. & Brabec, V. (2008). Binding of mismatch repair protein MutS to mispaired DNA adducts of intercalating ruthenium(II) arene complexes. *Journal of Biological Inorganic Chemistry*, Vol.13, No.6, (August 2008), pp. 993-9, ISSN 0949-8257

Chen, D.; Kolbanovskiy, A.; Shastry, A.; Ding, S.; Broyde, S.; Bolton, J.L.; Van Houten, B. & Geacintov, N.E. (2006). Nucleotide excision repair of DNA adducts derived from the binding of the equine estrogen metabolite 4-OHEN to dC and dA adducts in vitro. *Proceedings of the 97th Annual Meeting of the American Association for Cancer Research, 2006 Apr 1-5, Washington, DC. Philadelphia (PA): AACR*, Vol.47, Abstract #5255.

Choi, C.H.; Kalosakas, G.; Rasmussen, K.O.; Hiromura, M.; Bishop, A.R. & Usheva, A. (2004). DNA dynamically directs its own transcription initiation. *Nucleic Acids Research*, Vol.32, No.4, (March 2004), pp. 1584-90, ISSN 0305-1048

Chvalova, K.; Sari, M.A. Bombard, S. & Kozelka, J. (2008). LEF-1 recognition of platinated GG sequences within double-stranded DNA. Influence of flanking bases. *Journal of Biological Inorganic Chemistry*, Vol.102, No.2, (February 2008), pp. 242-50, ISSN 0949-8257

Clement, F.C.; Camenisch, U.; Fei, J.; Kaczmarek, N.; Mathieu, N. & Naegeli, H. (2010). Dynamic two-stage mechanism of versatile DNA damage recognition by xeroderma pigmentosum group C protein. *Mutation Research*, Vol.685, No.1-2, (March 2010), pp. 21-8, ISSN 0027-5107

Cosman, M.; De los Santos, C.; Fiala, R.; Hingerty, B.E.; Ibanez, V.; Luna, E.; Harvey, R.; Geacintov, N.E.; Broyde, S. & Patel, D.J. (1993). Solution conformation of the (+)-*cis-anti*-[BP]dG adduct in a DNA duplex: intercalation of the covalently attached benzo[*a*]pyrenyl ring into the helix and displacement of the modified deoxyguanosine. *Biochemistry*, Vol.32, No.16, (April 1993), pp. 4145–55, ISSN 0006-2960

Couvé-Privat, S.; Macé, G.; Rosselli, F & Saparbaev, M.K. (2007). Psoralen-induced DNA adducts are substrates for the base excision repair pathway in human cells. *Nucleic Acids Research*, Vol.35, No. 18, (March 2009), pp. 5672–5682, ISSN 0305-1048

Damia, G.; Silvestri, S.; Carrassa, L.; Filiberti, L.; Faircloth, G.T.; Liberi, G.; Foiani, M. & D'Incalci, M. (2001). Unique pattern of ET-743 activity in different cellular systems with defined deficiencies in DNA-repair pathways. *International Journal of Cancer*, Vol.92, No.4, (May 2001), pp. 583-8, ISSN 1097-0215

Darzynkiewicz, Z.; Evenson, D.; Kapuscinski, J. & Melamed, M.R. (1983). Denaturation of RNA and DNA in situ induced by acridine orange. *Experimental Cell Research*, Vol.148, No.1, (October 1983), pp. 31-46, ISSN 0014-4827

D'Atri, S.; Tentori, L.; Lacal, P.M.; Graziani, G.; Pagani, E.; Benincasa, E.; Zambruno, G.; Bonmassar, E. & Jiricny, J. (1998). Involvement of the mismatch repair system in temozolomide-induced apoptosis. *Molecular Pharmacology*, Vol.54, No.2, (August 1998), pp. 334–341, ISSN 0026-895X

David-Cordonnier, M.-H.; Gajate, C.; Olmea, O.; Laine, W.; de la Iglesia-Vicente, J.; Perez, C.; Cuevas, C.; Otero, G.; Bailly, C. & Mollinedo F. (2005). DNA and non-DNA targets in the mechanism of action of the antitumor drug Yondelis™ (trabectedin, ET-743). *Chemistry and Biology*, Vol.12, No.11, (November 2005), pp. 1201-10, ISSN 1074-5521

David, A.; Bleimling, N.; Beuck, C.; Lehn, J.M.; Weinhold, E.; Teulade-Fichou, M.P. (2003). DNA mismatch-specific base flipping by a bisacridine macrocycle. *Chembiochem*, Vol.4, No.12, (December 2003), pp. 1326-31, ISSN 1439-4227

David-Cordonnier, M.-H.; Laine, W.; Lansiaux, A.; Kouach, M.; Briand, G.; Pierré, A.; Hickman, J.A. & Bailly, C. (2002). Alkylation of guanine in DNA by S23906-1, a novel potent antitumor compound derived from the plant alkaloid acronycine. *Biochemistry*, Vol.41, No. 31, (August 2002), pp. 9911-20, ISSN 0006-2960

David-Cordonnier, M.-H.; Laine, W.; Lansiaux, A.; Rosu, F.; Colson, P.; de Pauw, E.; Michel, S.; Tillequin, F.; Koch, M.; Hickman, J.A.; Pierré, A. & Bailly, C. (2005). Covalent binding of antitumor benzoacronycines to double-stranded DNA induces helix opening and the formation of single-stranded DNA: unique consequences of a novel DNA-bonding mechanism. *Molecular Cancer Therapeutics*, Vol.4, No.1, (January 2005), pp. 71-80, ISSN 1535-7163

David-Cordonnier, M.-H.; Payet, D.; D'Halluin, J.-C.; Waring, M.J.; Travers, A.A. & Bailly, C. (1999). The DNA-binding domain of human c-Abl tyrosine kinase promotes the interaction of a HMG chromosomal protein with DNA. *Nucleic Acids Research*, Vol.27, No.11, (June 1999), pp. 2265-70, ISSN 0305-1048

David-Cordonnier, M.-H.; Hamdane, M.; Bailly, C.; D'Halluin, J.-C. (1998). The DNA binding domain of the human c-Abl tyrosine kinase preferentially binds to DNA sequences containing an AAC-motif and to distorted DNA structures. *Biochemistry*, Vol.37, No.17, (April 1998), pp. 6065-76, ISSN 0006-2960

Depauw, S.; Gaslonde, T.; Léonce, S.; Kraus-Berthier, L.; Laine, W.; Lenglet, G.; Chiaroni, A.; Pfeiffer, B.; Bailly, C.; Michel, S.; Tillequin, F.; Pierré, A. & David-Cordonnier, M.-H. (2009). Influence of the stereoisomeric position of the reactive acetate groups of the benzo[*b*]acronycine derivative S23906-1 on its DNA alkylation, helix opening, cytotoxic and anti-tumor activities. *Molecular Pharmacoly*, Vol.76, No.6, (December 2009), pp. 1172-85, ISSN 0026-895X

Ding, S.; Shapiro, R.; Geacintov, N.E. & Broyde, S. (2005). Equilenin-derived DNA adducts to cytosine in DNA duplexes: structures and thermodynamics. *Biochemistry*, Vol.44, No.44, (November 2005), pp. 14565-76, ISSN 0006-2960

Ding, S.; Shapiro, R.; Geacintov, N.E. & Broyde, S. (2007). 4-hydroxyequilenin-adenine lesions in DNA duplexes: stereochemistry, damage site, and structure. *Biochemistry*, Vol.46, No.1, (January 2007), pp. 182-91, ISSN 0006-2960

Dornberger, U.; Leijon, M. & Fritzsche, H. (1999). High base pair opening rates in tracts of GC base pairs. *Journal of Biological Chemistry*, Vol.274, No.11, (March 1999), pp. 6957-62, ISSN 0021-9258

Dronkert, M.L. & Kanaar, R. (2001). Repair of DNA interstrand cross-links. *Mutation Research*, Vol.486, No.4, (September 2001), pp. 217–47, ISSN 0027-5107

Embrechts, J.; Lemiere, F.; Van Dongen, W.; Esmans, E.L.; Buytaert, P.; Van Marck, E.; Kockx, M. & Makar, A. (2003). Detection of estrogen DNA-adducts in human breast tumor tissue and healthy tissue by combined nano LC-nano ES tandem mass spectrometry. *Journal of the American Society of Mass Spectrometry*, Vol.14, No.5 (May 2003), pp. 482–91, ISSN

Everhard, S.; Kaloshi, G.; Crinière, E.; Benouaich-Amiel, A.; Lejeune, J.; Marie, Y.; Sanson, M.; Kujas, M.; Mokhtari, K.; Hoang-Xuan, K.; Delattre, J.Y. & Thillet, J. (2006). MGMT methylation: a marker of response to temozolomide in low-grade gliomas. *Annals of neurology* , Vol.60, No.6, (December 2006), pp 740-3, ISSN 0364-5134

Fishel, M.L.; He, Y.; Smith, M.L.; Kelley, M.R. (2008). Manipulation of base excision repair to sensitize ovarian cancer cells to alkylating agent temozolomide. *Molecular Pharmacology*, Vol.74, No.1, (July 2008), pp 173-83, ISSN 0026-895X

Fourrier, L.; Brooks, P. & Malinge, J.M. (2003). Binding discrimination of MutS to a set of lesions and compound lesions (base damage and mismatch) reveals its potential role as a cisplatin-damaged DNA sensing protein. *Journal of Biological Chemistry*, Vol.278, No.23, (June 2003), pp. 21267-75, ISSN 1044-0305

Fridman, A.S.; Brabec, V.; Haroutiunian, S.G.; Wartell, R.M. & Lando, D.Y. (2003). Melting of cross-linked DNA v. cross-linking effect caused by local stabilization of the double helix. *Journal of Biomolecular Structure & Dynamics*, Vol.20, No.4, (February 2003), pp. 533-45, ISSN 0739-1102

Friedman, D.; Hu, Z.; Kolb, E.A.; Gorfajn, B. & Scotto, K.W. (2002). Ecteinascidin-743 inhibits activated but not constitutive transcription. *Cancer Research*, Vol.62, No. 12, (June 2002), pp. 3377-81, ISSN 0008-5472

Fukushima, T.; Takeshima, H. & Kataoka, H. (2009). Anti-glioma Therapy with Temozolomide and Status of the DNA-Repair Gene MGMT. *Anticancer Research*, Vol.29, No.11, (November 2009), pp 4845-54, ISSN 0250-7005

García-Nieto, R.; Manzanares, I.; Cuevas, C. & Gago, F. (2000). Increased DNA binding specificity for antitumor ecteinascidin 743 through protein-DNA interactions? *Journal of Medicinal Chemistry*, Vol.43, No.23, (November 2000), pp. 4367-9, ISSN ISSN 0022-2623

Guilbaud, N.; Kraus-Berthier, L.; Meyer-Losic, F.; Malivet, V.; Chacun, C.; Jan, M.; Tillequin, F.; Koch, M.; Pfeiffer, B.; Atassi, G.; Hickman, J. & Pierré, A. (2001). Marked antitumor activity of a new potent acronycine derivative in orthotopic models of human solid tumors. *Clinical Cancer Research*, Vol.7, No.8, (August 2001), pp. 2573-80, ISSN 1078-0432

Hägerlöf, M.; Papsai, P.; Chow, C.S. & Elmroth, S.K. (2006). More pronounced salt dependence and higher reactivity for platination of the hairpin r(CGCGUUGUUCGCG) compared with d(CGCGTTGTTCGCG). *Journal of Biological Inorganic Chemistry*, Vol.11, No.8, (November 2006), pp. 974-90, ISSN 0949-8257

Hartinger, C.G.; Jakupec, M.A.; Zorbas-Seifried, S.; Groessl, M.; Egger, A.; Berger, W.; Zorbas, H.; Dyson, P.J. & Keppler, B.K. (2008). KP1019, a new redox-active anticancer agent--preclinical development and results of a clinical phase I study in tumor patients. *Chemistry and Biodiversity*, Vol.5, No.10, (October 2008), pp. 2140-55, ISSN 1612-1880

Harvey, S.C. (1983). DNA structural dynamics: longitudinal breathing as a possible mechanism for B↔Z transition. *Nucleic Acids Research*, Vol.11, No.14, (July 1983), pp. 4867-78, ISSN 0305-1048

Herrero, A.B.; Martín-Castellanos, C.; Marco, E.; Gago, F. & Moreno, S. (2006). Cross-talk between nucleotide excision and homologous recombination DNA repair pathways in the mechanism of action of antitumor trabectedin. *Cancer Research*, Vol.66, No.16, (August 2006), pp. 8155-62, ISSN 0008-5472

Herrick, G. & Alberts, B. (1976). Nucleic acid helix-coil transitions mediated by helix-unwinding proteins from calf thymus. *Journal of Biological Chemistry*, Vol.251, No.7, (April 1976), pp. 2133-41, ISSN 0021-9258

Hornby, D.P. & Ford, G.C. (1998). Protein-mediated base flipping. *Current Opinion in Biotechnology*, Vol.9, No.4, (August 1998), pp. 354-8, ISSN 0958-1669

Huang, J.C.; Zamble, D.B.; Reardon, J.T.; Lippard, S.J. & Sancar, A. (1994). HMG-domain proteins specifically inhibit the repair of the major DNA adduct of the anticancer drug cisplatin by human excision nuclease. *Proceedings of the National Academy of Sciences USA*, Vol.91, No.22, (October 1994), pp. 10394-8, ISSN 0027-8424

Hurley, L.H. & Zewail-Foote, M. (2001). The antitumor agent ecteinascidin 743: characterization of its covalent DNA adducts and chemical stability. *Advances in Experimental Medicine and Biology*, Vol.500, pp. 289-99, ISSN 0065-2598

Jia, L.; Kropachev, K.; Ding, S.; Van Houten, B.; Geacintov, N.E. & Broyde, S. (2009). Exploring damage recognition models in prokaryotic nucleotide excision repair with a benzo[*a*]pyrene-derived lesion in UvrB. *Biochemistry*, Vol.48, No.38, (September 2009), pp. 8948-57, ISSN 0006-2960

Jin, S.; Gorfajn, B.; Faircloth, G. & Scotto, K.W. (2000). Ecteinascidin 743; a transcription-targeted chemotherapeutic that inhibits MDR1 activation. *Proceedings of the National Academy of Sciences USA*, Vol.97, No.12, (June 2000), pp. 6775-9, ISSN 0027-8424

Kachnic, L.A.; Li. L; Fournier. L & Willers. H. (2010) Fanconi anemia pathway heterogeneity revealed by cisplatin and oxaliplatin treatments. *Cancer Letters*, Vol.292, No.1, (June 2010), pp. 73-9, ISSN 0304-3835

Kapuscinski, J. & Darzynkiewicz, Z. (1983). Increased accessibility of bases in DNA upon binding of acridine orange. *Nucleic Acids Research*, Vol.11, No.21, (November 1983), pp. 7555-68, ISSN 0305-1048

Kapuscinski, J. & Darzynkiewicz, Z. (1984). Denaturation of nucleic acids induced by intercalating agents. Biochemical and biophysical properties of acridine orange-DNA complexes. *Journal of Biomolecular Structure & Dynamics*, Vol.1, No.6, (June 1984), pp. 1485-99, ISSN 0739-1102

Karpel, R.L & Burchard, A.C. (1981). A basic isozyme of yeast glyceraldehyde-3-phosphate dehydrogenase with nucleic acid helix-destabilizing activity. *Biochimica and Biophysica Acta*, Vol.654, No.2, (July 1981), pp. 256-67, ISSN 0006-3002

Kaspárková, J.; Nováková, O.; Vrána, O.; Farrell, N. & Brabec, V. (1999). Effect of geometric isomerism in dinuclear platinum antitumor complexes on DNA interstrand cross-linking. *Biochemistry*, Vol.38, No.34, (August 1999), pp. 10997-1005, ISSN 0006-2960

Kasparkova, J.; Marini, V.; Bursova, V. & Brabec, V. (2008a). Biophysical studies on the stability of DNA intrastrand cross-links of transplatin. *Biophysical Journal*, Vol.95, No.9, (November 2008), pp. 4361-71, ISSN 0006-3495

Kasparkova, J.; Vojtiskova, M.; Natile, G. & Brabec, V. (2008b). Unique properties of DNA interstrand cross-links of antitumor oxaliplatin and the effect of chirality of the carrier ligand. *Chemistry*, Vol.14, No.4, (January 2008), pp. 1330-41, ISSN 1521-3765

Kolbanovskiy, A.; Kuzmin, V.; Shastry, A.; Kolbanovskaya, M.; Chen, D.; Chang, M.; Bolton, J.L. & Geacintov, N.E. (2005). Base selectivity and effects of sequence and DNA secondary structure on the formation of covalent adducts derived from the equine estrogen metabolite 4-hydroxyequilenin. *Chemical Research in Toxicology*, Vol.18, No.11, (November 2005), pp. 1737-47, ISSN 0893-228X

Kondo, N.; Takahashi, A.; Mori, E.; Noda, T.; Zdzienicka, M.Z.; Thompson, L.H.; Helleday, T.; Suzuki, M.; Kinashi, Y.; Masunaga, S.; Ono, K.; Hasegawa, M. & Ohnishi, T. (2011). FANCD1/BRCA2 plays predominant role in the repair of DNA damage induced by ACNU or TMZ. *PLoS One*, Vol.6, No5, (May 2011), e19659, ISSN 1932-6203

Kostrhunova, H.; Vrana, O.; Suchankova, T.; Gibson, D.; Kasparkova, J. & Brabec, V. (2010). Different features of the DNA binding mode of antitumor *cis*-amminedichlorido(cyclohexylamine)platinum(II) (JM118) and cisplatin in vitro. *Chemical Research in Toxicology*, Vol.23, No.11, (November 2010), pp. 1833–42, ISSN 0893-228X

Krueger, A.; Protozanova, E. & Frank-Kamenetskii, M.D. (2006). Sequence-dependent base pair opening in DNA double helix. *Biophysical Journal*, Vol.90, No.9, (May 2006), pp. 3091-9, ISSN 0006-3495

Lai, T.C.; Chow, K.C.; Fang, H.Y.; Cho, H.C.; Chen, C.Y.; Lin, T.Y.; Chiang, I.P. & Ho, S.P. (2011). Expression of xeroderma pigmentosum complementation group C protein predicts cisplatin resistance in lung adenocarcinoma patients. *Oncology Report*, Vol.25, No.5, (May 2011), pp. 1243-51, ISSN 1021-335X

Lange, S.S.; Reddy, M.C. & Vasquez K.M. (2009). Human HMGB1 directly facilitates interactions between nucleotide excision repair proteins on triplex-directed psoralen interstrand crosslinks. *DNA Repair (Amst)*, Vol.8, No.7, (July 2009), pp. 865-72, ISSN 1568-7864

Lanuszewska, J. & Widlak, P. (2000). High mobility group 1 and 2 proteins bind preferentially to DNA that contains bulky adducts induced by benzo[*a*]pyrene diol epoxide and N-acetoxy-acetylaminofluorene. *Cancer Letters*, Vol.158, No.1, (September 2000), pp. 17–25, ISSN 0304-3835

Léonce, S.; Kraus-Berthier, L.; Golsteyn, R.; David-Cordonnier, M.-H.; Tardy, C.; Lansiaux, A.; Poindessous, V.; Larsen, A. K. & Pierré, A. (2006). Generation of replication-dependent double-strand breaks by the novel N^2-G-alkylator S23906-1. *Cancer Research*, Vol.66, No.14, (July 2006), pp. 7203-10, ISSN 0008-5472

Liu, L.; Taverna, P.; Whitacre CM, Chatterjee S. & Gerson S.L. (1999). Pharmacologic disruption of base excision repair sensitizes mismatch repair-deficient and -proficient colon cancer cells to methylating agents. *Clinical Cancer Research*, Vol.5, No.10, (October 1999), pp 2908-17, ISSN 1078-0432

Lum, B. L.; Srinivas, S.; Beck, J. T.; Vesole, D.; Largey, M.; Valone, F. H. & Sayre P. H. (2003). Phase I trial of oral gallium maltolate in refractory malignancies. 2003 ASCO Annual Meeting. *Proceedings - American Society of Clinical Oncology Program*, Vol.22, abstr 943, ISSN 1081-0641

Macé-Aimé, G.; Couvé, S.; Khassenov, B.; Rosselli, F. & Saparbaev, M.K. (2010). The Fanconi anemia pathway promotes DNA glycosylase-dependent excision of interstrand DNA crosslinks. *Environmental and Molecular Mutagenesis*, Vol.15, No.6, (July 2010), pp. 508-19, ISSN 0893-6692

Maillard, O.; Solyom, S. & Naegeli H. (2007). An aromatic sensor with aversion to damaged strands confers versatility to DNA repair. *PLoS Biology*, Vol.5, No.4, (April 2007), e79, ISSN 1544-9173

Malina, J.; Novakova, O.; Vojtiskova, M.; Natile, G. & Brabec, V. (2007). Conformation of DNA GG intrastrand cross-link of antitumor oxaliplatin and its enantiomeric analog. *Biophysical Journal*, Vol.93, No.11, (December 2007), pp. 3950-62, ISSN 0006-3495

Malinge, J.M.; Pérez, C. & Leng, M. (1994). Base sequence-independent distorsions induced by interstrand cross-links in *cis*-diamminedichloroplatinum (II)-modified DNA. *Nucleic Acids Research*, Vol.22, No.19, (September 1994), pp. 3834-9, ISSN 0305-1048

Maor-Shoshani, A.; Meira, L.B.; Yang, X. & Samson, L.D. (2008). 3-Methyladenine DNA glycosylase is important for cellular resistance to psoralen interstrand cross-links. *DNA Repair (Amst)*, Vol.7, No.8, (August 2008), pp. 1399-406, ISSN 1568-7864

McCormack; A.I.; McDonald, K.L.; Gill, A.J.; Clark, S.J.; Burt, M.G.; Campbell, K.A.; Braund, W.J.; Little, N.S.; Cook, R.J.; Grossman, A.B.; Robinson, B.G. & Clifton-Bligh, RJ. (2009). Low O6-methylguanine-DNA methyltransferase (MGMT) expression and response to temozolomide in aggressive pituitary tumours. *Clinical Endocrinology*, Vol.71, No.2, (August 2009), pp 226-33, ISSN 0300-0664

Mendes, F.; Groessl, M.; Nazarov, A.A.; Tsybin, Y.O.; Sava, G.; Santos, I.; Dyson, P.J. & Casini, A. (2011). Metal-Based Inhibition of Poly(ADP-ribose) Polymerase - The Guardian Angel of DNA. *Journal of Medicinal Chemistry*, Vol.54, No.7, (March 2011), pp. 2196–206, ISSN 0022-2623

Mirzoeva O.K.; Kawaguchi, T. & Pieper, R.O. (2006). The Mre11/Rad50/Nbs1 complex interacts with the mismatch repair system and contributes to temozolomide-induced G2 arrest and cytotoxicity. *Molecular Cancer Therapeutics*, Vol.5, No.11, (November 2006), pp. 2757-66, ISSN 1535-7163

Mocquet, V.; Kropachev, K.; Kolbanovskiy, M.; Kolbanovskiy, A.; Tapias, A.; Cai, Y.; Broyde, S.; Geacintov, N.E. & Egly, J.M. (2007). The human DNA repair factor XPC-HR23B distinguishes stereoisomeric benzo[*a*]pyrenyl-DNA lesions. *EMBO Journal*, Vol.26, No.12, (June 2007), pp. 2923-32, ISSN 0261-4189

Moldovan, G.L. & D'Andrea, A.D. (2009). How the fanconi anemia pathway guards the genome. *Annual Review of Genetic*, Vol.43, pp. 223-49, ISSN 0066-4197

Mura, C. & McCammon, J.A. (2008). Molecular dynamics of a kappaB DNA element: base flipping via cross-strand intercalative stacking in a microsecond-scale simulation. *Nucleic Acids Research*, Vol.36, No.15, (September 2008), pp. 4941-55, ISSN 0305-1048

Narayanan, N.; Gorelick, R.J & DeStefano, J.J. (2006). Structure/function mapping of amino acids in the N-terminal zinc finger of the human immunodeficiency virus type 1 nucleocapsid protein: residues responsible for nucleic acid helix destabilizing activity. *Biochemistry*, Vol.45, No.41, (October 2006), pp. 12617-28, ISSN 0006-2960

Neher, T.M.; Rechkunova, N.I.; Lavrik, O.I. & Turchi, J.J. (2010). Photo-cross-linking of XPC-Rad23B to cisplatin-damaged DNA reveals contacts with both strands of the DNA duplex and spans the DNA adduct. *Biochemistry*, Vol.49, No.4, (February 2010), pp. 669-78, ISSN 0006-2960

Newlands, E.S.; Stevens, M.F.G.; Wedge, S.R.; Wheelhouse, R.T. & Brock C. (1997). Temozolomide: a review of its discovery, chemical properties, pre-clinical development and clinical trials. *Cancer Treatment Reviews*, Vol.23, No.1, (January 1997), pp 35–61, ISSN 0305-7372

Notch, E.G. Miniutti, D.M. & Mayer, G.D. (2007). 17alpha-Ethinylestradiol decreases expression of multiple hepatic nucleotide excision repair genes in zebrafish (Danio rerio). *Aquatic Toxicology*, Vol.84, No.3, (October 2007), pp. 301-9, ISSN 0166-445X

Nováková, O.; Kasparkova, J.; Bursova, V.; Hofr, C.; Vojtiskova, M.; Chen, H.; Sadler, P.J. & Brabec, V. (2005). Conformation of DNA modified by monofunctional Ru(II) arene complexes: recognition by DNA binding proteins and repair. Relationship to cytotoxicity. *Chemistry & Biology*, Vol.12, No.1, (January 2005), pp. 121-9, ISSN 1074-5521

Nováková, O.; Nazarov, A.A.; Hartinger, C.G.; Keppler, B.K. & Brabec, V. (2009). DNA interactions of dinuclear RuII arene antitumor complexes in cell-free media. *Biochemical Pharmacology*, Vol.77, No.3, (February 2009), pp. 364-74, ISSN 0006-2952

Nováková, O.; Malina, J.; Suchankova, T.; Kasparkova, J.; Bugarcic, T.; Sadler, P.J. & Brabec, V. (2010). Energetics, conformation, and recognition of DNA duplexes modified by monodentate Ru(II) complexes containing terphenyl arenes. *Chemistry*, Vol.16, No.19, (May 2010), pp. 5744-54, ISSN 1521-3765

Park, S. & Lippard, S.J. (2011). Redox state-dependent interaction of HMGB1 and cisplatin-modified DNA. *Biochemistry*, Vol.50, No.13, (April 2011), pp. 2567-74, ISSN 0006-2960

Pisha, E.; Lui, X.; Constantinou, A. I. & Bolton, J. L. (2001). Evidence that a metabolite of equine estrogens, 4-hydroxyequilenin, induces cellular transformation in vitro. *Chemical Research in Toxicology*, Vol.14, No.1, (January 2001), pp. 82–90, ISSN 0893-228X

Planck, S.R. & Wilson, S.H. (1980). Studies on the structure of mouse helix-destabilizing protein-1. DNA binding and controlled proteolysis with trypsin. *Journal of Biological Chemistry*, Vol.255, No.23, (December 1980), pp. 11547-56, ISSN 0021-9258

Pommier, Y.; Kohlhagen, G.; Bailly, C.; Waring, M.J.; Mazumder, A. & Kohn, K.W. (1996). DNA sequence- and structure-selective alkylation of guanine N^2 in the DNA minor groove by ecteinascidin 743, a potent antitumor compound from the Caribbean tunicate Ecteinascidia turbinata. *Biochemistry*, Vol.35, No.41, (October 1996), pp. 13303-9, ISSN 0006-2960

Privalov, P.L.; Dragan, A.I. & Crane-Robinson, C. (2009). The cost of DNA bending. *Trends in Biochemical Sciences*, Vol.34, No.9, (September 2009), pp. 464-70, ISSN 0968-0004

Putnam, B.F.; Van Zandt, L.L.; Prohofsky, E.W. & Mei, W.N. (1981). Resonant and localized breathing modes in terminal regions of the DNA double helix. *Biophysical Journal*, Vol.35, No.2, (August 1981), pp. 271-87, ISSN 0006-3495

Rocca, C.J.; Poindessous, V.; Soares, D.G.; Ouadrani, K.E.; Sarasin, A.; Guérin, E.; de Gramont, A.; Henriques, J.A.; Escargueil, A.E. & Larsen, A.K. (2010). The NER proteins XPC and CSB, but not ERCC1, regulate the sensitivity to the novel DNA binder S23906: Implications for recognition and repair of antitumor alkylators. *Biochemical Pharmacology*, Vol.80, No.3, (August 2010), pp. 335-43, ISSN 0006-2952

Rodríguez, F.A.; Cai, Y.; Lin, C.; Tang, Y.; Kolbanovskiy, A.; Amin, S.; Patel, D.J.; Broyde, S. & Geacintov, N.E. (2007). Exocyclic amino groups of flanking guanines govern sequence-dependent adduct conformations and local structural distortions for minor groove-aligned benzo[*a*]pyrenyl-guanine lesions in a GG mutation hotspot context. *Nucleic Acids Research*, Vol.35, No.5, (March 2007), pp. 1555-68, ISSN 0305-1048

Rossouw, J.E.; Anderson, G.L.; Prentice, R.L.; LaCroix, A.Z.; Kooperberg, C.; Stefanick, M.L.; Jackson, R.D.; Beresford, S.A.; Howard, B.V.; Johnson, K.C.; Kotchen, J.M. & Ockene, J. (2002). Risks and benefits of estrogen plus progestin in healthy postmenopausal women: principal results From the Women's Health Initiative randomized controlled trial. *Journal of the American Medical Association*, Vol.288, No.3, (July 2002), pp. 321–33, ISSN 0002-9955

Schneider, T.D. (2001). Strong minor groove base conservation in sequence logos implies DNA distortion or base flipping during replication and transcription initiation. *Nucleic Acids Research*, Vol.29, No.23, (December 2001), pp. 4881-91, ISSN 0305-1048

Schwartz, A.; Marrot, L. & Leng, M. (1989). Conformation of DNA modified at a d(GG) or a d(AG) site by the antitumor drug *cis*-diamminedichloroplatinum(II). *Biochemistry*, Vol.28. No.20, (October 1989), pp. 7975-9, ISSN 0006-2960

Sharma, A.; Ramanjaneyulu, A.; Ray, R. & Rajeswari, M.R. (2009). Involvement of high mobility group B proteins in cisplatin-induced cytotoxicity in squamous cell carcinoma of skin. *DNA and Cell Biology*, Vol.28, No.7, (July 2009), pp. 311-8, ISSN 1044-5498

Slama-Schwok, A.; Peronnet, F.; Hantz-Brachete, E.; Taillandier, E.; Teulade-Fichou, M.P.; Vigneron, J.P.; Baudoin, O.; Best-Belpomme, M. & Lehn J.M. (1997). A macrocyclic bis-acridine shifts the equilibrium from duplexes towards DNA hairpins. *Nucleic Acids Research*, Vol.25, No.13, (July 1997), pp. 2574-81, ISSN 0305-1048

Soares, D.G.; Battistella, A.; Rocca, C.J.; Matuo, R.; Henriques, J.A.; Larsen, A.K. & Escargueil, A.E. (2011). Ataxia telangiectasia mutated- and Rad3-related kinase drives both the early and the late DNA-damage response to the monofunctional antitumour alkylator S23906. *Biochemical Journal*, Vol.47, No.1, (July 2011), pp. 63-73, ISSN 0264-6021

Soares, D.G.; Escargueil, A.E.; Poindessous, V.; Sarasin, A.; de Gramont, A.; Bonatto, D.; Henriques, J.A. & Larsen A.K. (2007). Replication and homologous recombination repair regulate DNA double-strand break formation by the antitumor alkylator ecteinascidin 743. *Proceedings of the National Academy of Sciences USA*, Vol.104, No32, (August 2007), pp. 13062-7; ISSN 0027-8424

Sundheim, O.; Talstad, V.A.; Vågbø, C.B.; Slupphaug, G. & Krokan, H.E. (2008). AlkB demethylases flip out in different ways. *DNA Repair (Amst)*, Vol.7, No. 11, (November 2008), pp. 1916-23, ISSN 1568-7864

Takahashi, M.; Koi, M.; Balaguer, F.; Boland, C.R. & Goel, A. (2011). MSH3 mediates sensitization of colorectal cancer cells to cisplatin, oxaliplatin and a poly(ADP-ribose) polymerase inhibitor. *Journal of Biological Chemistry*, Vol.286, No.14, (April 2011), pp. 12157-65, ISSN 0021-9258

Takebayashi, Y.; Pourquier, P.; Zimonjic, D.B.; Nakayama, K.; Emmert, S.; Ueda, T.; Urasaki, Y.; Kanzaki, A.; Akiyama, S.I.; Popescu, N.; Kraemer, K.H. & Pommier, Y. (2001). Antiproliferative activity of ecteinascidin 743 is dependent upon transcription-coupled nucleotide-excision repair. *Nature Medicine*, Vol.7,No.8, (August 2001), pp. 961-6, ISSN 1078-8956

Tang, J.B.; Svilar, D.; Trivedi, R.N.; Wang, X.H.; Goellner, E.M.; Moore, B.; Hamilton, R.L.; Banze, L.A.; Brown, A.R. & Sobol, R.W. (2011). N-methylpurine DNA glycosylase and DNA polymerase {beta} modulate BER inhibitor potentiation of glioma cells to temozolomide, *Neuro-Oncology*, (April 2011), online, ISSN 1522-8517

Tavecchio, M.; Simone, M.; Erba, E.; Chiolo, I.; Liberi, G.; Foiani, M.; D'Incalci, M. & Damia, G. (2008). Role of homologous recombination in trabectedin-induced DNA damage. *European Journal of Cancer*, Vol.44, No4, (March 2008), pp. 609-18, ISSN 1359-6349

Teicher, BA. (1996). Cancer therapeutics: Experimental and clinical agents. *Cancer Drug Discovery and Development*, Beverly A. Teicher Editor.

Teulade-Fichou, M.P; Vigneron, J.P & Lehn, J.M. (1995). Molecular recognition of nucleosides and nucleotides by a water soluble cyclo-bis-intercaland type receptor molecule based on acridine subunits. *Supramolecular Chemistry*, Vol.5, No.2, (February 1995), pp. 139-47, ISSN 1061-0278

Thoma, B.S.; Wakasugi, M.; Christensen, J.; Reddy, M.C. & Vasquez, K.M. (2005). Human XPC-hHR23B interacts with XPA-RPA in the recognition of triplex-directed psoralen DNA interstrand crosslinks. *Nucleic Acids Research*, Vol.33, No.9, (May 2005), pp. 2993-3001, ISSN 0305-1048

Todd, R.C. & Lippard S.J. (2010). Structure of duplex DNA containing the cisplatin 1,2-{$Pt(NH_3)_2$}$_2$+-d(GpG) cross-link at 1.77 A resolution. *Journal of Inorganic Biochemistry*, Vol.104, No.9, (September 2010), pp. 902-8, ISSN 0162-0134

Treiber, D.K; Zhai, X.; Jantzen, H.M. & Essigmann, J.M. (1994). Cisplatin-DNA adducts are molecular decoys for the ribosomal RNA transcription factor hUBF (human upstream binding factor). *Proceedings of the National Academy of Sciences USA*, Vol.91, No.12, (June 1994), pp. 5672-6, ISSN 0027-8424

Triantafillidi, K.; Karidi, K.; Novakova., O; Malina, J. & Garoufis, A. (2011). DNA binding selectivity of oligopyridine-ruthenium(II)-lysine conjugate. *Dalton Transactions*, Vol.40, No.2, (January 2011), pp. 472-83, ISSN 0022-4944

Trimmer, E.E.; Zamble, D.B.; Lippard, S.J. & Essigmann, J.M. (1998). Human testis-determining factor SRY binds to the major DNA adduct of cisplatin and a putative target sequence with comparable affinities. *Biochemistry*, Vol.37, No.1, (January 1998), pp. 352-362, ISSN 0006-2960

Trivedi, R.N.; Wang X.; Jelezcova, E.; Goellner, E.M.; Tang, J. & Sobol R.W. (2008). Human methyl purine DNA glycosylase and DNA polymerase β expression collectively predict sensitivity to Temozolomide. *Molecular Pharmacology*, Vol.74, No.2, (August 2008), pp 505–516, ISSN 0026-895X

Tubbs, J.L.; Pegg, A.E. & Tainer, J.A. (2007). DNA binding, nucleotide flipping, and the helix-turn-helix motif in base repair by O6-alkylguanine-DNA alkyltransferase and its implications for cancer chemotherapy. *DNA Repair (Amst)*, Vol.6, No8, (August 2007), pp. 1100-15, ISSN 1568-7864

Vasquez, K.M.; Christensen, J.; Li, L.; Finch, R.A. & Glazer, P.M. (2002). Human XPA and RPA DNA repair proteins participate in specific recognition of triplex-induced helical distortions. *Proceedings of the National Academy of Sciences USA*, Vol.99, No.9, (April 2002), pp. 5848–53, ISSN 0027-8424

Wold, M.S. (1997). Replication protein A: a heterotrimeric, single-stranded DNA-binding protein required for eukaryotic DNA metabolism. *Annual Review of Biochemistry*, Vol.66, (July 1997), pp. 61-92, ISSN 1545-4509

Wu, M.; Yan, S.; Patel, D.J.; Geacintov, N.E. & Broyde, S. (2002). Relating repair susceptibility of carcinogen-damaged DNA with structural distortion and thermodynamic stability. *Nucleic Acids Research*, Vol.30, No.15, (August 2002), pp. 3422-32, ISSN 0305-1048

Wu, Q.; Christensen, L.A.; Legerski, R.J. & Vasquez, K.M. (2005). Mismatch repair participates in error-free processing of DNA interstrand crosslinks in human cells. EMBO Reports, Vol.6, No.6, (June 2005), pp. 551–7, ISSN 1469-221X.

Wu, Q & Vasquez, K.M. (2008). Human MLH1 protein participates in genomic damage checkpoint signaling in response to DNA interstrand crosslinks, while MSH2 functions in DNA repair. PLoS Genetics, Vol.4, No.9 (September 2008), e1000189, ISSN 1553-7390

Yang, C.G.; Garcia, K. & He, C. (2009). Damage detection and base flipping in direct DNA alkylation repair. *Chembiochem*, Vol.10, No.3, (February 2009), pp. 417-423, ISSN 1439-4227

Yang, J.; Liu, X.; Niu, P.; Zou, Y. & Duan, Y. (2009). Correlations and co-localizations of Hsp70 with XPA, XPG in human bronchial epithelia cells exposed to benzo[*a*]pyrene. *Toxicology*, Vol. 265, No.1-2, (November 2009), pp. 10-4, ISSN 0300-483X

Yang, W. (2006). Poor base stacking at DNA lesions may initiate recognition by many repair proteins. *DNA Repair (Amst)*, Vol.5, No6, (June 2006), pp. 654-66, ISSN 1568-7864

Yuqin, C.; Dinshaw, J.P.; Nicholas, E.G. & Suse, B. (2009). Differential nucleotide excision repair susceptibility of bulky DNA adducts in different sequence contexts: Hierarchies of recognition signals. *Journal of Molecular Biology*, Vol.385, No.1, (January 2009), pp. 30-44, ISSN 0022-2836

Zhang, C.X. & Lippard, S.J. (2003). New metal complexes as potential therapeutics. *Current Opinion in Chemical Biology*, Vol.7, No.4, (August 2003), pp. 481-9, ISSN 1367-5931

Zhang, J.; Stevens, M.F.; Laughton, C.A.; Madhusudan, S. & Bradshaw, T.D. (2010). Acquired resistance to temozolomide in glioma cell lines: molecular mechanisms and potential translational applications. *Oncology*. Vol.78, No.2, (March 2010), pp 103-14, ISSN 0030-2414

Zhang, Y.; Rohde, L.H. & Wu, H. (2009). Involvement of nucleotide excision and mismatch repair mechanisms in double strand break repair. *Current Genomics*, Vol.10, No.4, (June 2009), pp 250–8, ISSN 1389-2029

Zhao, J.; Jain, A.; Iyer, R.R.; Modrich, P.L. & Vasquez, K.M. (2009). Mismatch repair and nucleotide excision repair proteins cooperate in the recognition of DNA interstrand crosslinks. *Nucleic Acids Research*, Vol.37, No.13, (July 2009), pp. 4420-9, ISSN 0305-1048

Zheng, H.; Cai, Y.; Ding, S.; Tang, Y.; Kropachev, K.; Zhou, Y.; Wang, L.; Wang, S.; Geacintov, N.E.; Zhang, Y. & Broyde, S. (2010). Base flipping free energy profiles for damaged and undamaged DNA. *Chemical Research in Toxicology*, Vol.23, No.12, (November 2010), pp. 1868–70, ISSN 0893-228X

Zhu, G.Y.; Chang, P. & Lippard, S.J. (2010). Recognition of Pplatinum- DNA damage by poly(ADP-ribose) polymerase-1. *Biochemistry*, Vol.49, No12, (November 2010), pp. 6177–83, ISSN 0006-2960

Zhu, L.B.; Xu, Q.; Hong, C.Y.; Yue, Z.; Zhang, Y.; Ye, H.N. & Yuan, Y. (2010). XPC gene intron 11 C/A polymorphism is a predictive biomarker for the sensitivity to NP chemotherapy in patients with non-small cell lung cancer. *Anticancer Drugs*, Vol.21, No.7, (August 2010), pp. 669-73, ISSN 0959-4973

Zou, Y. & Van Houten, B. (1999). Strand opening by the UvrA(2)B complex allows dynamic recognition of DNA damage. *EMBO Journal*, Vol.18, No.17, (September 1999), pp. 4889–901, ISSN 0261-4189

Zunino, F.; Gambetta, R.; Di Marco, A. & Zaccara, A. (1972). Interaction of daunomycin and its derivatives with DNA. *Biochimica and Biophysica Acta*, Vol.277, No.3, (September 1972), pp. 489-98, ISSN 0006-3002

10

Effect of Oxidative Stress on DNA Repairing Genes

Bedia Cakmakoglu, Zeynep Birsu Cincin and Makbule Aydin
Istanbul University, Institute for Experimental Medicine Research, Turkey

1. Introduction

Oxidative DNA damage has been thought to contribute to the general decline in cellular functions that are associated with a variety of diseases including Alzheimer disease, amyotrophic lateral sclerosis (ALS), Parkinson's disease, atherosclerosis, ischemia/reperfusion neuronal injuries, degenerative disease of the human temporomandibular-joint, cataract formation, macular degeneration, degenerative retinal damage, rheumatoid arthritis , multiple sclerosis , muscular dystrophy, diabetes mellitus, human cancers as well as the aging process itself. Oxidative stress occurs when the production of the reactive oxygen species (ROS) exceeds natural antioxidant defence mechanisms. There are several sources that form the ROS. Most of ROS come from the endogenous sources as by-products of normal and essential metabolic reactions, such as energy generation from mitochondria or the detoxification reactions involving the liver cytochrome *P-450* enzyme system. There are also exogenous ROS sources including exposure to cigarette smoke, environmental pollutants such as emission from automobiles and industries, consumption of alcohol in excess, asbestos, exposure to ionizing radiation, and bacterial, fungal or viral infections. ROS cause damage to biomolecules such as lipid, proteins and DNA by attaching. ROS may directly attack DNA, either the sugar, phosphate or purine and pyrimidine bases. On the other hand, oxidative damage may be indirect by rising of intracellular Ca^{+2} ions. Free radical-mediated reactions can cause structural alterations in DNA (e.g., nicking, base-pair mutations, rearrangement, deletions insertions and sequence amplification). Degradation of the bases will produce numerous products, including 8-OH-Gua, hydroxymethylurea, urea, thymine glycol; thymine and adenine ring opened and saturated products. Most oxidized bases in DNA are repaired by base excision repair (BER). BER consists of four main steps. The first step involves the removal of the oxidised base by a specific DNA glycosylase, yielding an apurinic/apyrimidinic (AP) site. In the second step, an AP endonuclease removes the deoxyribose phosphate group from the AP site generating a single nucleotide gap. A DNA polymerase, thought to be predominantly DNA polymerase b, fills this gap. Finally, a DNA ligase, probably DNA ligase III, seals the stand break and completes the repair process.

This chapter mainly deals with: (i) formation of ROS in physiological and pathological conditions, (ii) ROS-mediated DNA damage, leading to cellular pathology and ultimately to cell death (iii) Oxidative DNA damage repair systems, (iv) The molecular mechanism of ROS-mediated diseases such as cancer, cardiovascular disease, neurodegenerative diseases, inflammatory disease, ischemia-reperfusion injury and aging.

If the mechanisms of oxidative DNA damage and DNA repairing system are well understood, the diseases resulting from oxidative DNA damage or inefficient DNA repairing could be treated in future and a better understanding of these mechanisms would also allow biomarkers of DNA damage to become potentially useful clinical tools.

2. Formation of reactive oxygen species

Oxygen (O_2) is an element obligatory for life and living systems have evolved to survive in the presence of molecular O_2. Oxidative properties of O_2 play a vital role in diverse biological phenomena. O_2 has double-edged properties, being essential for life; it can also aggravate the damage within the cell by oxidative events. This situation is referred to as the "Oxygen Paradox" [Sen et al., 2010; Khanna & Shiloh, 2009].

Aerobic organisms are constantly subjected to a variety of reactive entities derived from molecular O_2, often collectively referred to as reactive oxygen species (ROS). Some ROS contain unpaired electrons and are therefore referred to as free radicals. A radical is an atom or group of atoms that have one or more unpaired electrons. Radicals can have positive, negative or neutral charge. A prominent feature of radicals is that they have extremely high chemical reactivity, which explains not only their normal biological activities, but also how they inflict damage on cells. There are many types of radicals, but in biological systems most significant are those derived from O_2 [Khanna & Shiloh, 2009, Colton & Gilbert, 1999]. The radicals derived from the reduction of molecular oxygen: superoxide/hydroperoxyl radicals hydrogen peroxide and the hydroxyl radical ($^{\bullet}OH$) the species derived from the reaction of carbon-centered radicals with molecular oxygen: peroxyl radicals alkoxyl radicals and organic hydroperoxides (ROOH); and other oxidants resulting in free radical formation such as hypochlorous acid (HOC1), peroxynitrite and singlet O_2 [Khanna & Shiloh, 2009, Colton & Gilbert, 1999].

The **diatomic oxygen** molecule qualifies as a radical, because it possesses two unpaired electrons, each located at a different orbital. Since both electrons have the same quantum spin number, O_2 itself has relatively low reactivity. Another radical derived from O_2 is singlet oxygen, $^1O_2$. This is an excited form of O_2 in which one of the electrons jumps to a superior orbital following absorption of energy. For O_2 to oxidize a molecule directly, it would have to accept a pair of electrons with a spin opposite to that of the O_2. In biological systems, O_2 can accept an electron and form one of the following species: superoxide anion ($^{\bullet}O_2^-$), $^{\bullet}OH$, or hydrogen peroxide (H_2O_2). These molecules possess various degrees of reactivity with nonradical compounds [Colton & Gilbert, 1999, Kohen & Nyska, 2002].

The mitochondrial respiratory chain is the major source of $^{\bullet}O_2^-$, [Colton & Gilbert, 1999, Kohen & Nyska, 2002, Bielski & Cabelli, 1995, Halliwell & Gutteridge, 1999, Schafer & Buettner, 2001, Forman & Boveris, 1982]. $^{\bullet}O_2^-$ is abundant and can reach an intracellular concentration of about 10^{-11} M [Halliwell & Gutteridge, 1999, Schafer & Buettner, 2001, Forman & Boveris, 1982, Babior, 2000, Nohl & Hegner, 1978]. $^{\bullet}O_2^-$ is not highly reactive for biological molecules however once formed it quickly undergoes dismutation to generate hydrogen peroxide, which is highly reactive. This reaction is markedly accelerated by a family of enzymes, the superoxide dismutases (SODs). $^{\bullet}O_2^-$ can react with H+ to form $HO_2^{\bullet}$ (hydroperoxy radical) which is much more reactive than $^{\bullet}O_2^-$. NADPH oxidase, primarily located in phagocytes, neutrophils and monocytes, can generate $^{\bullet}O_2^-$ and other reactive oxidants that are used for fighting invading microorganisms [Sohal, 1997].

The $^{\bullet}$**OH** is an extremely reactive oxidant [Halliwell & Gutteridge, 1999, Khanna & Shiloh, 2009]. It is also a short-lived molecule with an estimated half-life of nanoseconds at 37°C, traveling only a few Ångstroms. Despite its short life span, $^{\bullet}$OH is capable of inducing considerable damage to nuclear and mitochondrial DNA. This radical alone can cause over 100 types DNA modifications [Khanna & Shiloh, 2009, Michalik et al., 1995]. In addition, $^{\bullet}$OH can lead to lipid peroxidation and oxidation of amino acids, sugars, and metals. The $^{\bullet}$OH is a major product of irradiation due to radiation-induced dissociation of water molecules.

Although $\mathbf{H_2O_2}$ itself is not a radical, it is included in ROS due to producing highly reactive free radical, $^{\bullet}$OH. H_2O_2 is one of the most stable ROS and acts as a messenger in cellular signaling pathways [Khanna & Shiloh, 2009, Kamata & Hirata, 1999]. There are some enzymes that can produce H_2O_2 directly or indirectly, including SOD, monoamine oxidase (MAO), diamine and polyamine oxidase, and glycolate oxidase. Under normal conditions, H_2O_2 is not toxic up to a cellular concentration of about 10^{-8} M [Imlay et al., 1988] H_2O_2 molecules are freely dissolved in aqueous solution and can easily penetrate biological membranes. Their deleterious chemical effects can be divided into the categories of direct activity, originating from their oxidizing properties, and indirect activity in which they serve as a source for more deleterious species, such as OH· or HClO. In the presence of transition metals such as Fe^{2+} or Cu^{+}, H_2O_2 it can be converted to highly reactive $^{\bullet}$OH, either by Fenton or Harber- Weiss reactions [Yamasaki & Piette, 1991, Halliwell & Gutteridge, 1999, Khanna & Shiloh, 2009]. H_2O_2 is detoxified by a set of enzymes that includes the selenium-dependent glutathione peroxidase (GPx) and catalase.

The nitric oxide (NO), or nitrogen monoxide, which is a radical (NO$^{\bullet}$), is produced by the oxidation of one of the terminal guanido nitrogen atoms of L-arginine. In this reaction, L-arginine is converted to NO and L-citrulline by nitric oxide synthase (NOS) which has three isoforms: neuronal NOS, endothelial NOS (eNOS), and inducible NOS (iNOS). NO is quite stable and benign for a free radical, with a lifetime of several seconds. Under normal conditions, NO has many physiological functions such as a neuronal messenger and modulator of smooth muscle contraction. NO can interact with $^{\bullet}O_2-$ to form the peroxynitrite anion (ONOO−) that induces a cascade of events that can eventually lead to cell death [Radi et al., 1991a]. This molecule accounts for much of the NO toxicity. The reactivity of ONOO− is roughly the same as that of $^{\bullet}$OH and N $O_2^{\bullet}$. Its toxicity is derived from its ability to directly nitrate and hydroxylate the aromatic rings of amino acid residues [Schafer & Buettner, 2001] and to react with sulfahydryls [Beckman et al., 1992], lipids [Radi, 1991b], proteins [Moreno & Pryor, 1992] and DNA [King et al., 1992]. Under physiological conditions, ONOOH can react with other components present in high concentrations, such as H_2O_2 or CO_2, to form an adduct that might be responsible for many of the deleterious effects seen in biological sites. Peroxynitrite anion can also affect cellular energy status by inactivating key mitochondrial enzymes [Radi et. Al, 1994], and it may trigger calcium release from the mitochondria [Packer & Murphy, 1994].

3. Classification of reactive oxygen species

ROS generated in response to both endogenous and exogenous stimuli can be divided into Endogenous ROS and exogenous ROS. (Figure 1) [Ziech et al., 2010, Fukai & Nakamura, 2008, Klaunig & Kamendulis, 2004, Galaris et al., 2008].

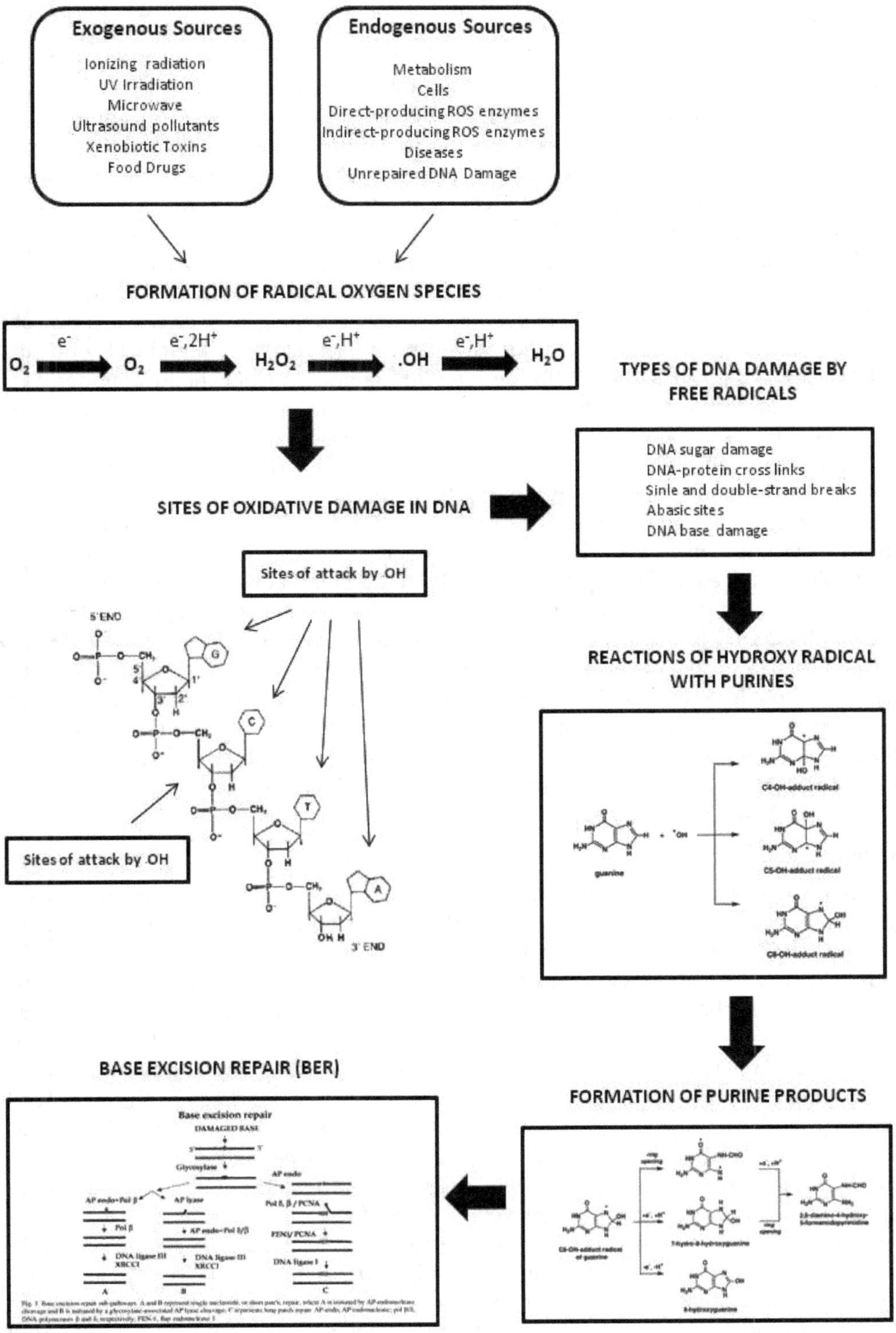

Fig. 1. Oxidative damage and repair of DNA.

Endogenous ROS

In eukaryotic cells, aerobic respiration in the mitochondria is the main source for the generation of ROS. ROS are also produced by peroxisomal oxidation of fatty acids, microsomal cytochrome P450 metabolism of xenobiotic compounds, stimulation of phagocytosis by pathogens or lipopolysaccharides, arginine metabolism and tissue specific enzymes [Adly, 2010]. Enzymes in the cytosol, such as oxygenases, peroxidases and oxidases, generate small amounts of ROS. It is estimated that more than 95% of $^{\bullet}O_2^-$ produced during normal metabolism are generated as a by-product from the electron transfer reactions at the inner mitochondrial membrane. Approximately 1-2% of the O_2 consumed by mitochondria is converted into $^{\bullet}O_2^-$ [Cadenas & Davies, 2000, Hashiguchi et al., 2004].Because of such a highly oxidative environment, mitochondria are also one of the main cellular targets of ROS induced damage, and in fact relatively high levels of oxidized proteins, lipids and nucleic acids are detected in mammalian mitochondria under normal metabolic conditions [Hashiguchi et al., 2004, Raha & Robinson, 2000].

Another significant endogenous source of ROS production is via the reduction of molecular O_2 by inflammatory cells [Klaunig & Kamendulis, 2004, Ziech et al., 2010, Fukai & Nakamura, 2008]. In this reaction, phagocytes produce $^{\bullet}O_2^-$ via oxygen's monovalent reduction. In order to counterbalance ROS-mediated injury, endogenous antioxidant defense systems exist and function by quenching and clearing intracellular ROS activity and accumulation and maintaining redox equilibrium [Ziech et al., 2010, Dizdaroğlu et al., 1993]. Generated chronic oxidative stress damage to cellular macromolecules like DNA, lipids and proteins [Klaunig & Kamendulis, 2004, Ziech et al., 2010]. The endogenous enzymatic antioxidant defenses (SOD, GPx and catalase) can counterbalance oxidative microenvironments by chelating superoxide and various other peroxides. Also, the non-enzymatic endogenous antioxidants (Vitamins E and C, coenzyme Q, B-carotene and glutathione) have the ability to eliminate ROS activity. Thus, ROS can be considered as critical determinants of intracellular redox states and thus serve as important cellular regulatory mechanism(s) in both health and disease [Klaunig & Kamendulis, 2004, Ziech et al., 2010].

Exogenous ROS

Environmental agents like radiation, xenobiotics and chlorinated compounds are significant inducers of cellular damage via ROS mediated toxicity [Galaris et al., 2008]. In addition, anticancer drugs, anesthetics, analgesics, trauma; radiation; electromagnetic fields; alcohol; cigarette smoke; medications; stress; allergens; cold, excessive exercise; dietary factors such as excess sugar, saturated fat and fried oils; malnutrition and various disease states have been considered as most established environmental sources of ROS [Cadenas & Davies, 2000]. Furthermore, exposure to ionizing and ultraviolet radiations also induces ROS-mediated alterations in major pathways associated with the control of cellular growth and survival. For instance, ultraviolet B rays can damage DNA directly and also increase ROS concentrations in epidermal cells [Mena et al., 2009]. In addition, urban air contains a mixture of oxidizing gases and particulates arising from a variety of sources, such as power plants, motor vehicles, wildfires and waste incinerators. Chronic exposure to polluted air induces irreversible damage to cellular macromolecules (DNA, proteins, lipids etc.) via ROS production and their accumulation in cells and tissues [Moller et al., 2008]. Metabolism of exogenous sources of ethanol and phenobarbital contributes to ROS generation through changes in the cytochrome P450 pathway [Wu & Cederbaum, 2003].

4. ROS-mediated DNA damage

Although DNA is a stable and well-protected molecule, ROS can interact with it and cause several types of damage: modification of DNA bases, single- and double-DNA breaks, loss of purines (apurinic sites), damage to the deoxyribose sugar, DNA-protein cross-linkage, and damage to the DNA repair system (Figure 1) [Kohen & Nyska, 2002].

Of the ROS, the highly reactive •OH reacts with DNA by addition to double bonds of DNA bases and by abstraction of an H atom from the methyl group of thymine and each of the C-H bonds of 2′-deoxyribose. Addition of •OH to the C5-C6 double bond of pyrimidines leads to C5-OH and C6-OH adduct radicals of cytosine and thymine and H atom abstraction from thymine results in the allyl radical. Adduct radicals differ in terms of their redox properties, C5-OH- and C6-OH-adduct radicals of pyrimidines possess reducing and oxidising properties, respectively [Sonntag, 1987, Steenken, 1987, Teoule, 1987, Cooke et al., 2003].

Pyrimidine OH-adduct radicals and the allyl radical are oxidised or reduced depending on their redox environment, redox properties and reaction partners, yielding a variety of products [Dizdaroglu, 1992, Evans et al., 2004]. Product types and yields depend on absence and presence of O_2 and on other conditions [Cooke et al., 2003, Breen & Murphy, 1995]. In the absence of O_2, the oxidation of C5-OH adduct radicals, followed by addition of OH_ (or addition of water followed by deprotonation), leads to cytosine glycol and thymine glycol. The oxidation of the allyl radical of thymine yields 5-hydroxymethyluracil (5-OHMeUra) when molecular O_2 adds to C5-OH-adduct radicals at diffusion-controlled rates generating C5-OH-6-peroxyl radicals, which subsequently eliminate O_2•− followed by reaction with water (addition of OH^-) to yield thymine and cytosine glycols [Evans et al., 2004, Sonntag, 1987, Teoule, 1987].

Addition of O_2 to the allyl radical leads to 5-OHMeUra and 5-formyluracil (5-FoUra). Pyrimidine peroxyl radicals are also reduced and then protonated to give hydroxyhydroperoxides [Teoule, 1987], which decompose and yield thymine glycol, 5-OHMeUra, 5-FoUra, and 5-hydroxy-5-methylhydantoin [Wagner et al., 1994, Dizdaroglu et al., 1993a].

Cytosine products may deaminate and dehydrate. Cytosine glycol deaminates to give uracil glycol, 5-hydroxycytosine (5-OH-Cyt), and 5-hydroxyuracil (5-OH-Ura) that are unique in that they can deaminate and dehydrate. However, there is evidence that these four compounds (cytosine glycol, uracil glycol, 5-OH-Cyt, and 5-OH-Ura) may simultaneously be existed damaged DNA [Wagner et al., 1994, Dizdaroglu et al., 1993a]. In the absence of O_2, C5-OH adduct radicals may be reduced, followed by protonation to give rise to 5-hydroxy-6-hydropyrimidines. 5-Hydroxy-6-hydrocytosine (5-OH-6-HCyt) readily deaminates into 5-hydroxy-6-hydrouracil (5-OH-6-HUra). Similarly, C6-OH adduct radicals of pyrimidines are reduced yielding 6-hydroxy-5-hydropyrimidines. Formation of these products are inhibited in the presence of O_2, because O_2 reacts with their precursors C5-OH- and C6-OH-adduct radicals at diffusion-controlled rates to yield peroxyl radicals and then other products.

Further reactions of C5-OH-6-peroxyl and C6-OH-5-peroxyl radicals of cytosine result in formation of 4-amino-5-hydroxy-2, 6(1H, 5H)-pyrimidinedione and 4-amino-6-hydroxy-2, 5(1H, 6H)-pyrimidinedione, respectively. The former deaminates to give dialuric acid, which is readily oxidised to yield alloxan [Dizdaroglu et al., 1993a, Behrend et al., 1989, Dizdaroglu 1993b]. The presence of alloxan in damaged DNA has been shown by its release from DNA by *E. coli* Nth [Dizdaroglu et al., 1993a].

Decarboxylation of alloxan yields 5-hydroxyhydantoin (5-OH-Hyd) upon acidic treatment. Isodialuric acid is formed by deamination of 4-amino-6-hydroxy-2, 5(1H, 6H)-pyrimidinedione. However, these two compounds may simultaneously exist in DNA as evidenced from the detection of their enol forms (5, 6-dihydroxycytosine (5, 6-diOH-Cyt) and 5, 6-dihydroxyuracil (5, 6-diOH-Ura), respectively) [11, 13]. 5-OH-6-hydroperoxide of cytosine undergoes intramolecular cyclisation to yield *trans*-1-carbamoyl-2-oxo-4, 5-dihydroxyimidazolidine as a major product in cytosine [Kohen & Nyska, 2002] However, this compound is formed as a minor product in DNA [Dizdaroglu et al., 1993a, Behrend et al., 1989, Dizdaroglu 1993b].

Hydroxyl adduct radicals of guanine are formed by addition of •OH to the C4-, C5- and C8-positions of guanine, generating C4-OH-, C5-OH- and C8-OH-adduct radicals [O'Neill, 1983, Steenken, 1989, Candeisas & Steenken, 2000]. The 6-substituted purines such as adenine undergo analogous reactions, yielding at least two OH adducts, are formed: C4-OH and C8-OH adduct radicals [Steenken, 1989, Candeisas & Steenken, 2000]. C4-OH and C5-OH adduct radicals of purines differ in their redox properties, with C4-OH-adduct radicals being oxidising, and C5-OH- and C8-OH-adduct radicals being primarily reducing.

On the other hand, different mesomeric structures of these radicals may be oxidizing or reducing, a phenomenon called "redox ambivalence" [Vieira & Steenken, 1990]. Dehydration of C4-OH- and C5-OH-adduct radicals of purines reconstitutes the purine by first yielding a purine (–H)• radical, followed by reduction and protonation [Melvin et al., 1996]. The C4-OH-adduct radical of guanine also eliminates OH− to give rise to the guanine radical cation (guanine•+), which may deprotonate depending on pH to give guanine(-H)• [Moreno & Pryor, 1992]. Furthermore, on the basis of product analysis, the radical cation does not hydrate to lead to the C8-OH adduct radical and then to 8-hydroxyguanine by oxidation. However, it may react with 2′-deoxyribose in DNA by H abstraction, leading to DNA strand breaks [O'Neill & Chapman, 1985].

This diversity has been explained by the notion that the hydration of guanine•+ in ds-DNA may be much faster than that of monomeric guanine•+ [Candeias & Steenken, 2000]. O_2 readily reacts with guanine(-H)•; however, its reaction with the C4-OH-adduct radical of guanine is rather slow [Candeias & Steenken, 2000]. The reaction of guanine(-H)• with O_2 leads to imidazolone and oxazolone derivatives [Cadet et al., 1991]. However, this suggestion has not been confirmed by pulse radiolysis data and an alternative mechanism has been proposed [Melvin et al., 1996]. The C4-OH-adduct radical of adenine readily reacts with O_2, however, final products of this reaction are not known [O'Neill & Chapman, 1985]. C8-OH adduct radicals of purines may be oxidized by oxidants including O_2. In contrast to C4-OH adduct radicals, their reaction with O_2 is diffusion controlled [Vieira & Steenken, 1990].

8-Hydroxypurines are formed in DNA by the one-electron oxidation of C8-OH-adduct radicals [Bielski & Cabelli, 1995, Halliwell & Gutteridge, 1999] This reaction competes with the unimolecular opening of the imidazole ring by scission of the C8–N9 bond [Steenken, 1989, Candeias & Steenken, 2000]. The one-electron reduction of the ring-opened radical leads to 2, 6-diamino-4-hydroxy-5-formamidopyrimidine (FapyGua) from guanine and 4, 6-diamino-5-formamidopyrimidine (Fapy- Ade) from adenine [O'Neill, 1983, Breen & Murphy, 1995]. The C8-OH adduct radicals may also be reduced without ring opening to give rise to 7-hydro-8-hydroxypurines, which, as hemiorthoamides, are converted into formamidopyrimidines. However, 8-Hydroxypurines and formamidopyrimidines are unique in that they are formed in DNA both in the absence and presence of O_2, although O_2 increases the yields of 8-hydroxypurines. Moreover, other experimental conditions highly affect the yields of these compounds, such as the presence of reducing or oxidizing agents [Dizdaroglu, 1992, Breen & Murphy, 1995]. In the case of adenine, the •OH attack at the C2-position has also been proposed to take place and yield 2-hydroxyadenine (2-OH-Ade) when oxidation of the thus-formed C2-OH-adduct radical [Nackerdien et al., 1991]. Reactions of pyrimidines and purines result in multiple products in DNA. Most of these modified bases were identified in DNA in vitro and in vivo upon exposure to free radical generating systems [Dizdaroglu, 1998].

Reactions of •OH with the sugar moiety of DNA by H abstraction give rise to sugar modifications. Some sugar products are released from DNA as free modified sugars, whereas others remain within DNA or constitute end groups of broken DNA strands. A unique reaction of the C5′-centered sugar radical is the addition to the C8- position of the purine ring of the same nucleoside. This intramolecular cyclisation followed by oxidation yields 8, 5′-cyclopurine-2′-deoxynucleosides [Dizdaroglu, 1986, Dirksen et al., 1988]. Both 5′R- and 5′S-diastereomers of 8, 5′-cyclo-2′-deoxyguanosine (cyclo-dG) and 8, 5′-cyclo-2′-deoxyadenosine (cyclo-dA) are generated in DNA[Dizdaroglu, 1986, Dirksen et al., 1988]. (5′R)-and (5′S)- cyclo-dGs were also identified in human cells exposed to ionizing radiation [Dizdaroglu, 1987]. These tandem lesions represent a concomitant damage to both the base and sugar moieties of DNA. O_2 inhibits their formation by reacting with the C5′ centered sugar radical before cyclization.

Another reaction of base radicals is the addition to an aromatic amino acid of proteins or combination with an amino acid radical, leading to DNA–protein cross-linking [Dizdaroglu, 1988]. Covalent DNA–protein cross-links are formed in cells in vivo or in chromatin in vitro by exposure to free radical-generating systems, e.g., ionising radiation. The formation of a thymine–tyrosine cross-link has been observed in mammalian chromatin in vitro and in living cells upon exposure to ionising radiation, H_2O_2, metal ions and carcinogenic compounds [Dizdaroglu et al. 1989, Nackerdien et al., 1991, Olinski et al., 1992, Altman et al., 1995]. The formation mechanism of DNA–protein cross-link has been proposed to involve the addition of the allyl radical of thymine in DNA to tyrosine in a protein, followed by oxidation. Chemical structures of other DNA base-amino acid cross-links have been identified in mammalian chromatin in vitro, but not in vivo [Dizdaroglu, 1998]

5. Mechanism of oxidative DNA base damage: The BER pathway

As mentioned above, excess ROS may induce oxidative DNA damage, DNA strand breaks, base modifications and chromosomal aberrations [Marnett, 2000]. For repair of the DNA damage, human cells have five DNA repair systems: Direct reversal, mismatch repair, double-strand break repair, base excision repair (BER) and nucleotide excision repair (NER) [Wood et al., 2001]. DNA lesions resulting from oxidative stress, as well as single strand breaks, are repaired via the BER pathway in organisms ranging from E. coli to mammals (Figure 1) [Hazra et al., 2007, Krokan et al., 2003].

It is believed that DNA-BER is the major pathway for repairing deaminated bases and bases with oxidative damage generated by ROS and can be used to repair alkylated bases [Hazra et al., 2007, Hedge et al., 2008]. BER has 4 main steps (i.e. base removal, AP site incision, synthesis, and ligation) and involves 4 major classes of DNA repair enzymes: DNA glycosylases, APE, DNA polymerases, and DNA ligases.

The proteins involved in this reaction function in concert to remove a damaged DNA base and replace it with the correct base. A currently accepted model for the BER pathway reveals five distinct enzymatic steps for the repair of damaged bases.

Glycosylases at the initial step of BER. DNA glycosylases make BER possible - glycosylases recognize specific damaged bases and excise them from the genome, effectively initiating both longpatch and short-patch BER. To date, 11 different mammalian glycosylases have been characterized. The primary function of most DNA glycosylases is to recognize their substrate (the damaged base) and catalyze the cleavage of an N-glycosidic bond, releasing a free base and creating an abasic site [Lindahl, 1974]. In addition to catalyzing the cleavage of N-glycosydic bonds, some glycosylases are bifunctional having an additional AP lyase activity [O'Connor & Laval, 1989]. The uracil-DNA glycosylase (UNG) was the first DNA glycosylase identified and cloned [Lindahl, 1974]. MPG, N-methylpurine-DNAglycosylase, and 8-oxoguanine-DNA glycosylase (OGG1)represent some extensively studied DNA glycosylases [Sedgwick et al., 2007, Kavli et al., 2007, Klungland & Bjelland, 2007, Robertson et al., 2009]. After recognition of the damaged base by the appropriate DNA glycosylase, this glycosylase catalyzes the cleavage of an N-glycosidic bond, effectively removing the damaged base and creating an apurinic or apyrimidinic site (AP site). The DNA backbone is cleaved by either a DNA AP endonuclease or a DNA AP lyase - an activity present in some glycosylases. AP endonuclease activity creates a single-stranded DNA nick 5′ to the AP site, contrasting with the nick being created 3′ to the AP site as a result of activity (β-elimination or β, δ-elimination).

Repair can then proceed through one of two subpathways: short or long-patch BER. The short-patch BER involves the incorporation of a single nucleotide into the gap by DNA polymerase followed by strand ligation by DNA ligase. The long-patch BER involves incorporation of several nucleotides, typically two to seven, followed by cleavage of the resulting 5′ flap and ligation. Mitochondria possess independent BER machinery, the components of which are coded by nuclear genes.

Most DNA glycosylases have broad substrate specificities but can have preferences for either purines or pyrimidines. The major bifunctional glycosylase for purines is 8-oxoguanine DNA glycosylase 1, which removes OHdG and 8-oxoG. Most oxidized pyrimidines are removed by endonuclease III-like protein, uracil DNA glycosylase (UNG), and Nei-like DNA glycosylase (NEIL-1 and NEIL-2). In human cells, there are at least 2 isoforms of OGG1 (α and β) that arise from alternative splicing of products of the OGG1 gene [Boeiteux & Radicella, 2000]. α-OGG1 is a 345-amino acid (~39 kd) protein that localizes to the nucleus and mitochondria, whereas β-OGG1 is a 424-amino acid protein (47 kd) that seems to localize exclusively to mitochondria [Boeiteux & Radicella, 2000]. Because of the absence of an αO helix domain, β-OGG1 seems to lack glycosylase activity [Hashiguchi et al., 2004]. Endonuclease III-like protein 1 is a 312-amino acid (~34 kd) protein that localizes to the nucleus. OGG1 and endonuclease III-like protein require duplex DNA for efficient repair. After the glycosylase reaction, the newly created nick is processed by the Apurinic/apyrimidinic endonuclease (APE), creating a single-nucleotide gap in the DNA. Importantly, the gap created contains a 3′- hydroxyl and a 5′-phosphate, substrates compatible with the downstream enzymatic reactions in BER.

APE cleaves intact AP sites by making a single nick 5′ to the AP site to create 3′-OH and 5′-deoxyribose phosphate termini that are removed by the activity of 3′-OH and 5′-deoxyribose phosphatase proteins such as DNA Polβ. The 3-phosphate removal activity of APE is, however, approximately 70-fold lower than the AP endonuclease activity of APE [Winters et al., 1994], suggesting that other enzymes are important for the processing of damaged 3′ ends [Takahashi et al., 2007] APE is a 317-amino acid (~37 kd) multifunctional protein localized to the nucleus [Demple et al., 1991]. In addition to its role in BER, APE is required for the redox activation of transcription factors (e.g. p53) spontaneously oxidized at cysteine residues in DNA binding domains to establish DNA binding activity [Jayaraman et al., 1997]. Deletion of APE in mice causes embryonic lethality [Jayaraman et al., 1997]. Cells from mice with APE haploinsufficiency respond poorly to oxidative stress [Meira et al., 2001].

The nick generated by the cleavage of the abasic site is filled in by either Pol β or Pol δ/ε in the nucleus, and Pol γ in the mitochondria. Pol γ is the only DNA polymerase identified so far in vertebrate mitochondria and functions both as the replicative and the repair polymerase [Weissman et al., 2007, Kaguni, 2004]. Relevant to its role in BER, Pol γ has a dRP-lyase activity and can catalyze the 3′-end-processing necessary for short-patch BER [Longley et al., 1998].

The final step in the BER pathway is ligation of the nick with the correct nucleotide by DNA polymerases. An adenosine triphosphate-dependent DNA ligase (Ligase [Lig]I or III) completes the repair process and restores the integrity of the helix by sealing the nick. In the nucleus, two distinct DNA ligases participate in BER, ligase I, which has been implicated in long-patch BER, and ligase III, implicated in short-patch. The human ligase III gene (*LIG3*) also encodes for a mitochondrial variant, with a putative MTS generated by an alternative downstream translation initiation site [Lakshmipathy & Campbell, 1999, Lakshmipathy & Campbell, 2001]. The localization of ligase III protein to mitochondria suggests, then, that this enzyme may perform the ligation step in mtBER. Accordingly, reduction of ligase III expression using an antisense strategy resulted in an increase in breaks in mtDNA [Lakshmipathy & Campbell, 2001].

6. Diseases associated with defects of oxidative DNA damage repair systems

It is quite new and non conclusive that oxidative DNA damage might result in diseases. Increasing numbers of oxidatively modified DNA lesions are proposed to be appropriate, intermediate biomarkers of a disease endpoint. For this reason alone, the association between oxidative DNA damage and disease should be determined. As seen above , it is clear that oxidative DNA damage has effects upon cells other than mutation. Nevertheless, DNA mutation is perhaps one of the most important consequences of lesion persistence, evidenced by the presence of multiple systems to prevent lesion formation and, should damage occur, ensure rapid lesion removal; with the DNA repair systems responsible for the latter having much overlap of substrates, as discussed previously [Evans et al., 2004].

Cumulative oxidative DNA damage have a significant effect of the impairment on normal cellular repair mechanisms. In fact, one of the main etiological hypotheses linking genomic instability, mutagenesis and tumorigenesis is that of deficient cellular repair mechanisms due to extensive oxidative DNA damage and cellular injury [Ziech, 2011]. Clearly, reduced repair will result in elevated lesions and an increased risk of disease [Cooke et al., 2003]. ROS-mediated DNA damage in addition to ineffective DNA repair mechanisms are well established lesions common to many life threatening human diseases, including neurodegenerative diseases, atherosclerosis, cancer, and aging has invoked free radical reactions as an underlying mechanism of injury [Ziech, 2011]. Given the importance of mutation in carcinogenesis, cancer will be the first disease in which a role for oxidative DNA damage in its aetiology is considered [Evans et al., 2004].

Cancer

The carcinogenicity of oxidative stress is primarily attributed to the genotoxicity of ROS in diverse cellular processes [Ziech, 2011]. Oxidative mechanisms have been demonstrated to possess a potential role in the initiation, promotion, and malignant conversion (progression) stages of carcinogenesis [Cooke et al., 2003] . It has been suggested that some signaling system induces ROS that exhibit dual roles, cancer promoting and cancer suppresing, in tumorogenesis. ROS participate simultaneously in two signaling pathways that have inverse functions in tumorigenesis, Ras-Raf-MEK1/2-ERK1/2 signaling and the p38 mitogen-activated protein kinases (MAPK) pathway. Ras-Raf-MEK1/2-ERK1/2 signaling plays a role in oncogenesis, while the p38 MAPK pathway contributes to cancer suppression. The accumulation of intracellular ROS induced by oncogenic Ras is ERK-dependent during the activation of p38a [Pan et al., 2009)

Increased intracellular levels of ROS, induced by the Ras-Raf-MEK-ERK signaling cascade, may mediate the activation of the p38 pathway and act as an intermediate signal between the MEK-ERK and MKK3/6-p38 pathways. On the one hand, the activation of p38 mitogen-activated protein kinase (MAPK) is a prerequisite for ROS-mediated functions such as apoptotic cell death in cancer cells. On the other hand, inhibiting or scavenging ROS may attenuate the activation of p38-dependent pathways. Human cancer cell lines with high ROS levels display enhanced tumorigenicity and impaired p38α activation by ROS [Pan et al., 2009].

The effect of ROS by Ras may occur at the transcription level. GATA-6 is a component of the specific protein-DNA complexes at the nicotinamide adenine dinucleotide phosphate oxidase (Nox) 1 promoter, and is able to trans-activate the Nox1 promoter. GATA-6 is phosphorylated at serine residues by MEK-activated extracellular signal regulated kinase (ERK), which enhances GATA-6 DNA binding. The activity of the ROS-generating enzyme Nox1 is required for vascular endothelial growth factor (VEGF), a potent stimulator of tumor angiogenesis. Ras signaling enhances the transcription of Nox1 [Adachi et al., 2008]. A regulatory subunit, Rac, of the NADPH oxidase complex also involves the regulation of ROS [Heyworth et al., 1993, Kadara et al., 2008]. However, if extracellular signal-regulated kinase (ERK)-dependent phosphorylation of the transcription factor Sp1 and Sp1 binding to a VEGF promoter is inhibited, this activity does not occur [Pan et al., 2009].

Although some studies suggested that increased intracellular ROS elevate the activation of p38, these results have not been confirmed yet by the other researchers. It seems that further studies are needed to understand the mechanism of ROS in cancer.

Since the main purpose of this chapter is not to deal with the effect of ROS in tumorogenesis, we will explain the effect of ROS on DNA and DNA repair enzymes. ROS can cause direct oxidative DNA damage by increasing a cell's mutation.

Major oxidative DNA damage products including those of 8-oxo-7, 8-dihydroadenine (8-oxoAde), 8-oxo-7, 8-dihydroguanine (8-oxoGua), 8-oxo-7, 8-dihydro-2′-deoxyguanosine (8-oxodG), and 5, 6-dihydroxy-5, 6-dihydrothymine as well as the ring-open lesions of 4, 6-diamino-5-formamido-pyrimidine and 2, 6-diamino-4-hydroxy-5-formamido-pyrimidine [Kohen & Nyska, 2002]. Of these oxidative products, 8-oxoGua is known to be a biomarker of oxidative stres and its mutagenicity in mammalian cells demonstrates an additional potential as an intermediate marker of a disease endpoint (e.g. cancer). Elevated levels of such DNA lesions have been noted in many tumor types and are strongly implicated in the etiology of cancer [Valko et al., 2006]. Approximately 50%

higher rates of 8-oxoGua levels have been observed in lung, breast or prostate cancer patients when compared to otherwise healthy individuals [Tudek et al., 2010]. In addition, recent investigations have showed higher endogenous levels of 8-oxoGua in tumor tissues when compared to controls, thus suggesting oxidative DNA damage as a contributing factor in cancer development [Trachootham et al., 2009]. In addition, high levels of 8-oxoGua and possibly other DNA lesions are suggested as reliable risk factors associated with the transformation of benign to malignant tumors [Chen et al., 2007]. Furthermore, 8-oxoGua lesions are known to induce aberrant modifications in adjacent DNA a hypothesized mechanism that significantly contributes to the genetic instability and metastatic potential of tumor cells [Valko et al., 2006]. For example, formation of 8-oxoGua lesions has been shown to induce a cascade of adjacent DNA base mutations, such as GC $\rightarrow$ TA transversions in the *ras* oncogene [Bos, 1988] and *p53* tumour suppressor gene in lung and liver cancer [Valko et al.2006, Mos, 1988, Takahashi et al., 1989]. Under normal conditions, DNA repair mechanisms include OGG1, nei-like glycosylase 1 (NEIL1), APE1, and MutY homologue (MUTYH) (Evans et al. 2004). In addition, nucleotide excision repair (NER) may also participate in the process of removing the 8-OHdG lesion [Klaunig, 2010]. Several genes involved in the processing of oxidative DNA damage have been analysed in relation to human cancer risk in molecular epidemiological studies . Among these genes, allele polymorphic variants have been found in OGG1, XRCC1, Pol b, APE1 and MUTYH, which are associated with a varying extent increased cancer risk [Canbay et al., 2010, Agachan et al., 2009, Narter et al., 2009, Attar et al., 2010]. Several SNPs within hOGG1 have been reported [Kohno et al., 1998]. As polymorphisms in this gene alter glycosylase function and an individual's ability to repair oxidatively damaged DNA, they may contribute to carcinogenesis [Boiteaux & Radicella, 2000, Ide & Kotera, 2004, Shao et al., 2006]. Epidemiologic studies investigating the association between the SNPs of OGG1 have led to conflicting results. The variant allele of this SNP was shown to be associated with significantly increased risk of a number of human cancers, including lung [Hung et al., 2005, Li & Kong, 2008], esophageal [Xing et al., 2001], prostate [Xu et al., 2002], and gastric [Farinati et al., 2008] cancer but not with squamous cell carcinoma of the head and neck (SCCHN) [Zhang et al., 2004] or pancreatic cancer [McWilliams et al., 2008]. A total of eighteen polymorphisms in APE1 have been reported, among which Gln51His and Asp148Glu are the two most common SNPs. Associations between polymorphisms in APE1 and increased risk of lung, colon, breast, SCCHN, prostate, and pancreatic cancer have been reported, but with mixed results [Hung et al., 2005, Zhang et al., 2004, Goode et al., 2002, Jiao et al., 2006].

Studies relating to lung cancer and smoking have supported a potential role for ROS in cancer. Cigarette smoking is strongly linked to the aetiology of lung cancer [Hoffman & Wynder, 1986], being shown to increase the generation of free radical species [Church & Pryor, 1985] and elevate levels of oxidative DNA damage in human lungs [Asami et al., 1997, Agachan et al., 2009,] and white blood cells [Kiyosawa et al., 1990, Lodovici et al., 2000], as well as to increase the repair of 8-OH-Gua [Asami et al., 1996] and lead to an increased urinary excretion of 8-OH-dG and 5-OHMeUra in smokers compared to non-smokers [Loft et al., 1994, Pourcelot et al., 1999].

Recently ROS-mediated mutations in mitochondrial DNA (mtDNA) have emerged as an important contributor to human carcinogenesis [Freuhaug & Meyskens, 2007]. Mutations in mitochondrial genes encoding complexes I, III, IV and V, as well as within the hypervariable region of mtDNA, have been identified in various human cancers. In general, mtDNA is more susceptible to oxidative damage than nuclear DNA because (i) mitochondrial DNA is not protected by histones, (ii) mitochondrial DNA repair capacity is limited, and (iii) under physiological conditions, the mitochondria converts roughly 3–5% of O_2 consumed into $\bullet O_2^-$ and subsequently H_2O_2. In addition, mtDNA is located in close proximity to the respiratory chain and thus is consequently readily exposed to ROS-induced oxidative damage. As a result, mtDNA has more than two orders of magnitude higher frequency of oxidative damage than that of nuclear DNA and significantly correlates with the development of cancer [Ralph et al., 2010].

Cardiovascular disease

It is known that DNA alterations exist in atherosclerotic tissues and may play a fundamental role in the pathogenesis of this disease [Olinski et al., 2002, De Flora et al., 1997, Lee et al., 2001]. Elevated level of 8-OH-Gua found in the lesion of the aorta wall in atherosclerotic patients may be one of the events directly involved in the development of the disease [De Flora et al., 1997]. Oxidized low-density lipoprotein (LDL) might play an important role in the development of atherosclerotic lesions [Ross, 1993]. Interestingly, it has been found that oxidized LDL downregulates enzymes that take part in the BER pathways [Chen et al., 2000]. This DNA repair mechanism is responsible for the removal of 8-OH-Gua from cellular DNA [Dianov et al., 1998]. Therefore, it is possible that oxidized LDL that contributes directly to the development of atherosclerosis, may also be responsible for the high level of 8-OH-Gua observed in blood lymphocytes [Chen et al., 2000].

Neurodegenerative diseases

Alzheimer's disease (AD), Huntington's disease and Parkinson's disease (PD) are neurodegenerative conditions, thought to be the result, in part, of chronic exposure to environmental neurotoxins, coupled with a genetic component. These diseases all have oxidative stress implicated in their pathogenesis [Lovell et al., 1999, Lezza et al., 1999, Alam et al., 1997, Zhang et al., 1999], and elevated levels of oxidative DNA damage have been measured in a broad range of neurological conditions [Koppele et al., 1996, Alam et al., 2000]. Supportive of the studies showing elevated lesion levels are data derived from in vitro studies demonstrating that neurotransmitters such as dopamine and serotonin can generate DNA-damaging, free radical species [Spencer et. al., 1994, Wrona et al., 1998]. Overall, the role of oxidative stress in neurodegenerative disease appears undisputed. However, damage to lipid and protein, rather than DNA, appears to have been apportioned the greatest significance [Markesbery, 1999, Christen, 2000, Smith et al., 2000].

Inflammatory disease

The association between inflammation and oxidative stress is well documented [Wiseman et al., 1996, Khanna & Shiloh, 2009], with numerous studies of inflammatory conditions or infections reporting elevated levels of 8-OH-dG: hepatitis [Shimoda et al., 1994], hepatitis C infection [Farinati et al., 1999], and atopic dermatitis. An important source of the ROS are the bactericidal species ($O_2^{\bullet-}$ and H_2O_2), generated from the respiratory burst of invading neutrophils, macrophages, and eosinophils damaging surrounding tissue. Chronic inflammation, and the accompanying oxidative stress, has been closely linked to the pathogenesis of autoimmune diseases such as rheumatoid arthritis [Bashir et.al, 1993] and systemic lupus erythematosus [Lunec et.al., 1994], with free radical production resulting, not only in connective tissue damage, but also modified biomolecules being exposed to the systemic circulation, postulated to be the antigen driving autoantibody production [Weitzman & Gordon, 1990].

Elevated DNA levels of 8-OH-dG have been reported in lymphocytes from patients with RA, SLE, vasculitis or Behcet's disease. These same lymphocytes, from RA and SLE patients, also display increased sensitivity to hydrogen peroxide-induced cytotoxicity [Bashir et al., 1993].

Ischemia-reperfusion injury

The literature provides a growing number of reports in which levels of oxidative DNA damage are elevated in post-ischaemia-reperfusion. Elevated levels of urinary 8-OH-dG or dTg were reported following liver transplantation, which proposed to be due to ischemia-reperfusion or reoxygenation injury [Thier et al., 1999, Loft et al., 1995]. Ischaemia-reperfusion injury is a significant factor affecting morbidity and mortality following bypass and transplantation surgery, haemorrhagic or septic shock, myocardial infarction and multiple organ failure. During the period of ischaemia, xanthine dehydrogenase is converted to xanthine oxidase. Upon reperfusion, there is a "burst" of xanthine oxidase activity which, rather than transferring electrons to NAD+, transfers them to O_2, generating superoxide, with the subsequent potential for generating other ROS and hence DNA damage. Endogenous levels of xanthine dehydrogenase vary from organ to organ and hence ischemia-reperfusion injury might be more relevant to some tissues than others. Human leukocytes appear to be sensitive to the genotoxic effects of ischemia-reperfusion (163) and therefore represent a potential surrogate tissue in which to study the effects of ischemia-reperfusion that have affected a less accessible tissue.

Aging

Major theories of aging are grouped under two categories: damage accumulation aging and developmentally programmed aging. However, a developing (emerging) hypothesis described as the free radical theory of aging appears to have adopted elements of the former theories. The basis of the Harman's theory [Harman, 1956] suggested that aging occurs through the gradual accumulation of free radical damage to biomolecules. With age, antioxidant defences fail to scavenge all potentially damaging radical species that result in the insidious accumulation of damage and gradual loss of function [Beckman et al., 1998]. One of the few focussing upon DNA damage, is a report of an age-related increase in serum 8-OH-dG in apparently disease-free individuals over an age range of 15–91 years [Rattan et al., 1995]. Although this same trend was not evident in the urinary 8-OH-dG output of infants, a gradual increase was noted over the first month postpartum, which mirrored the velocity growth curve [Drury et al., 1998].

The accumulation of lesions can, in part, be explained by the discovery that DNA repair capability correlates with species-specific life span [168]. Furthermore, repair activity appears to decline with age, resulting in the persistence of damage and a subsequent increase in replication errors [Hirano et al., 1995].

7. Conclusion

Although there is association between oxidative DNA damage and diseases, elucidation of the role of oxidative DNA damage requires much more work. It is well known that DNA repair enzymes are important for oxidative DNA damage. If individual spesific biomarkers related DNA repair enzyme are found, new treatmant strategies would be developed to cure disease related oxidative DNA damage.

8. References

Adachi Y, Shibai Y, Mitsushita J, Shang WH, Hirose K, Kamata T. 2008. Oncogenic Ras upregulates NADPH oxidase 1 gene expres s ion through MEK-ERK-dependent phosphorylation of GATA-6. *Oncogene* 27: 4921-4932

Adly, AAM. 2010. Oxidative stress and disease: An updated review. *Res. J. Immunol.*, 3: 129-145.

Agaçhan B, Küçükhüseyin O, Aksoy P, Turna A, Yaylim I, Görmüs U, Ergen A, Zeybek U, Dalan B, Isbir T. 2009. Apurinic/apyrimidinic endonuclease (APE1) gene polymorphisms and lung cancer risk in relation to tobacco smoking. *Anticancer Res.*, 29(6):2417-20.

Alam ZI, Jenner A, Daniel SE, Lees AJ, Cairns N, Marsden CD, Jenner P, Halliwell B. 1997. Oxidative DNA damage in the Parkinsonian brain: an apparent selective increase in 8-hydroxyguanine levels in substantia nigra, J. *Neurochem.* , 1196–1203.

Alam ZI, Halliwell B, Jenner P. 2000. No evidence for increased oxidative damage to lipids, proteins, or DNA in Huntington's disease. J. *Neurochem.*, 840–846

Altman SA, Zastawny TH, Randers-Eichhorn L, Cacciuttolo MA, Akman SA, Dizdaroglu M., Rao G. 1995. Formation of DNA-protein cross-links in cultured mammalian cells upon treatment with iron ions. *Free Radical Biol. Med.*, 897–902.

Asami S, Manabe H, Miyake J, Tsurudome Y, Hirano T, Yamaguchi R, Itoh H, Kasai H. 1997. Cigarette smoking induces an increase in oxidative DNA damage, 8-hydroxydeoxyguanosine, in a central site of the human lung. *Carcinogenesis,* 18;1763–1766.

Asami S, Hirano T, Yamaguchi R, Tomioka Y, Itoh H, Kasai H. 1996. Increase of a type of oxidative DNA damage, 8-hydroxyguanine, and its repair activity in human leukocytes by cigarette smoking. *Cancer Res.*, 56; 2546–2549.

Attar R, Cacina C, Sozen S, Attar E, Agachan B. 2010. DNA repair genes in endometriosis. *Genet Mol Res.*, 6;9(2):629-36.

Babior BM.2000. The NADPH oxidase of endothelial cells. *IUBMB Life,* 50;267–269.

Bashir S, Harris G, Denman MA, Blake DR, Winyard PG. 1993. Oxidative DNA damage and cellular sensitivity to oxidative stress in human autoimmune diseases. *Ann. Rheum. Dis.*, 52; 659–666.

Beckman JS, Ischiropoulos H, Zhu L, van der Woerd M, Smith C, Chen J, Harrison J, Martin JC, Tsai M.1992. Kinetics of superoxide dismutase- and iron-catalyzed nitration of phenolics by peroxynitrite. *Arch Biochem Biophys.*, 298:438–445.

Beckman KB and Ames BN. 1998. The free radical theory of aging matures. *Physiol. Rev.*, 78, 547–581.

Behrend, R. and Roosen, O. 1889. Synthese der Harnsa¨ure. *Liebigs Ann.Chem.*, 251, 235–256.

Bielski BHJ and Cabelli DE. 1995. Superoxide and hydroxyl radical chemistry in aqueous solution. In: *Active Oxygen in Chemistry*, Foote CS, Valentine JS, Greenberg A, Liebman JF (eds). Chapman and Hall, London, pp. 66–104.

Boiteux S and Radicella JP.2000. The human OGG1 gene: Structure, functions, and its implication in the process of carcinogenesis. *Arch Biochem Biophys.*, 377, 1–8.

Bos JL. 1988. The ras gene family and human carcinogenesis.*Mutat. Res.*, 195;255–271.

Breen AP and Murphy JA.1995. Reactions of hydroxyl radicals with DNA. *Free Radic. Biol. Med.*, 18, 1033–1077

Cadenas E and Davies KJ. 2000. Mitochondrial free radical generation, oxidative stress, and aging. *Free Radic Biol Med.*, 29(3-4):222-30.

Cadet J, Berger M, Decarroz C, Mouret JF, Vanlier JE, Wagner RJ. 1991.Photoinduced and radio-induced radical oxidation of the purine and pyrimidine bases of nucleic acids. *J. Chim. Phys. Phys.-Chim. Biol.* 88;1021–1042.

Cadet J, Berger M, Buchko GW, Joshi PC, Raoul S., Ravanat J-L. 1994.2, 2-Diamino-4-[3, 5-di-*O*-acetyl-2-deoxy-betad-erythrosepentofuranosyl) amino]-5-(2H)-oxazolone—a novel and predominant radical oxidation product of 3_, 5_-di-*O*-acetyl-2_-deoxyguanosine. *J. Am. Chem. Soc.* 116;7403–7404.

Canbay E, Agachan B, Gulluoglu M, Isbir T, Balik E, Yamaner S, Bulut T, Cacina C, Eraltan IY, Yilmaz A, Bugra D. 2010.Possible associations of APE1 polymorphism with susceptibility and HOGG1 polymorphism with prognosis in gastric cancer. *Anticancer Res.*, 30(4):1359-64.

Candeias LP, Steenken S. 2000. Reaction of HO. with Guanine Derivatives in Aqueous Solution: Formation of Two Different Redox-Active OH-Adduct Radicals and Their Unimolecular Transformation Reactions. Properties of G(-H).*Chemistry - A European Journal*, 6: 475–484

Chen HI, Liou SH, Ho SF, Wu KY, Sun CW, Chen MF, Cheng LC, Shih TS, Loh CH.2007. Oxidative DNA damage estimated by plasma 8-hydroxyxeoxyguanosine (8-OHdG): influence of 4, 4'-methylenebis (2-chloroaniline) exposure and smoking. *J. Occup. Health.* 49, pp. 389–398

Chen KH, Srivastava DK, Singhal RK, Jacob S, Ahmed AE, Wilson SH. 2000.Modulation of base excision repair by low density lipoprotein, oxidized low density lipoprotein and antioxidants in mouse monocytes. *Carcinogenesis*, 21:1017–1022.

Christen Y. 2000.Oxidative stress and Alzheimer disease. *Am. J. Clin. Nutr.* 71;621S–629S.

Church DF, Pryor WA. 1985. Free-radical chemistry of cigarette smoke and its toxicological implications. *Environ. Health Perspect.* 64;111–126.

Colton CA , Gilbert DL. 1999. Reactive Oxygen Species in Biological Systems: An Interdisciplinary Approach. *Springer US. 740. Hardcover*

Cooke MS, Evans MD, Dizdaroglu M, Lunec J. 2003.Oxidative DNA damage: mechanisms, mutation, and disease. *FASEB J.*, 17(10):1195-214.

De Flora S, Izzotti A, Walsh D, Degan P, Petrilli GL, Lewtas J. 1997.Molecular epidemiology of atherosclerosis. *FASEB J*, .11:1021–1031.

Demple B, Herman T, Chen DS. 1991.Cloning and expression of APE, the cDNA encoding the major human apurinic enodnuclease: Definition of a family of DNA repair enzymes. *Proc Natl Acad Sci U S A*, 88:11450–54.

Dianov G, Bischoff C, Piotrowski J, Bohr VA.1998. Repair pathways for processing of 8-oxoguanine in DNA by mammalian cell extracts. *J. Biol. Chem.*, 273:33811–33816.

Dirksen ML, Blakely WF, Holwitt E, Dizdaroglu, M.1988.Effect of DNA conformation on the hydroxyl radicalinduced formation of 8, 5_-cyclopurine 2_-deoxyribonucleoside residues in DNA. *Int. J. Radiat. Biol.*, 54, 195–204

Dizdaroglu M, Bauche C, Rodriguez H, Laval J. 2000.Novel substrates of *Escherichia coli* Nth protein and its kinetics for excision of modified bases from DNA damaged by free radicals. *Biochemistry*, 39;5586–5592.

Dizdaroglu M, Gajewski E, Reddy P, Margolis SA.1989. Structure of a hydroxyl radical induced DNA-protein cross-link involving thymine and tyrosine in nucleohistone.*Biochemistry*, 28; 3625–3628.

Dizdaroglu M.1998.Mechanisms of free radical damage to DNA, in: O.I. Aruoma (Ed.), DNA & Free Radicals: Techniques, Mechanisms & Applications, *OICA International, Saint Lucia*, pp. 3–26.

Dizdaroglu M.1993. Quantitative determination of oxidative base damage in DNA by stable isotope-dilution mass spectrometry, *FEBS Lett.*, 315;1–6.

Dizdaroglu M.1986.Free-radical-induced formation of an 8, 5_-cyclo-2_-deoxyguanosine moiety in deoxyribonucleic acid. *Biochem. J*, . 238, 247–254

Dizdaroglu M. 1992. Oxidative damage to DNA in mammalian chromatin. *Mutat. Res*, 275, 331–342.

Dizdaroglu M, Dirksen, ML, Jiang HX, Robbins JH. 1987. Ionizing-radiation-induced damage in the DNA of cultured human cells. Identification of 8, 5-cyclo-2-deoxyguanosine. *Biochem. J.*, 241, 929–932

Dizdaroglu M, Laval J, Boiteux S.1993.Substrate specificity of the *Escherichia coli* endonuclease III: excision of thymine- and cytosine-derived lesions in DNA produced by radiation-generated free radicals. *Biochemistry*, 32, 12105–12111.

Drury JA, Jeffers G, Cooke RW.1998.Urinary 8-hydroxydeoxyguanosine in infants and children. *Free Radic. Res.* 28, 423–428

Duarte V, Gasparutto D, Jaquinod M, Cadet J.2000. In vitro DNA synthesis opposite oxazolone and repair of this DNA damage using modified oligonucleotides. *Nucl. Acids Res.* 28;1555–1563.

Evans MD, Dizdaroglu M, Cooke MS. 2004.Oxidative DNA damage and disease: induction, repair and significance. *Mutat Res.* 567(1):1-61.

Farinati F, Cardin R, Bortolami M, Nitti D, Basso D., de Bernard M., Cassaro M., Sergio A, Rugge, M. 2008. Oxidative DNA damage in gastric cancer: CagA status and OGG1 gene polymorphism. *Int J Cancer.* , 123, 51–5.

Farinati, F., Cardin, R., Degan, P., De Maria, N., Floyd, R. A., Van Thiel, D. H., and Naccarato, R. (1999) Oxidative DNA damage in circulating leukocytes occurs as an early event in chronic HCV infection. *Free Radic. Biol., Med.* 27, 1284–1291

Forman HJ, Boveris A. 1982. Superoxide radical and hydrogen peroxide in mitochondria, in: WA Pryor (Ed.), *Free Radicals in Biology*, Vol. V, New York: Academic Press, pp. 65–90

Frenkel K. 1992. Carcinogen-mediated oxidant formation and oxidative DNA damage. *Pharmacol. Ther.* 53, 127–166

Fruehaug JP, Meyskens FL. 2007.Reactive oxygen species: a breath of life of death? *Clin. Cancer Res.* 13;789–794.

Galaris D, Skiada V, Barbouti A.2008. Redox signaling and cancer: the role of 'labile' iron, Cancer Lett. 266;21–29.

Goode EL, Ulrich CM, Potter JD.2002. Polymorphisms in DNA repair genes and associations with cancer risk. *Cancer Epidemiol Biomarkers Prev.*, 11, 1513–30.

Halliwell B, Gutteridge JM. 1999.Free Radicals in Biology and Medicine, third edition. *Oxford University Press,* Midsomer Norton, Avon, England.

Harman D.1956. Aging: a theory based on free radical and radiation chemistry. *J. Gerontol,* . 11, 298–300

Hart RW, Setlow RB.1974. Correlation between deoxyribonucleic acid excision-repair and life-span in a number of mammalian species. *Proc. Natl. Acad. Sci. USA,* 71;2169–2173.

Hashiguchi K, Bohr VA, de Souza-Pinto NC. 2004.Oxidative stress and mitochondrial DNA repair: implications for NRTIs induced DNA damage. *Mitochondrion.,* 4(2-3):215-22.

Hashiguchi K, Stuart JA, de Souza-Pinto NC, Bohr VA. 2004.The C-terminal αO helix of human Ogg1 is essential for 8-oxoguanine DNA glycosylase activity: The mitochondrial β-Ogg1 lacks this domain and does not have glycosylase activity. *Nucleic Acids Res.,* 32:5596–5608.

Hazra TK, Das A, Das S.2007.Oxidative DNA damage repair in mammalian cells: A new perspective. *DNA Repair,* 6: 470–480.

Hedge ML, Hazra TK, Mitra S. 2008.Early steps in the DNA base excision/single-strand interruption repair pathway in mammalian cells. *Cell Res.* 18:27–47.

Heyworth PG, Knaus UG, Settleman J, Curnutte JT, Bokoch GM. Regulation of NADPH oxidase activity by Rac GTPase activating protein(s). *Mol Biol Cell* 1993; 4: 1217-1223

Hirano T, Yamaguchi Y, Hirano H, Kasai H. 1995.Ageassociated change of 8-hydroxyguanine repair activity in cultured human fibroblasts.*Biochem. Biophys. Res.Commun.,* 214;1157–1162.

Hoffmann D, Wynder EL. 1986. Chemical constituents and bioactivity of tobacco smoke, *IARC Sci. Publ.,* 74; 145–165.

Hsu IC, Metcalf RA, Sun T, Welsh JA, Wang NJ, Harris CC.1991. Mutational hotspot in the p53 gene in human hepatocellular carcinomas.*Nature,* 350;427–428.

Hung RJ, Hall J, Brennan P, Boffetta P. 2005. Genetic polymorphisms in the base excision repair pathway and cancer risk: A HuGE review.*Am J Epidemiol,* 162, 925–42.

Ide H., Kotera M. 2004. Human DNA glycosylases involved in the repair of oxidatively damaged DNA. *Biol Pharm Bull,* 27, 480–5.

Imlay JA, Chin SM, Linn S. 1988. Toxic DNA damage by hydrogen peroxide through the Fenton reaction in vivo and in vitro. *Science,* 240; 640-642.

Jayaraman L, Murthy KGK, Zhu C.1997. Identification of redox/repair protein Ref-1 as a potent activator of p53. *Genes Dev.,* 11:558–70.

Jiao L., Bondy ML, Hassan MM, Wolff RA, Evans DB, Abbruzzese JL., Li D. 2006. Selected polymorphisms of DNA repair genes and risk of pancreatic cancer. *Cancer Detect Prev,* 30, 284–91

Kadara H, Tahara E, Kim HJ, Lotan D, Myers J, Lotan R. Involvement of Rac in fenretinide-induced apoptosis. *Cancer Res* 2008; 68: 4416-4423

Kaguni LS.2004. DNA polymerase gamma, the mitochondrial replicase.*Annu Rev Biochem,* 73:293–320.

Kamata H, Hirata H.1999.Redox regulation of cellular signalling. *Cell Signal,* 11:1–14.

Kavli B, Otterlei M, Slupphaug G, Krokan HE. 2007. Uracil in DNA – general mutagen, but normal intermediate in acquired immunity. *DNA Repair (Amst),* 6, 505–516.

Khanna KK, Shiloh Y.2009.The DNA Damage Response: Implications on Cancer Formation and Treatment. *Springer Publication.* XII, 449 p.

King PA, Anderson VE, Edwards JO, Gustafson G, Plumb RC, Sugas JW. 1992. A stable solid that generates hydroxyl radical upon dissolution in aqueous solution: reaction with proteins and nucleic acids. *J Am Chem Soc*, 114:5430 -5432.

Kiyosawa H, Suko M, Okudaira H, Murata K, Miyamoto T, Chung MH, Kasai H, Nishimura S.1990. Cigarette smoking induces formation of 8-hydroxydeoxyguanosine, one of the oxidative DNA damages in human peripheral leukocytes. *Free Radical Res. Commun.* 11;23–27.

Klaunig J, Kamendulis LM.2004. The role of oxidative stress in carcinogenesis.*Annu.Rev. Pharmacol. Toxicol.* 44; 239–267.

Klaunig JE, Kamendulis LM, Hocevar BA.2010. Oxidative stress and oxidative damage in carcinogenesis. *Toxicol Pathol.*, 38(1):96-109.

Klungland A, Bjelland S. 2007.Oxidative damage to purines in DNA: role of mammalian Ogg1. *DNA Repair (Amst)*, 6, 481–488.

Kohen R, Nyska A. 2002. Oxidation of biological systems: oxidative stress phenomena, antioxidants, redox reactions, and methods for their quantification. *Toxicol Pathol.* , 30(6):620-50.

Kohno T, Shinmura K, Tosaka M, Tani M, Kim, SR, Sugimura H, Nohmi T, Kasai H, Yokota J. 1998. Genetic polymorphisms and alternative splicing of the hOGG1 gene, that is involved in the repair of 8-hydroxyguanine in damaged DNA. *Oncogene*, 16, 3219–25.

Koppele J, Lucassen PJ, Sakkee AN, van Asten JG, Ravid R, Swaab DF, van Bezooijen CFA.1996. 8-OHdG levels in brain do not indicate oxidative DNA damage in Alzheimer's disease. *Neurobiol. Aging*, 17, 819–826

Krokan HE, Nilsen H, Skorpen F, et al.2000 Base excision repair of DNA in mammalian cells. *FEBS Lett*, 476: 73–77.

Lakshmipathy U, Campbell C.1999.The human DNA ligase III gene encodes nuclear and mitochondrial proteins. *Mol Cell Biol*, 19: 3869–3876.

Lakshmipathy U, Campbell C.2001.Antisense-mediated decrease in DNA ligase III expression results in reduced mitochondrial DNA integrity. *Nucleic Acids Res.*, 29:668–676.

Lee KW, Lee HJ.2006. Biphasic effects of dietary antioxidants on oxidative stress- mediated carcinogenesis.*Mech. Ageing Dev.* 127; 424–431.

Lee SH, Blair IA.2001. Oxidative DNA damage and cardiovascular disease. *Trends Cardiovasc. Med.*, 11:148–155.

Lezza A, Mecocci P, Cormio A, Flint Beal M, Cherubini A, Cantatore P, Senin U, Gadaleta MN. 1999.Areaspecific differences in OH8dG and mtDNA4977 levels in Alzheimer disease patients and aged controls.J. Anti-aging Med. 2 ;209–215.

Li W, Kong AN. 2008. Molecular mechanisms of Nrf2-mediated antioxidant response. *Mol Carcinog*, 48, 91–104.

Lindahl T.1974. An N-glycosidase from Escherichia coli that releases free uracil from DNAcontaining deaminated cytosine residues. *Proc. Natl. Acad. Sci. USA*, 71, 3649–3653

Lodovici M, Casalini C, Cariaggi R, Michelucci L, Dolara P.2000.Levels of 8-hydroxydeoxyguanosine as a marker of DNA damage in human leukocytes.*Free Radical Biol. Med.*, 28;13–17.

Loft S, Astrup A, Buemann B, Poulsen HE.1994. Oxidative DNA damage correlates with oxygen consumption in humans, *Faseb J.* 8;534–537.

Loft S, Larsen PN, Rasmussen A, Fischer-Nielsen A, Bondesen S, Kirkegaard P, Rasmussen LS, Ejlersen E, Tornoe K, Bergholdt, R. 1995. Oxidative DNA damage after transplantation of the liver and small intestine in pigs. *Transplantation,* 59, 16–20

Longley MJ, Prasad R, Srivastava DK, Wilson SH, Copeland WC. 1998. Identification of 5=-deoxyribose phosphate lyase activity in human DNA polymerase gamma and its role in mitochondrial base excision repair in vitro. *Proc Natl Acad Sci U S A* , 95:12244–12248.

Lovell MA, Gabbita SP, . Markesbery WR.1999. Increased DNA oxidation and decreased levels of repair products in Alzheimer's disease ventricular CSF. *J. Neurochem.* 72; 771–776.

Lunec J, Herbert K, Blount S, Griffiths HR, Emery P.1994. 8-Hydroxydeoxyguanosine. A marker of oxidative DNA damage in systemic lupus erythematosus. *FEBS Lett.* 348 ; 131–138.

Markesbery WR. 1999.The role of oxidative stress in Alzheimer disease.*Arch. Neurol.* 56; 1449–1452.

Marnett LJ.2000. Oxyradicals and DNA damage. *Carcinogenesis,* 21:361–70.

McWilliams RR., Bamlet WR, Cunningham JM, Goode EL, de Andrade M, Boardman LA, Petersen, GM. 2008. Polymorphisms in DNA repair genes, smoking, and pancreatic adenocarcinoma risk. *Cancer Res.* 68, 4928–35.

Meira LB, Devaraj S, Kisby GE.2001.Heterozygosity for the mouse Apex gene result in phenotypes associated with oxidative stress. *Cancer Res,* 61:5552–57.

Mena S, Ortega A, Estrela J.2009. Oxidative stress in environmental-induced carcinogenesis. *Mutat. Res.* 674 ;36–44.

Michalik V, Spotheim Maurizot M, Charlier M.1995. Calculation of hydroxyl radical attack on different forms of DNA. *J Biomol Struct Dyn,* 13:565–575.

Moller P, Folkmann JK, Forchhammer L, Brauner EV, Danielsen P, Rison L, Loft S. 2008.Air pollution, oxidative damage to DNA, and carcinogenesis. *Cancer Lett.*;266;84–97.

Moreno JJ, Pryor WA (1992) Inactivation of alpha 1-proteinase inhibitor by peroxynitrite. Chem Res Toxicol 5:425–431.

Nackerdien Z, Rao G., Cacciuttolo MA, Gajewski E, Dizdaroglu M.1991. Chemical nature of DNA-protein cross-links produced in mammalian chromatin by hydrogen peroxide in the presence of iron or copper ions, *Biochemistry* 30; 4873–4879.

Nackerdien Z, Kasprzak KS, Rao G, Halliwell B, Dizdaroglu M.1991. Nickel(II)- and cobalt(II)-dependent damage by hydrogen peroxide to the DNA bases in isolated human chromatin. *Cancer Res.* 51, 5837–5842.

Narter KF, Ergen A, Agaçhan B, Görmüs U, Timirci O, Isbir T. 2009.Bladder cancer and polymorphisms of DNA repair genes (XRCC1, XRCC3, XPD, XPG, APE1, hOGG1). *Anticancer Res.,* 29(4):1389-93.

Nohl H, Hegner D.1978. Do mitochondria produce oxygen radicals in vivo? *Eur J Biochem,* 82:563–567.

O'Connor TR, Laval J. 1989. Physical association of the 2, 6-diamino-4-hydroxy-5N-formamidopyrimidine-DNA glycosylase of Escherichia coli and an activity nicking DNA at apurinic/apyrimidinic sites. *Proc. Natl. Acad. Sci. USA,* 86, 5222–5226.

O'Neill P.1983. Pulse radiolytic study of the interaction of thiols and ascorbate with OH adducts of dGMP and dG: implications for DNA repair processes. *Radiat. Res.*, 96 ; 198–210.

Olinski R, Gackowski D, Foksinski M, Rozalski R, Roszkowski K, Jaruga P.2002.Oxidative DNA damage: assessment of the role in carcinogenesis, atherosclerosis, and acquired immunodeficiency syndrome. *Free Radic Biol Med.* 33(2):192-200.

Olinski R, Nackerdien Z, Dizdaroglu M.1992. DNA–protein cross-linking between thymine and tyrosine in chromatin of gamma-irradiated or H_2O_2-treated cultured human cells.*Arch. Biochem. Biophys.* 297; 139–143.

O'Neill P, Chapman PW. 1985. Potential repair of free radical adducts of dGMP and dG by a series of reductants. A pulse radiolytic study. *Int. J. Radiat. Biol. Relat. Stud. Phys. Chem. Med.*, 47, 71–80

Packer MA, Murphy MP. 1994. Peroxynitrite causes calcium efflux from mitochondria which is prevented by Cyclosporin A. *FEBS Lett.*, 345:237–240.

Pan JS, Hong MZ, Ren JL. Reactive oxygen species: a double-edged sword in oncogenesis. World J Gastroenterol. 2009 Apr 14;15(14):1702-7.

Pourcelot S, Faure H, Firoozi F, Ducros V, Tripier M, Hee J, Cadet J, Favier A.1999. Urinary 8-oxo-7, 8-dihydro-2_-deoxyguanosine and 5-(hydroxymethyl) uracil in smokers. *Free Radical Res.*, 30; 173–180.

Radi R, Beckman JS, Bush KM, Freeman BA. 1991a. Peroxynitrite-induced membrane lipid peroxidation: the cytotoxic potential of superoxide and nitric oxide. *Arch Biochem Biophys.*, 288:481–487.

Radi R, Beckman JS, Bush KM, Freeman BA. 1991b. Peroxynitrite oxidation of sulfhydryls. The cytotoxic potential of superoxide and nitric oxide. *J Biol Chem.*, 266:4244–4250.

Radi R, RodriguezM, Castro L, Telleri R.1994. Inhibition of mitochondrial electron transport by peroxynitrite. *Arch Biochem Biophys.*, 308:89–95.

Raha S, Robinson BH. 2000. Mitochondria, oxygen free radicals, disease and ageing. *Trends Biochem. Sci.* 25, 502–508.

Ralph SJ, Enríquez SR, Neuzil J, Saavedra E, Sánchez RM. 2010. The causes of cancer revisited: "mitochondrial malignancy" and ROS-induced oncogenic transformation -Why mitochondria are targets for cancer therapy. *Mol. Aspects Med.* 31; 145–170.

Raoul S, Berger M, Buchko GW, Joshi PC, Morin B, Weinfeld M, Cadet J.1996. H-1, C-13 and N-15 nuclear magnetic resonance analysis and chemical features of the two main radical oxidation products of 2_-deoxyguanosine: oxazolone and imidazolone nucleosides. *J. Chem. Soc. Perkin Trans.*, 371–381.

Rattan S, Siboska GE, Wikmar FP, Clark BFC, Woolley P. 1995. Levels of oxidative DNA damage product 8-hydroxy-2_-deoxyguanosine in human serum increases with age. *Med. Sci. Res.* 23, 469–470

Robertson AB, Klungland A, Rognes T, Leiros I. 2009.DNA repair in mammalian cells: Base excision repair: the long and short of it. *Cell Mol Life Sci.*, 66(6):981-93.

Ross R. 1993. *Rous-Whipple Award Lecture.* Atherosclerosis: a defense mechanism gone awry. *Am J Pathol., 143: 987–1002*

Schafer FQ, Buettner GR. 2001. Redox environments of the cell as viewed through the redox state of the glutathione disulfide/glutathione couple. *Free Rad Biol Med.*, 30: 1191–1212.

Sedgwick B, Bates PA, Paik J, Jacobs SC, Lindahl T. 2007. Repair of alkylated DNA: recent advances. *DNA Repair* (Amst) 6, 429–442.

Sen S , Chakraborty R, Sridhar C, Reddy YSR, De B. 2010. Free Radicals, Antioxidants, Diseases and Phytomedicines: Current Status and Future Prospect. *International Journal of Pharmaceutical Sciences Review and Research*, Volume 3, Issue 1, p.91-100

Shao L, Hittelman WN, Lin J, Yang H, Ajani JA., Wu X. 2006.Deficiency of cell cycle checkpoints and DNA repair system predispose individuals to esophageal cancer. *Mutat Res.*, 602, 143–50.

Shimoda R, Nagashima M., Sakamoto M, Yamaguchi N, Hirohashi S, Yokota J, Kasai H. 1994. Increased formation of oxidative DNA damage, 8-hydroxydeoxyguanosine, in human livers with chronic hepatitis. *Cancer Res.*, 54, 3171–3172

Smith MA, Rottkamp CA, Nunomura A, Raina AK, Perry G.2000. Oxidative stress in Alzheimer's disease. *Biochim.Biophys. Acta,* 1502;139–144.

Sohal RS.1997. Mitochondria generate superoxide anion radicals and hydrogen peroxide. FASEB J 11:1269–1270.

von Sonntag C. 1987. The Chemical Basis of Radiation Biology. *Taylor* and *Francis,* London, *1987,* p. 57

Spencer JP, Jenner A, Aruoma OI, Evans P J, Kaur H., Dexter DT, Jenner P, Lees AJ, Marsden DC, Halliwell B. 1994.Intense oxidative DNA damage promoted by L-dopa and its metabolites. Implications for neurodegenerative disease. *FEBS Lett.,* 353, 246–250

Steenken S.1989. Purine bases, nucleosides, and nucleotides:aqueous solution redox Chemistry and transformation reactions of their radical cations and e− and OH adducts.*Chem. Rev.* 89;503–520.

Steenken S. 1987. Addition-elimination paths in electrontransfer reactions between radicals and molecules. *J. Chem. Soc. Faraday Trans. I,* 83, 113–124

Sultan SM, Ioannou Y, Isenberg DA. 2000. Is there an association of malignancy with systemic lupus erythematosus? An analysis of 276 patients under long-term review. *Rheumatology (Oxford),* 39, 1147–1152

Takahashi T, Tada M, Igarashi S, et al. Aprataxin, causative gene product for EAOH/AOA1, repairs DNA single-strand breaks with damaged 3'-phosphate and 3'-phosphoglycolate ends. Nucleic Acids Res 2007;35:3797–3809.

Takahashi T, Nau MM, Chiba I, Birrer MJ, Rosenberg RK, Vinocour M, Levitt M, Pass H, Gazdar AF, . Minna JD.1989. p53: a frequent target for genetic abnormalities in lung cancer.*Science,* 246 ;491–494.

Teoule R. 1987. Radiation-induced DNA damage and its repair. *Int. J. Radiat. Biol. Relat. Stud. Phys. Chem. Med.,* 51, 573–589

Thier R, Bruning T, Kocher K, Blaszkewicz M, Makropoulos V, Sundberg A, Bolt HM.1999. Determination of urinary thymidine glycol using affinity chromatography, HPLC and post-column reaction detection: a biomarker of oxidative DNA damage upon kidney transplantation. *Arch. Toxicol.,* 73, 479–484

Toyokuni S, Mori T, Hiai H, Dizdaroglu M.1995.Treatment of Wistar rats with a renal carcinogen, ferric nitrilotriacetate, causes DNA-protein cross-linking between thymine and tyrosine in their renal chromatin. *Int. J. Cancer,* 62;309–313.

Trachootham D, Alexander J, Huang P.2009. Targeting cancer cells by ROS-mediated mechanism: a radical therapeutic approach? *Nat. Rev.* 8;579–591.

Tudek B, Winczura A, Janik J, Siomek A, Foksinski M, Olinski R.2010. Involvement of oxidatively damaged DNA and repair in cancer development and aging. *Am. J. Transl. Res.*, 2; 254–284.

Ushio-Fukai M, Nakamura Y.2008. Reactive oxygen species and angiogenesis:NADPH oxidase as target for cancer therapy. *Cancer Lett.* 266; 37–52.

Valko M, Rhodes CJ, Moncol J, Izakovic M, Mazur M.2006. Free radicals, metals and antioxidants in oxidative stress-induced cancer, Chem. Biol. Interact. 160 ;1–40.

Vieira AJSC, Steenken S. 1990. Pattern of OH radical reaction with adenine and its nucleosides and nucleotides. Characterisation of two types of isomeric OH adduct and their unimolecular transformation reactions. *J. Am. Chem. Soc.*, 112, 6986–6994

Wagner JR, Van Lier JE, Berger M, Cadet, J. 1994. Thymidine hydroperoxides: structural assignments, conformational features and thermal decomposition in water. *J. Am. Chem. Soc*, . 116, 2235–2242

Weissman L, de Souza-Pinto NC, Stevnsner T, Bohr VA. 2007. DNA repair, mitochondria, and neurodegeneration. *Neuroscience*, 145(4):1318-29.

Weitzman SA, Gordon LI. 1990. Inflammation and cancer: role of phagocyte-generated oxidants in carcinogenesis. *Blood*, 76, 655–663

Willy C, Dahouk S, Starck C, Kaffenberger W, Gerngross H, Plappert UG. 2000. DNA damage in human leukocytes after ischemia/reperfusion injury. *Free Radic. Biol. Med*, . 28, 1–12

Winters TA, Henner WD, Russel PS, et al. 1994.Removal of 3′-phosphoglycolate from DNA strand-break damage in an oligonucleotide substrate by recombinant human apurinic/apyrimidinic endonuclease. *Nucleic Acids Res*, 22:18866–73.

Wiseman H, Halliwell B.1996. Damage to DNA by reactive oxygen and nitrogen species: role in inflammatory disease and progression to cancer. *Biochem. J.* , 313, 17–29

Wood RD, Mitchell M, Sgouros J, Lindahl T. 2001.Human DNA repair genes. *Science*, 291:1284–9.

Wrona MZ, Dryhurst G. 1998. Oxidation of serotonin by superoxide radical: implications to neurodegenerative brain disorders. *Chem. Res. Toxicol.*, 11, 639–650

Wu D, Cederbaum AI.2003.Alcohol, oxidative stress and free radical damage. *Alcohol Res. Health*, 27; 277–284.

Xing DY, Tan W, Song N, Lin DX. 2001. Ser326Cys polymorphism in hOGG1 gene and risk of esophageal cancer in a Chinese population.*Int J Cancer*, 95, 140–43.

Xu J, Zheng SL, Turner A, Isaacs SD, Wiley KE, Hawkins GA, Chang BL, Bleecker ER., Walsh PC, Meyers, DA, Isaacs WB.2002. Associations between hOGG1 sequence variants and prostate cancer susceptibility. *Cancer Res*, 62, 2253–57.

Yamasaki I, Piette LH.1991. EPR spin trapping study on the oxidizing species formed in the reaction of the ferrous ion with hydrogen peroxide. *J Am Chem Soc* , 113:7588–7593.

Zhang J, Perry G, Smith MA, Robertson D, Olson SJ, Graham DG, Montine TJ.1999. Parkinson's disease is associated with oxidative damage to cytoplasmic DNA and RNA in substantia nigra neurons. *Am. J. Pathol.* 154 ;1423– 1429.

Zhang Z, Shi Q, Sturgis EM, Spitz MR, Hong WK., Wei, Q.2004. Thymidylate synthase 5′- and 3′-untranslated region polymorphismsassociated with risk and progression of squamous cell carcinoma of the head and neck. *Clin Cancer Res*, 10, 7903–10.

Ziech D, Franco R, Georgakilas AG, Georgakila S, Malamou-Mitsi V, Schoneveld O, Pappa A, Panayiotidis MI. 2010.The role of reactive oxygen species and oxidative stress in environmental carcinogenesis and biomarker development. *Chem Biol Interact.* , 188(2):334-9.

Ziech D, Franco R, Pappa A, Panayiotidis MI.2011. Reactive Oxygen Species (ROS)--Induced genetic and epigenetic alterations in human carcinogenesis. *Mutat Res.*, Mar 16.

11

DNA Damage Response and Repair: Insights into Strategies for Radiation Sensitization

Joshua D. Lawson[1], Kristopher T. Kahle[2], Kimberly Ng[3], Bob Carter[4], Santosh Kesari[5] and Clark C. Chen[3]
[1]*Department of Radiation Oncology, Moores Cancer Center, University of California, San Diego, La Jolla, CA*
[2]*Department of Neurosurgery, Massachusetts General Hospital and Harvard Medical School, Boston, MA*
[3]*Department of Radiation Oncology, Division of Genomic Stability and DNA Repair, Dana-Farber Cancer Institute, Boston, MA*
[4]*Center for Theoretical and Applied Neuro-Oncology, Moores Cancer Center, University of California, San Diego, La Jolla, CA*
[5]*Department of Neurosciences, Moores Cancer Center, University of California, San Diego, La Jolla, CA*
USA

1. Introduction

Glioblastoma is the most common form of primary brain tumors [1]. About 10,000 new patients each year in the US are diagnosed with GBM. Despite its comparatively low incidence of about 2-3 new cases per 100,000 people per year (for comparison, the incidence of colon cancer in the US is approximately 1 new case per 1,800 people per year), the total number of deaths per year attributable to glioblastoma rivals that of other major cancers. This disparity reflects the lethal nature of the disease. If untreated, patients with glioblastoma generally die within 3 months of their diagnosis [2]. Diffuse invasion into the surrounding normal cerebral parenchyma is a cardinal feature of glioblastoma, preventing surgical cure. In this context, it is not surprising that surgical resection alone does not significantly prolong patient survival [2]. When maximal surgical resection is combined with radiation and the chemotherapeutic agent, temozolomide, the median survival of patients improved to 14.6 months [3]. While this regimen achieves an approximate 10% five-year progression free survival [4], the majority of the afflicted patients succumb to the disease within a year of diagnosis. Effective therapeutic strategies are desperately needed.

Despite the abundance of strategies and agents that have been tested over the last half-century for the treatment of GBM, the single most efficacious modality and significant advance has been the use of post-resection radiation therapy. In 1966, the Montreal Neurology Institute published the first large case series that suggested a survival advantage in patients who received an average total post-resection IR dose of 5,000–6,000 cGy [5]. Over the next decade, other case series corroborated those data, suggesting an improvement in patient survival with post-resection IR [6-9]. Although interpretation of these case series is confounded by their retrospective, non-randomized nature, and wide variations in radiation dose regimen, an overall trend of improved patient survival was seen.

The efficacious nature of radiation therapy in glioblastoma was subsequently confirmed in three subsequent randomized control trials. *BTSG 66-01*, the first of the initial three clinical studies that randomized patients with newly-diagnosed malignant gliomas to with Whole-Brain RadioTherapy (WBRT) with or without mithramycin [10]. While mithramycin did not significantly impact survival, the survival of patients who received adjuvant WBRT were extended to about 5 months on average. *BTSG 69-01* randomized patients post-surgical resection to best supportive care or chemotherapy (BCNU), with or without WBRT. Overall patient *survival* was improved with radiation therapy (with or without BCNU) when compared to supportive care alone. The median survival for the surgery only patient was 14 weeks. The median survival for patients who underwent surgery followed by radiation therapy was 36 weeks ($p<0.05$). Similar results were seen in another randomized trial, *BTSG72-01*.

A meta-analysis of *66-01, 69-01,* and *72-01* [11]showed that patients who did not receive radiation or were treated with less than 4,500 cGy exhibited poor survival (median survival of 4.2 and 3.1 months, respectively). On the other hand, patients treated with 5,000, 5,500, and 6,000 cGy showed improved survival (median survival of 6.5, 8.4, and 9.8 months, respectively). Subsequent dose escalation beyond 6,000 cGy revealed increased neuro-toxicity without significant therapeutic gain [12]. These studies collectively established the dosimetry for modern glioblastoma therapy.

It is important to note that, as a single agent, the efficacy of radiation therapy as a glioblastoma therapeutic has yet been matched by any chemotherapy [12]. For this reason, radiation therapy remains a universal component in clinical trials with curative intent for treatment of newly diagnosed glioblastomas. Identification of agents that augment the efficacy of radiation therapy remains a promising strategy for glioblastoma therapy. In this context, we will review the molecular mechanism underlying cellular response to radiation.

2. DNA repair and damage response following ionizing radiation

While Ionizing Radiation (IR) has been shown to induce a plethora of cellular effects, it is widely held that its tumoricidal activity is largely related its effect on DNA [13]. IR induces multiple types of DNA lesions, including damages to the nucleobase, sugar, and phosphate back bone [13]. Ultimately, these lesions, if unrepaired, are converted into Double Stranded DNA Breaks (DSBs). DSBs are highly cytotoxic as the presence of a single DSB in a cell is sufficient to induce death [14-19]. Our understanding of DNA damage response and DSB repair has expanded exponentially in the past decade. To make this vast information more accessible to the reader, we will organize the information into the following sections: 1) general mechanism of DSB repair, 2) mechanism by which DNA damage response activates DSB repair, and 3) effect of DNA damage on cell cycle progression.

2.1 General mechanism of DSB repair

DSBs are repaired by two major mechanisms: Non-Homologous End Joining (NHEJ) or Homologous Recombination (HR) [20, 21]. The simplest way of repairing DSB is by re-ligation. This process is termed NHEJ since no significant DNA sequence homology at the broken ends is required. Instead, the NHEJ enzymatic machinery relies on limited processing of the DNA ends followed by annealing short stretches of complementary DNA sequences.

Because short stretches of complementary sequences occur at some regularity in the human genome, NHEJ is prone to the generation of mutations, deletions, as well as chromosomal rearrangements[22].

The second major DSB repair process is termed HR. HR initiates with extensive 5′ to 3′ end processing of the broken ends into large regions of single stranded tails. The resultant 3′ single stranded tail invades a homologous donor sequence. This strand invasion is mediated by enzyme(s) termed "recombinase" that coats the single stranded tail. Subsequent strand extension and Holliday junction resolution result in restoration of DNA continuity. The resolution is mediated by specific enzymes(s) termed "resolvase" [21]. Because the process cannot proceed without extensive sequence homology, HR tends to be less prone to mutagenesis relative to NHEJ. Because of the requirement for a homologous donor sequence, HR occurs only in the S/G2/M phases of the cell cycle while NHEJ occurs throughout the cell cycle. Both HR and NHEJ contribute to the repair of RT induced DSBs, suggesting that these pathways may be functionally compensatory [23-25]. Given the critical role of these two processes, it is not surprising they are subject to complex regulation.

In mammalian cells, both are carried out by multi-step processes facilitated by a large number of proteins. The mechanistic details of these processes remain an active area of investigation. Working models are described as follows.

For NHEJ, upon DNA damage response activation (see below), the Ku70/Ku 80 heterodimer is recruited to the break site. This protein complex forms a ring shaped structure to protect the broken DNA ends [26]. Additionally, the heterodimer serves as a platform for binding of the critical kinase, DNA-PK [27], and the XRCC4-Ligase IV-XLF4 complex [28]to the site of damage. DNA-PK performs two important functions: 1) it phosphorylates the Ligase IV complex to facilitate the joining of DNA ends; and 2) in cases where DNA end processing is required before rejoining, DNA-PK binds to and recruits the Artemis endonuclease to perform this function. While other proteins also participate in NHEJ [21], *in vitro* reconstitution of NHEJ with these seven proteins (Ku70, Ku80, DNA-PK, XRCC4-Ligase IV-XLF4 complex, and Artemis) suggest that they are essential for this process.

In comparison, the genetics of HR is more complex and far less well understood. Upon DNA damage response activation, it is thought that the BRCA1 and BRCA2 protein are recruited to the site of DNA damage. These two proteins were cloned by virtue of their inactivation in familial breast cancer cohorts (BReast CAncer genes 1 and 2) [29-31]. Both proteins encode large molecular weight proteins that mediate multiple cellular processes to suppress tumor formation. One of these critical functions involves HR. It's proposed that BRCA1 and 2 bind to aberrant DNA structures related to DSB ends [32, 33]. Through BRCA2, the mammalian recombinase, RAD51, is recruited to the site of damage [34]. RAD51 coats the DNA and facilitates the strand exchange reaction in homologous recombination [35-37]. After strand invasion, resolution of the Holliday intermediate is mediated by a protein complex consisting of XRCC3 and RAD51C (two homologues of RAD51) [21, 38].

The mechanism by which HR and NHEJ is activated in response to DNA damage is discussed below.

2.2 DNA damage response

The DNA Damage Response (DDR) refers to the signal transduction cascades that are triggered by DNA damages. These cascades coordinate DNA repair, cell cycle progression, and cell death mechanisms to facilitate the faithful transmission of genetic material after

DNA damage. The process initiates with the recognition of DNA damage by specialized "sensor" proteins. These sensor proteins, in turn, recruit and/or activate "transducer" proteins required for subsequent signaling to "effector" responses, such as cell cycle arrest, apoptosis, transcription, and DNA repair [39]. Defects in DNA damage response have been associated with genomic instability, sensitivity to genotoxic agents, and cancer predisposition [40].

Upon DNA damage, the strand discontinuities trigger complex changes in DNA topology secondary to histone acetylation and phosphorylation of chromatin proteins [41]. The unveiled strand break is recognized by the Mre11-Rad50-Nbs1 (MRN) complex. In addition to serving as an exo/endonuclease to process the DSBs into single stranded DNA tails [42], the MRN complex also recruits the Ataxia Telangiectasia Mutated (ATM) protein kinase to the site of the DSB [43, 44]. When recruited to DSBs, ATM - normally existing in an inactive dimeric form - dissociates and autophosphorylates on multiple residues that are thought to be important for activation of ATM's kinase activity [45]. The activated ATM phosphorylates the histone protein, H2AX, over a region of megabases surrounding a DSB [46, 47]. The phosphorylated H2AX (also known as γ-H2AX), in turn, recruits the Mediator of DNA Checkpoint (MDC1) protein [48, 49]. The MDC1 protein serves as a scaffold protein for docking of the E3 ubiquitin ligase complex, UBC13-RNF8 [50], which serves to poly-ubiquitinate H2AX. Completion of this poly-ubiquitination reaction requires a second ubiquitin ligase, RNF168 [51]. RNF168 is recruited to the site of DNA damage through its interaction with HERC2 and RNF8 [52]. The poly-ubiquitination reaction alters local chromatin structure as well as provides docking site for the ubiquitin binding protein, RAP80. RAP80, in turn, recruits the BRCA1/BRCA2/RAD51 repair complex by direct physical interaction[53]. This complex initiates DSB repair by HR as well as arrests cell cycle progression in a process known as DNA damage checkpoint activation (see ensuing section).

It is important to note that while the above damage response is described in a linear manner, parallel interactions occur at each step. For instance, MDC1, in addition to recruiting UBC13-RNF8, also interacts with ATM [48] and MRN [54] to stabilize the repair complex. The aggregate effect of these other complex interactions induces chromatin state changes surrounding the DSB and the localization of numerous proteins required for coordinating DNA repair and checkpoint regulation.

Similar to HR, the NHEJ process can be initiated by the MRN complex upon DDR activation. The Mre11 protein in the complex can directly interact with the Ku70 subunit [55]. Moreover, the RAD50 protein in the MRN complex encodes a high-affinity DNA binding domain and a second domain that facilitates homodimeric interactions that holds DNA ends in close proximity [56] to facilitate subsequent NHEJ.

Since the MRN complex may initiate either HR or NHEJ, a central question in the field of DNA repair involves the mechanism of this regulation. Inappropriate activation of HR in the G1 phase of the cell cycle could lead to cell death. Similarly, activation of NHEJ during the S/G2 phases of the cell cycle could increase the rate of mutagenesis. One of the key mediators of this regulatory process involves the protein CTBP Interacting Protein (CTIP). In a landmark study [57], CTIP was found to interact with the MRN complex to promote its exo/endonuclease activity and process DSBs into single stranded DNA ends. Importantly, this activity is regulated by cell cycle dependent phosphorylation events mediated by Cyclin-Dependent Kinases (CDKs). In the S/G2 phase of the cell cycle, CTIP is phosphorylated. Thus, the MRN complex processes DSBs into single stranded tails required for the initiation of HR. On the other hand, in the G1 phase of the cell cycle, CTIP remains unphosphorylated, and the MRN complex remains inactive as an exo/endo-nuclease. Without this processing, HR cannot be initiated. Thus, NHEJ becomes the predominant repair process.

2.3 Effect of DNA damage on cell cycle progression

In addition to the assembly of repair complexes as above described, DNA damage triggers signaling to proteins required for cell cycle progression, such as the CDK/cyclin complex. Generally speaking, DNA damage checkpoint regulation occurs at three distinct phases of the cell cycle: the G1-S transition, the intra-S-phase, and the G2-M transition. Most of what we understand of this transduction process involves protein phosphorylation cascades, though the importance of other types of reversible modifications, such as ubiquitination and sumoylation, are become increasingly apparent [58]. Here, we will review an illustrative example of signal transduction between DNA damage sensors and cell cycle regulation. Upon recognition of DSB, the MRN complex recruits and activates the critical ATM kinase. The ATM kinase, in turn, phosphorylates the tumor suppressor p53 and another kinase termed Chk2 (Checkpoint Kinase 2) [59]. ATM phosphorylation of Chk2 activates its kinase activity which, in turn, phosphorylates both p53 and MDM2. These phosphorylation events stabilize p53 by interrupting its association with its negative regulator, MDM2 [60]. Activated p53 then induces the transcription of its target genes, which include the critical regulator of the G1-S transition, p21 [61]. The binding of p21 to the CDK-cyclin complexes and prevents phosphorylation of the retinoblastoma protein (pRb). When in a hypophosphorylated state, pRb blocks cell proliferation by sequestering and altering the function of E2F transcription factors that control transcription of genes required for progression from G1 into S phase. Disruption of the pRb pathway - as occurs with mutant p53 or p21 - liberates E2Fs and allows cell proliferation, which renders cells insensitive to DNA damage-induced anti-growth signals that normally operate to inhibit passage through G1 phase of the cell cycle [62]. With regards to the G2-M checkpoint, ATM release inhibition of p53 additionally results in the transcriptional induction of 14-3-3σ in addition to p21. The 14-3-3σ protein sequesters the cyclinB-cdc2 kinase complex in the cytoplasm and prevents nuclear phosphorylation events required for G2/M progression [63]. Additionally, p21 binds to any residual cdc2 that enters the nucleus to prevent its activation. These and other ATM events prevent progression through the G2/M transition and afford time for DSB repair [64].

3. Strategies for sensitization

A prediction of the above presented model is that inhibition of any of the proteins required for DDR or DSB repair should lead to radiation sensitization. In general, this prediction has been confirmed [65]. However, therapeutic agents that directly inhibit these critical proteins are still years from reaching clinical trial. Encouragingly, several FDA-approved agents have recently been shown to modulate DNA damage response. This property may be explored as therapeutic strategy.

3.1 Molecular rationale for therapeutic window

Before considering the strategy of radiation sensitization, one must first consider the molecular rationale for therapeutic window. After all, if normal and tumor cells were equally sensitized by the agent, then no therapeutic efficacy is gained.

A large body has yielded data suggesting that oncogene activation creates a tumor state that increases the accumulation of DNA damage [66-69]. This damage, if unrepaired, can be converted into DSBs that eventually lead to cell death. To compensate for this increased DNA damage, the tumor cells require increased utilization of DNA repair processes [69]. In this context, the administration of radiation introduces additional DNA damage that further taxes the already over-utilized repair process. This situation, in turn, increases the likelihood of an unrepaired DSB causing cell death. The same effect can be achieved by inhibition of DSB repair. The following sections will review FDA-approved agents with such properties. It is important to note that these agents induce pleiotropic effects beyond DSB repair inhibition.

3.2 DNA damaging agents

Conventional chemotherapy involves DNA damaging agents that are often used in conjunction with radiation. In this context, these FDA-approved agents often sensitize the tumoricidal effects of radiation. The mechanism of this sensitization is thought to be related to the generation of DNA damages that sequester critical DNA repair proteins. For instance, lesions generated by cisplatin bind to and sequester the Ku70/80 heterodimer and thereby compromise the efficiency of NHEJ [70]. Further, most DNA damages induced by conventional chemotherapy are ultimately converted to DSBs [71]. These DSBs will titrate away the repair proteins available to repair the DSBs induced by subsequent radiation. These types of mechanisms likely account for the increased glioblastoma patient survival observed in the context of concurrent radiation/ temozolomide treatment relative to radiation treatment alone [3, 4].

3.3 Proteasome inhibitors

As a result of extreme aneuploidy, copy-number variation, and transcriptional alteration that are present in many cancer cells, there is increased stress on the chaperone pathways (such as heat shock proteins) to maintain folding of over-expressed proteins. When the capacity of these chaperone proteins becomes saturated, the unfolded proteins require degradation by the proteasome complex [72]. Thus, tumor cells exhibit increased dependency on proteasome function. Indeed, proteasome inhibition has been demonstrated to selectively ablate cancer cells both *in vitro* and *in vivo* [73]. The proteasome inhibitor bortezomib has attained FDA-approval as a treatment for multiple myeloma and mantle cell lymphoma.

Recent studies implicate proteasome function in DSB repair. The yeast Sem1 protein is a subunit of the 19S proteasome that is required for efficient HR [74]. The human Sem1 homologue, DSS1, physically interacts with the HR protein, BRCA2, and is required for its stability and function [75-77]. Using the DR-GFP assay to directly assess HR efficiency, Murakawa et al. demonstrated that HR efficiency is significantly reduced by proteasome inhibition [78]. As a whole, these studies suggest proteasome inhibition as a means to target HR in cancer therapy.

The mechanism by which proteasome inhibition modulates HR remains an area of investigation. One hypothesis frequently put forth is the following. The proteins destined for proteasome degradation are typically modified by attachment of multiple ubiquitin moieties [74]. Processing of the tagged protein releases the tagged ubiquitin to replete the intracellular pool. Proteasome inhibition, thus, leads to accumulation of ubiquitinated proteins. This accumulation, in turn, depletes the intracellular ubiquitin pool. Since free ubiquitins are required to activate HR, the repair process is compromised by proteasome inhibition.

3.4 Epidermal Growth Factor Receptor (EGFR) inhibitors

EGFR is frequently amplified or mutated in several cancer types, including Non-Small Cell Lung Cancer (NSCLC) and glioblastomas [79-81]. As aberrant EGFR signaling is required to sustain tumor survival and proliferation in some cancers, targeted inhibition has led to selective tumor ablation [79]. Clinical trial success has led to FDA-approval for treatment of NSCLC.

Several studies have demonstrated that EGFR inhibition sensitized tumor cells to radiation [65]. Insights into the mechanism underlying this sensitization have been provided by several recent studies. One series of studies demonstrate that a subset of EGFR travels to the nucleus where it binds to and enhances DNA-PK activity to enhance NHEJ [82, 83}. Indeed, glioblastomas over-expressing an over-active form of EGFR (termed EGFRvIII) exhibit radiation resistance that can be abridged by treatment with DNA-PK inhibitors [84]. Another series of studies reveal that EGFR inhibition leads to retention of BRCA1 in the cytoplasm, thereby causing defective HR [85]. Finally, other downstream effectors of EGFR, including the Extracellular signal Regulated Kinase (ERK1/2) also modulates HR efficiency [86]. It is likely that the radiation sensitization effect of EGFR inhibition represents a culmination of these individual effects.

3.5 Other late stage clinical trial agents

There are several other agents that are in mid- to late- clinical trial testing that have also been shown to inhibit DNA damage response. For instance, Histone DeACetylase (HDAC) inhibitors have been shown to down regulate the transcript level of BRCA1 [87]. These agents have also been shown to disrupt the chromatin re-organization required for ATM activation [41]. As another example, Heat Shock Protein 90 (HSP90, the prototypical chaperone protein) inhibitor treatment inhibits ATM autophosphorylation upon DNA damage [88] and destabilizes the MRN complex [89, 90], thereby inhibiting HR. Finally, CDK1 inhibition causes the loss of a critical phosphorylation event on BRCA1 required for its HR function [91].

There are additional modulators of DDR and DNA repair not described here [65]. Indeed, the number of pharmacologic inhibitors that either directly or indirectly inhibit DSB repair is being uncovered at a rapid pace. Careful consideration should be given for combination with radiation therapy in clinical trial design.

4. Closing remarks

Radiotherapy is the most effective post-surgical treatment modality in the management of glioblastoma. Adjuvant radiotherapy alone provides a more than doubling of median survival. Incremental gains with additional medical therapy have proven elusive, with most agents showing moderate activity *in vitro* or with encouraging early clinical experience only to demonstrate a lack of benefit in larger trials. Attempts at treatment intensification with radiotherapy have been similarly disappointing. Molecular understanding of DNA damage response and repair, on the other hand, has now afforded novel therapeutic targets. These targets are particularly attractive in the context that oncogenes induce increased DNA damage accumulation and cause tumors to become hyper-dependent on DNA damage response pathways. Encouragingly, several FDA-approved agents modulate critical proteins in DNA damage response/repair, including conventional DNA damaging agents, proteasome inhibitors, and EGFR inhibitors. Clinical trials involving these and other agents modulating DNA damage response should be designed with this consideration.

5. References

[1] Louis DN. Molecular pathology of malignant gliomas. *Annu Rev Pathol.* 2006;1:97-117.

[2] Walker MD, Alexander E, Jr., Hunt WE, et al. Evaluation of BCNU and/or radiotherapy in the treatment of anaplastic gliomas. A cooperative clinical trial. *J Neurosurg.* Sep 1978;49(3):333-343.

[3] Stupp R, Mason WP, van den Bent MJ, et al. Radiotherapy plus concomitant and adjuvant temozolomide for glioblastoma. *N Engl J Med.* Mar 10 2005;352(10):987-996.

[4] Stupp R, Hegi ME, Mason WP, et al. Effects of radiotherapy with concomitant and adjuvant temozolomide versus radiotherapy alone on survival in glioblastoma in a randomised phase III study: 5-year analysis of the EORTC-NCIC trial.

[5] Uihlein A, Colby MY Jr, Layton DD. Comparisons of surgery and surgery plus irradiation in the treatment of supratentorial gliomas. *Acta Radiol Ther Phys Biol.* 1966;3:67-78.

[6] Stage WS, Stein JJ. Treatment of malignant astrocytomas. *Am J Roentgenol Radium Ther Nucl Med.* Jan 1974;120(1):7-18.

[7] Sheline GE. Radiation therapy of brain tumors. *Cancer.* Feb 1977;39(2 Suppl):873-881.

[8] Sheline G. Conventional radiation therapy of gliomas. *Recent Results in Cancer Research. Gliomas: Current Concepts in Biology, Diagnosis, and Therapy.* New York: Springer-Verlag; 1975:125-134.

[9] Kramer S. Radiation therapy in the management of malignant gliomas. *Cancer of the Central Nervous System: Seventh National Cancer Conference Proceedings.* Philadelphia: Lippincott Company; 1973:823-826.

[10] Walker MD, Alexander E, Jr., Hunt WE, et al. Evaluation of mithramycin in the treatment of anaplastic gliomas. *J Neurosurg.* Jun 1976;44(6):655-667.

[11] Walker MD, Strike TA, Sheline GE. An analysis of dose-effect relationship in the radiotherapy of malignant gliomas. *Int J Radiat Oncol Biol Phys.* Oct 1979;5(10):1725-1731.

[12] Chang JE, Khuntia D, Robins HI, Mehta MP. Radiotherapy and radiosensitizers in the treatment of glioblastoma multiforme. *Clin Adv Hematol Oncol.* Nov 2007;5(11):894-902, 907-815.

[13] Hall E, ed *Radiobiology for the radiologist.* 6th ed. Philadelphia, PA: Lippincott Williams and Wilkins; 2006.

[14] Bennett CB, Lewis AL, Baldwin KK, Resnick MA. Lethality induced by a single site-specific double-strand break in a dispensable yeast plasmid. *Proc Natl Acad Sci U S A.* Jun 15 1993;90(12):5613-5617.

[15] Bennett CB, Westmoreland TJ, Snipe JR, Resnick MA. A double-strand break within a yeast artificial chromosome (YAC) containing human DNA can result in YAC loss, deletion or cell lethality. *Mol Cell Biol.* Aug 1996;16(8):4414-4425.

[16] Dugle DL, Gillespie CJ, Chapman JD. DNA strand breaks, repair, and survival in x-irradiated mammalian cells. *Proc Natl Acad Sci U S A.* Mar 1976;73(3):809-812.

[17] Game JC, Mortimer RK. A genetic study of X-ray sensitive mutants in yeast. *Mutat Res.* 1974;24:281-292.

[18] Lee SE, Moore JK, Holmes A, Umezu K, Kolodner RD, Haber JE. Saccharomyces Ku70, mre11/rad50 and RPA proteins regulate adaptation to G2/M arrest after DNA damage. *Cell.* Aug 7 1998;94(3):399-409.

[19] Sandell LL, Zakian VA. Loss of a yeast telomere: arrest, recovery, and chromosome loss. *Cell.* Nov 19 1993;75(4):729-739.

[20] Hartlerode AJ, Scully R. Mechanisms of double-strand break repair in somatic mammalian cells. *Biochem J.* Oct 15 2009;423(2):157-168.

[21] Wyman C, Kanaar R. DNA double-strand break repair: all's well that ends well. *Annu Rev Genet.* 2006;40:363-383.

[22] Lieber MR, Ma Y, Pannicke U, Schwarz K. Mechanism and regulation of human non-homologous DNA end-joining. *Nat Rev Mol Cell Biol.* Sep 2003;4(9):712-720.

[23] Ristic D, Modesti M, Kanaar R, Wyman C. Rad52 and Ku bind to different DNA structures produced early in double-strand break repair. *Nucleic Acids Res.* Sep 15 2003;31(18):5229-5237.

[24] Schar P, Herrmann G, Daly G, Lindahl T. A newly identified DNA ligase of Saccharomyces cerevisiae involved in RAD52-independent repair of DNA double-strand breaks. *Genes Dev.* Aug 1 1997;11(15):1912-1924.

[25] Takata M, Sasaki MS, Sonoda E, et al. Homologous recombination and non-homologous end-joining pathways of DNA double-strand break repair have overlapping roles in the maintenance of chromosomal integrity in vertebrate cells. *EMBO J.* Sep 15 1998;17(18):5497-5508.

[26] Walker JR, Corpina RA, Goldberg J. Structure of the Ku heterodimer bound to DNA and its implications for double-strand break repair. *Nature.* Aug 9 2001;412(6847):607-614.

[27] Gottlieb TM, Jackson SP. The DNA-dependent protein kinase: requirement for DNA ends and association with Ku antigen. *Cell.* Jan 15 1993;72(1):131-142.

[28] Nick McElhinny SA, Snowden CM, McCarville J, Ramsden DA. Ku recruits the XRCC4-ligase IV complex to DNA ends. *Mol Cell Biol.* May 2000;20(9):2996-3003.

[29] Futreal PA, Liu Q, Shattuck-Eidens D, et al. BRCA1 mutations in primary breast and ovarian carcinomas. *Science.* Oct 7 1994;266(5182):120-122.

[30] Miki Y, Swensen J, Shattuck-Eidens D, et al. A strong candidate for the breast and ovarian cancer susceptibility gene BRCA1. *Science.* Oct 7 1994;266(5182):66-71.

[31] Wooster R, Bignell G, Lancaster J, et al. Identification of the breast cancer susceptibility gene BRCA2. *Nature.* Dec 21-28 1995;378(6559):789-792.

[32] Paull TT, Cortez D, Bowers B, Elledge SJ, Gellert M. Direct DNA binding by Brca1. *Proc Natl Acad Sci U S A.* May 22 2001;98(11):6086-6091.

[33] Yang H, Jeffrey PD, Miller J, et al. BRCA2 function in DNA binding and recombination from a BRCA2-DSS1-ssDNA structure. *Science.* Sep 13 2002;297(5588):1837-1848.

[34] Powell SN, Kachnic LA. Roles of BRCA1 and BRCA2 in homologous recombination, DNA replication fidelity and the cellular response to ionizing radiation. *Oncogene.* Sep 1 2003;22(37):5784-5791.

[35] Galkin VE, Esashi F, Yu X, Yang S, West SC, Egelman EH. BRCA2 BRC motifs bind RAD51-DNA filaments. *Proc Natl Acad Sci U S A.* Jun 14 2005;102(24):8537-8542.

[36] Shin DS, Chahwan C, Huffman JL, Tainer JA. Structure and function of the double-strand break repair machinery. *DNA Repair (Amst).* Aug-Sep 2004;3(8-9):863-873.

[37] Shivji MK, Venkitaraman AR. DNA recombination, chromosomal stability and carcinogenesis: insights into the role of BRCA2. *DNA Repair (Amst).* Aug-Sep 2004;3(8-9):835-843.

[38] Liu Y, Masson JY, Shah R, O'Regan P, West SC. RAD51C is required for Holliday junction processing in mammalian cells. *Science.* Jan 9 2004;303(5655):243-246.

[39] Harper JW, Elledge SJ. The DNA damage response: ten years after. *Mol Cell.* Dec 14 2007;28(5):739-745.

[40] Jackson SP, Bartek J. The DNA-damage response in human biology and disease. *Nature.* Oct 22 2009;461(7267):1071-1078.

[41] van Attikum H, Gasser SM. The histone code at DNA breaks: a guide to repair? *Nat Rev Mol Cell Biol.* Oct 2005;6(10):757-765.

[42] D'Amours D, Jackson SP. The Mre11 complex: at the crossroads of dna repair and checkpoint signalling. *Nat Rev Mol Cell Biol.* May 2002;3(5):317-327.

[43] Lee JH, Paull TT. ATM activation by DNA double-strand breaks through the Mre11-Rad50-Nbs1 complex. *Science.* Apr 22 2005;308(5721):551-554.

[44] Paull TT, Lee JH. The Mre11/Rad50/Nbs1 complex and its role as a DNA double-strand break sensor for ATM. *Cell Cycle.* Jun 2005;4(6):737-740.

[45] Bakkenist CJ, Kastan MB. DNA damage activates ATM through intermolecular autophosphorylation and dimer dissociation. *Nature.* Jan 30 2003;421(6922):499-506.

[46] Paull TT, Rogakou EP, Yamazaki V, Kirchgessner CU, Gellert M, Bonner WM. A critical role for histone H2AX in recruitment of repair factors to nuclear foci after DNA damage. *Curr Biol.* Jul 27-Aug 10 2000;10(15):886-895.

[47] Rogakou EP, Boon C, Redon C, Bonner WM. Megabase chromatin domains involved in DNA double-strand breaks in vivo. *J Cell Biol.* Sep 6 1999;146(5):905-916.

[48] Lou Z, Minter-Dykhouse K, Franco S, et al. MDC1 maintains genomic stability by participating in the amplification of ATM-dependent DNA damage signals. *Mol Cell.* Jan 20 2006;21(2):187-200.

[49] Stucki M, Clapperton JA, Mohammad D, Yaffe MB, Smerdon SJ, Jackson SP. MDC1 directly binds phosphorylated histone H2AX to regulate cellular responses to DNA double-strand breaks. *Cell.* Dec 29 2005;123(7):1213-1226.

[50] Huen MS, Grant R, Manke I, et al. RNF8 transduces the DNA-damage signal via histone ubiquitylation and checkpoint protein assembly. *Cell.* Nov 30 2007;131(5):901-914.

[51] Doil C, Mailand N, Bekker-Jensen S, et al. RNF168 binds and amplifies ubiquitin conjugates on damaged chromosomes to allow accumulation of repair proteins. *Cell.* Feb 6 2009;136(3):435-446.

[52] Bekker-Jensen S, Rendtlew Danielsen J, Fugger K, et al. HERC2 coordinates ubiquitin-dependent assembly of DNA repair factors on damaged chromosomes. *Nat Cell Biol.* Jan 2010;12(1):80-86; sup pp 81-12.

[53] Kim H, Chen J, Yu X. Ubiquitin-binding protein RAP80 mediates BRCA1-dependent DNA damage response. *Science.* May 25 2007;316(5828):1202-1205.

[54] Chapman JR, Jackson SP. Phospho-dependent interactions between NBS1 and MDC1 mediate chromatin retention of the MRN complex at sites of DNA damage. *EMBO Rep.* Aug 2008;9(8):795-801.

[55] Goedecke W, Eijpe M, Offenberg HH, van Aalderen M, Heyting C. Mre11 and Ku70 interact in somatic cells, but are differentially expressed in early meiosis. *Nat Genet.* Oct 1999;23(2):194-198.

[56] Dinkelmann M, Spehalski E, Stoneham T, et al. Multiple functions of MRN in end-joining pathways during isotype class switching. *Nat Struct Mol Biol.* Aug 2009;16(8):808-813.

[57] Sartori AA, Lukas C, Coates J, et al. Human CtIP promotes DNA end resection. *Nature.* Nov 22 2007;450(7169):509-514.

[58] Abraham RT. Cell cycle checkpoint signaling through the ATM and ATR kinases. *Genes Dev.* Sep 1 2001;15(17):2177-2196.

[59] Peters M, DeLuca C, Hirao A, et al. Chk2 regulates irradiation-induced, p53-mediated apoptosis in Drosophila. *Proc Natl Acad Sci U S A.* Aug 20 2002;99(17):11305-11310.

[60] Cheng Q, Chen J. Mechanism of p53 stabilization by ATM after DNA damage. *Cell Cycle.* Feb 1 2010;9(3):472-478.

[61] Waldman T, Kinzler KW, Vogelstein B. p21 is necessary for the p53-mediated G1 arrest in human cancer cells. *Cancer Res.* Nov 15 1995;55(22):5187-5190.

[62] Shapiro GI, Harper JW. Anticancer drug targets: cell cycle and checkpoint control. *J Clin Invest.* Dec 1999;104(12):1645-1653.

[63] Bunz F, Dutriaux A, Lengauer C, et al. Requirement for p53 and p21 to sustain G2 arrest after DNA damage. *Science.* Nov 20 1998;282(5393):1497-1501.

[64] Chan TA, Hermeking H, Lengauer C, Kinzler KW, Vogelstein B. 14-3-3Sigma is required to prevent mitotic catastrophe after DNA damage. *Nature.* Oct 7 1999;401(6753):616-620.

[65] Ljungman M. Targeting the DNA damage response in cancer. *Chem Rev.* Jul 2009;109(7):2929-2950.

[66] Denko NC, Giaccia AJ, Stringer JR, Stambrook PJ. The human Ha-ras oncogene induces genomic instability in murine fibroblasts within one cell cycle. *Proc Natl Acad Sci U S A.* May 24 1994;91(11):5124-5128.

[67] Lee AC, Fenster BE, Ito H, et al. Ras proteins induce senescence by altering the intracellular levels of reactive oxygen species. *J Biol Chem.* Mar 19 1999;274(12):7936-7940.

[68] Lo HW, Hsu SC, Ali-Seyed M, et al. Nuclear interaction of EGFR and STAT3 in the activation of the iNOS/NO pathway. *Cancer Cell.* Jun 2005;7(6):575-589.

[69] Nitta M, Kozono D, Kennedy R, et al. Targeting EGFR induced oxidative stress by PARP1 inhibition in glioblastoma therapy. *PLoS One.* 2010;5(5):e10767.

[70] Turchi JJ, Henkels KM, Zhou Y. Cisplatin-DNA adducts inhibit translocation of the Ku subunits of DNA-PK. *Nucleic Acids Res.* Dec 1 2000;28(23):4634-4641.

[71] Stojic L, Mojas N, Cejka P, et al. Mismatch repair-dependent G2 checkpoint induced by low doses of SN1 type methylating agents requires the ATR kinase. *Genes Dev.* Jun 1 2004;18(11):1331-1344.

[72] Luo J, Solimini NL, Elledge SJ. Principles of cancer therapy: oncogene and non-oncogene addiction. *Cell.* Mar 6 2009;136(5):823-837.

[73] Rajkumar SV, Richardson PG, Hideshima T, Anderson KC. Proteasome inhibition as a novel therapeutic target in human cancer. *J Clin Oncol.* Jan 20 2005;23(3):630-639.

[74] Krogan NJ, Lam MH, Fillingham J, et al. Proteasome involvement in the repair of DNA double-strand breaks. *Mol Cell.* Dec 22 2004;16(6):1027-1034.

[75] Gudmundsdottir K, Lord CJ, Witt E, Tutt AN, Ashworth A. DSS1 is required for RAD51 focus formation and genomic stability in mammalian cells. *EMBO Rep.* Oct 2004;5(10):989-993.

[76] Li J, Zou C, Bai Y, Wazer DE, Band V, Gao Q. DSS1 is required for the stability of BRCA2. *Oncogene.* Feb 23 2006;25(8):1186-1194.

[77] Marston NJ, Richards WJ, Hughes D, Bertwistle D, Marshall CJ, Ashworth A. Interaction between the product of the breast cancer susceptibility gene BRCA2 and DSS1, a protein functionally conserved from yeast to mammals. *Mol Cell Biol.* Jul 1999;19(7):4633-4642.

[78] Murakawa Y, Sonoda E, Barber LJ, et al. Inhibitors of the proteasome suppress homologous DNA recombination in mammalian cells. *Cancer Res.* Sep 15 2007;67(18):8536-8543.

[79] da Cunha Santos G, Shepherd FA, Tsao MS. EGFR mutations and lung cancer. *Annu Rev Pathol.* Feb 28 2011;6:49-69.

[80] Parsons DW, Jones S, Zhang X, et al. An integrated genomic analysis of human glioblastoma multiforme. *Science.* Sep 26 2008;321(5897):1807-1812.

[81] TCGA. Comprehensive genomic characterization defines human glioblastoma genes and core pathways. *Nature.* Oct 23 2008;455(7216):1061-1068.

[82] Dittmann K, Mayer C, Fehrenbacher B, et al. Radiation-induced epidermal growth factor receptor nuclear import is linked to activation of DNA-dependent protein kinase. *J Biol Chem.* Sep 2 2005;280(35):31182-31189.

[83] Liccardi G, Hartley JA, Hochhauser D. EGFR nuclear translocation modulates DNA repair following cisplatin and ionizing radiation treatment. *Cancer Res.* Feb 1 2011;71(3):1103-1114.

[84] Mukherjee B, McEllin B, Camacho CV, et al. EGFRvIII and DNA double-strand break repair: a molecular mechanism for radioresistance in glioblastoma. *Cancer Res.* May 15 2009;69(10):4252-4259.

[85] Li L, Wang H, Yang ES, Arteaga CL, Xia F. Erlotinib attenuates homologous recombinational repair of chromosomal breaks in human breast cancer cells. *Cancer Res.* Nov 15 2008;68(22):9141-9146.

[86] Golding SE, Rosenberg E, Neill S, Dent P, Povirk LF, Valerie K. Extracellular signal-related kinase positively regulates ataxia telangiectasia mutated, homologous recombination repair, and the DNA damage response. *Cancer Res.* Feb 1 2007;67(3):1046-1053.

[87] Burkitt K, Ljungman M. Phenylbutyrate interferes with the Fanconi anemia and BRCA pathway and sensitizes head and neck cancer cells to cisplatin. *Mol Cancer.* 2008;7:24.

[88] Koll TT, Feis SS, Wright MH, et al. HSP90 inhibitor, DMAG, synergizes with radiation of lung cancer cells by interfering with base excision and ATM-mediated DNA repair. *Mol Cancer Ther.* Jul 2008;7(7):1985-1992.

[89] Camphausen K, Tofilon PJ. Inhibition of Hsp90: a multitarget approach to radiosensitization. *Clin Cancer Res.* Aug 1 2007;13(15 Pt 1):4326-4330.

[90] Dote H, Burgan WE, Camphausen K, Tofilon PJ. Inhibition of hsp90 compromises the DNA damage response to radiation. *Cancer Res.* Sep 15 2006;66(18):9211-9220.

[91] Johnson N, Cai D, Kennedy RD, et al. Cdk1 participates in BRCA1-dependent S phase checkpoint control in response to DNA damage. Mol Cell. Aug 14 2009;35(3):327-339.

Permissions

All chapters in this book were first published in STDNAR, by InTech Open; hereby published with permission under the Creative Commons Attribution License or equivalent. Every chapter published in this book has been scrutinized by our experts. Their significance has been extensively debated. The topics covered herein carry significant findings which will fuel the growth of the discipline. They may even be implemented as practical applications or may be referred to as a beginning point for another development.

The contributors of this book come from diverse backgrounds, making this book a truly international effort. This book will bring forth new frontiers with its revolutionizing research information and detailed analysis of the nascent developments around the world.

We would like to thank all the contributing authors for lending their expertise to make the book truly unique. They have played a crucial role in the development of this book. Without their invaluable contributions this book wouldn't have been possible. They have made vital efforts to compile up to date information on the varied aspects of this subject to make this book a valuable addition to the collection of many professionals and students.

This book was conceptualized with the vision of imparting up-to-date information and advanced data in this field. To ensure the same, a matchless editorial board was set up. Every individual on the board went through rigorous rounds of assessment to prove their worth. After which they invested a large part of their time researching and compiling the most relevant data for our readers.

The editorial board has been involved in producing this book since its inception. They have spent rigorous hours researching and exploring the diverse topics which have resulted in the successful publishing of this book. They have passed on their knowledge of decades through this book. To expedite this challenging task, the publisher supported the team at every step. A small team of assistant editors was also appointed to further simplify the editing procedure and attain best results for the readers.

Apart from the editorial board, the designing team has also invested a significant amount of their time in understanding the subject and creating the most relevant covers. They scrutinized every image to scout for the most suitable representation of the subject and create an appropriate cover for the book.

The publishing team has been an ardent support to the editorial, designing and production team. Their endless efforts to recruit the best for this project, has resulted in the accomplishment of this book. They are a veteran in the field of academics and their pool of knowledge is as vast as their experience in printing. Their expertise and guidance has proved useful at every step. Their uncompromising quality standards have made this book an exceptional effort. Their encouragement from time to time has been an inspiration for everyone.

The publisher and the editorial board hope that this book will prove to be a valuable piece of knowledge for researchers, students, practitioners and scholars across the globe.

List of Contributors

Sascha Biedermann
Washington State University Pullman, United States of America
Angewandte Genetik, Berlin, Germany

Sutton Mooney and Hanjo Hellmann
Washington State University Pullman, United States of America

Patrick E. Gygli, J. Scott Lockhart and Linda C. DeVeaux
Idaho State University, USA

Simona Catalani and Pietro Apostoli
Department of Experimental and Applied Medicine, Section of Occupational Health and Industrial Hygiene, University of Brescia, Italy

Keiji Suzuki, Motohiro Yamauchi, Masatoshi Suzuki, Yasuyoshi Oka and Shunichi Yamashita
Nagasaki University Graduate School of Biomedical Sciences, Atomic Bomb Disease Institute, Department of Radiation Medical Sciences, Japan

Ashwin L. Ganpudi and Dana F. Schroeder
University of Manitoba, Canada

Balam Muñoz and Arnulfo Albores
Departamento de Toxicología, Centro de Investigación y de Estudios Avanzados del I.P.N. México

Maddalena Mognato, Mauro Grifalconi, Sabrina Canova, Cristina Girardi and Lucia Celotti
University of Padova, Department of Biology, Italy

Haïtham Sghaier
Research Unit UR04CNSTN01 "Medical and Agricultural Applications of Nuclear Techniques", National Center for Nuclear Sciences and Technology (CNSTN), Sidi Thabet Technopark, Sidi Thabet, Tunisia

Gaëlle Lenglet, Sabine Depauw, Denise Mendy-Belaiche and Marie-Hélène David-Cordonnier
INSERM, Jean-Pierre Aubert Research Center (JPARC), Team 4 Molecular and Cellular Targeting for Cancer Treatment and University of Lille, Grand Nord, Institut pour la Recherche sur le Cancer de Lille, Place de Verdun, Lille France

Bedia Cakmakoglu, Zeynep Birsu Cincin and Makbule Aydin
Istanbul University, Institute for Experimental Medicine Research, Turkey

Joshua D. Lawson
Department of Radiation Oncology, Moores Cancer Center, University of California, San Diego, La Jolla, CA, USA

Kristopher T. Kahle
Department of Neurosurgery, Massachusetts General Hospital and Harvard Medical School, Boston, MA, USA

Kimberly Ng and Clark C. Chen
Department of Radiation Oncology, Division of Genomic Stability and DNA Repair, Dana-Farber Cancer Institute, Boston, MA, USA

Bob Carter
Center for Theoretical and Applied Neuro-Oncology, Moores Cancer Center, University of California, San Diego, La Jolla, CA, USA

Santosh Kesari
Department of Neurosciences, Moores Cancer Center, University of California, San Diego, La Jolla, CA, USA

Index

www.ingramcontent.com/pod-product-compliance
Lightning Source LLC
LaVergne TN
LVHW080636210926
848485LV00003B/274